AF361336

REVITALIZING HEALTH FOR ALL

Case Studies of the Struggle for Comprehensive Primary Health Care

While impressive medical and technological developments have improved health care around the world, improvements in *health* have been moderate and inconsistent across countries and communities. In response to this challenge, the World Health Organization outlined the concept of comprehensive primary health care, which involves not only providing a range of medical care from prevention to treatment, but also working to improve equity in health care access, community empowerment, the participation of marginalized groups, and collaboration across sectors beyond health.

Revitalizing Health for All examines 13 cases of efforts to implement comprehensive primary health care reforms in communities around the globe, including in Australia, Brazil, Democratic Republic of Congo, South Africa, and Iran. The case studies originated from an international research-to-action initiative that brought researchers and research-users from national public health systems together to design, implement, and assess local projects. This volume reveals the similarities among comprehensive primary health care projects in diverse national contexts and offers a rich evidence base from which future reform initiatives can draw.

RONALD LABONTÉ is a professor in the Faculty of Medicine at the University of Ottawa and the Faculty of Health Sciences at Flinders University.

DAVID SANDERS is a professor emeritus and founding director of the School of Public Health at the University of the Western Cape.

CORINNE PACKER is a senior researcher in the Faculty of Medicine at the University of Ottawa.

NIKKI SCHAAY is a senior researcher in the School of Public Health at the University of the Western Cape.

Revitalizing Health for All

Case Studies of the Struggle for
Comprehensive Primary Health Care

EDITED BY RONALD LABONTÉ,
DAVID SANDERS, CORINNE PACKER,
AND NIKKI SCHAAY

UNIVERSITY OF TORONTO PRESS
Toronto Buffalo London

INTERNATIONAL DEVELOPMENT RESEARCH CENTRE
Ottawa • Cairo • Montevideo •Nairobi • New Delhi

© International Development Research Centre 2017
Published by University of Toronto Press
Toronto Buffalo London
www.utppublishing.com
and
International Development Research Centre
PO Box 8500, Ottawa, ON, Canada K1G 3H9
www.idrc.ca/ info@idrc.ca
Printed in Canada

ISBN 978-1-4875-0175-4 (cloth)   ISBN 978-1-4875-2162-2 (paper)
ISBN 978-1-55250-592-2 (IDRC e-book)

♾ Printed on acid-free, 100% post-consumer recycled paper with vegetable-based inks.

Library and Archives Canada Cataloguing in Publication

Revitalizing health for all : case studies of the struggle for comprehensive primary
health care / edited by Ronald Labonté, David Sanders, Corinne Packer,
and Nikki Schaay.

Includes bibliographical references and index.
ISBN 978-1-4875-0175-4 (cloth). ISBN 978-1-4875-2162-2 (paper)

1. Primary health care – Case studies.   2. Health care reform – Case studies.
I. Labonté, Ronald N., author, editor   II. Sanders, David, 1945–, author, editor
III. Packer, Corinne, 1967–, author, editor   IV. Schaay, Nikki, author, editor

RA427.9.R48 2017   362.1   C2017-900121-3

The research presented in this publication was carried out with the aid of a grant from
the International Development Research Centre, Ottawa, Canada. The views expressed
herein do not necessarily represent those of IDRC or its Board of Governors.

University of Toronto Press acknowledges the financial assistance to its publishing
program of the Canada Council for the Arts and the Ontario Arts Council, an agency
of the Government of Ontario.

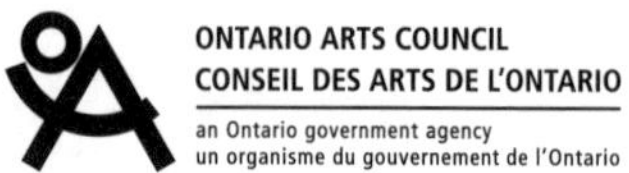

Canada

Contents

List of Figures and Tables

Tables

Abbreviations

ABS	Australian Bureau of Statistics
AHW	Aboriginal health worker
ANC	antenatal care
ANM	auxiliary nurse midwife
AOR	adjusted odds ratio
ASHA	accredited social health activist
CBHIS	community-based health information system
CBIS	community-based information system
CBRHA	community-based reproductive health agent
CHC	community health centre
CHEW	community health extension worker
CHV	community health volunteer
CHW	community health worker
CoHC	community health committee
CPHC	comprehensive primary health care
CSA	community strategy approach
CU	community health unit
DGHS	Directorate General of Health Services
DHS	district health system
DPT3	Diphtheria, Pertussis, and Tetanus – 3 doses
DRC	Democratic Republic of Congo
EDHS	Ethiopian Demographic and Health Survey
EOI	expression of interest
EPS	Health-Promoting Enterprise/Empresa Promotora de Salud
ESF	Family Health Strategy/Estratégia Saúde da Família
FGD	focus group discussion

FMOH	Federal Ministry of Health
FPO	family planning officer
GAVI	Global Alliance for Vaccines and Immunization
GLUK	Great Lakes University of Kisumu
GP	general practitioner
GRIFIA	Gender-Related Index for Indigenous Australians
HBC	home-based care
HEP	Health Extension Program, also referred to as Health Services Extension Program
HEW	health extension worker
HFMC	health facility management committee
HiAP	Health in All Policies
HSEP	Health Service Extension Program, also referred to as Health Extension Program
IAH	intersectoral action for health
ICDS	Integrated Child Development Service
IGA	income-generating activity
ISA	intersectoral action
ITN	insecticide treated net
KEPH	Kenya Essential Package for Health
KHC	Kebele Health Committee
LMIC	low- and middle-income countries
MHP	Male Health Program
MMR	maternal mortality rate
MoH	Ministry of Health
NGO	nongovernmental organization
NHM	National Health Mission
PHC	primary health care
PHCI	public health care coverage intensity
PHM	People's Health Movement
PIC	Collective Intervention Plan/Plan de Intervenciones Colectivas
PNC	postnatal care
POS	Compulsory Health Plan/Plan Obligatorio de Salud
PRA	participatory rapid appraisal
PSF	Family Health Program/Programa Saúde da Família
QLI	Quality of Life Index
RHFA	Revitalizing Health for All
SASC	Home Health/Salud a su Casa
SDG	Sustainable Development Goal

SDH	social determinant(s) of health
SGSSS	Social Security in Health/Sistema General de Seguridad Social en Salud
STI	sexually transmitted infection
SUS	Unified Health System/Sistema Único de Saúde
TBA	traditional birth attendant
TICH	Tropical Institute of Community Health and Development
UBS	Primary Care Unit/Unidade Básica de Saúde
UH	Union Health
UHC	universal health coverage
UpHC	Upazila Health Complex
USF	Family Health Clinic/Unidade de Saúde da Família
VAHS	Victorian Aboriginal Health Service
VIP	Violence Intervention Program
ZHD	Zonal Health Department

Foreword

This volume synthesizes evidence from comprehensive primary health care (CPHC) initiatives and reform from across the globe. The information was compiled through an innovative project entitled *Revitalizing Health for All: Towards Comprehensive Primary Health Care (RHFA)*. The project, which began in 2007 and ended in 2011, had approximately 50 collaborators from countries in Africa, Asia, Latin America, North America, and Europe. The aim of the *RHFA* project was to assess existing knowledge on CPHC and, based on this assessment, to pose new researchable questions that would advance CPHC as a functional, ethical, affordable, and equitable model for health-systems organization in low- and middle-income countries. Our work proceeded from three key propositions that informed our vision for this initiative:

1 Provision of effective, efficient, equitable, and sustainable health care (including disease prevention and health promotion) depends on a broad programmatic approach directed towards meeting the primary health care needs of communities (including vulnerable and marginalized people) while also addressing the social conditions threatening their health. CPHC provides the basis for such a programmatic approach, although the need to interrogate and expand upon the evidence base for its effectiveness remains.
2 CPHC principles have been sharply contested by other models of health care. The controversy results partly from a perception of an inadequate evidence base and from unresolved policy debates including selective versus comprehensive programming; the roles and interrelationships of the public and private sectors; the role or importance of popular participation and mobilization in programs

of care and prevention; and engagement with other policy sectors responsible for what are now frequently referred to as "social determinants of health" (e.g., housing, sanitation, environmental protection, social protection, and labour/employment, to name a few). There is an urgent need to synthesize and provide new evidence that addresses these areas of controversy.

3 Research to provide such evidence poses many methodological challenges, including the plurality of knowledge systems (e.g., technical, lay, culturally embedded) and methods for gathering the required evidence; issues of voice and power in defining, generating, and interpreting such evidence; the need to address the concerns of local practitioners and research users; and, above all, the need to integrate the context-specificity of CPHC implementation into general lessons about its impact and effectiveness.

The CPHC concept arose, in part, as a response to the increasing recognition of the limitations of a biomedical and technological approach to improving health. As outlined in the Declaration of Alma-Ata (World Health Organization and UNICEF, 1978), *comprehensive* primary health care combines not only first-line medical and allied health-care workers offering a range of care from prevention to treatment but also includes other elements such as equity of access, collaboration across sectors beyond health, and community empowerment and participation in the services made available. In 2008, on the thirtieth anniversary of the Alma-Ata Declaration, the World Health Organization issued its annual World Health Report (*Primary Health Care: Now More Than Ever*) addressing some of the successes and identifying many of the gaps in efforts to achieve the health system envisioned in Alma-Ata. Our own parallel project, recounted in this volume, was a "bottom-up" effort to support new research on struggles at different scales and in different parts of the world that have attempted to move towards the comprehensive vision of primary health care so evocatively pronounced more than 30 years ago – one that is no less relevant now than it was then.

Special Thanks

The research project *Revitalizing Health for All: Learning from Comprehensive Primary Health Care Experiences*, which enabled the teams contributing to the book to conduct their research, was kindly supported by the Global Health Research Initiative, a collaborative research funding partnership of the Canadian Institutes of Health Research, the Canadian International Development Agency, Health Canada, the International Development Research Centre (IDRC), and the Public Health Agency of Canada, through IDRC Grant No. 103460-041. Smaller additional grants supported the project, notably a grant from the World Health Organization's Alliance for Health Policy and Systems Research to promote capacity development for health policy and systems research, and IDRC Grant No. 103460-084 to introduce knowledge transfer and exchange as well as outcomes mapping to the project's teams. We are also grateful to the International Development Research Centre for their grant (107108-00020703-025) to collate and publish this volume on the research findings of the project and the individual teams.

We would like to acknowledge that the initial concept for this project was developed in the first International People's Health University, a training course on the political economy of health and primary health care, held in association with the Second People's Health Assembly of the People's Health Movement (www.phmovement.org) in Cuenca, Ecuador, in 2005. Particular thanks go to Francoise Barten, Fran Baum, Rakhal Gaitonde, Maija Kagis, David Legge, Thelma Narayan, and Claudio Schuftan.

We would also like to express our sincere appreciation to Shirley Sarfo, Margaret Frère, Mary Holshausen, and Elsa Michel at the University of Ottawa for their assistance in bringing this book to print. In addition, we wish to thank Nola Haddadian at IDRC for her editing assistance.

Finally, the editors on behalf of the contributors dedicate this book to the memories of Gwendolyn ("Lyn") Lusi, deceased 17 March 2012, and Dr. Christa ("Victoria") Baatz, deceased 17 April 2015. Ms. Lusi (Chapter 4) cofounded a charity providing medical and social services in Goma, DRC, and committed herself to supporting women victims of violent rape. Dr. Baatz played a major and inspiring role in the development of the comprehensive primary health care system in Guarjila, El Salvador, described in Chapter 15.

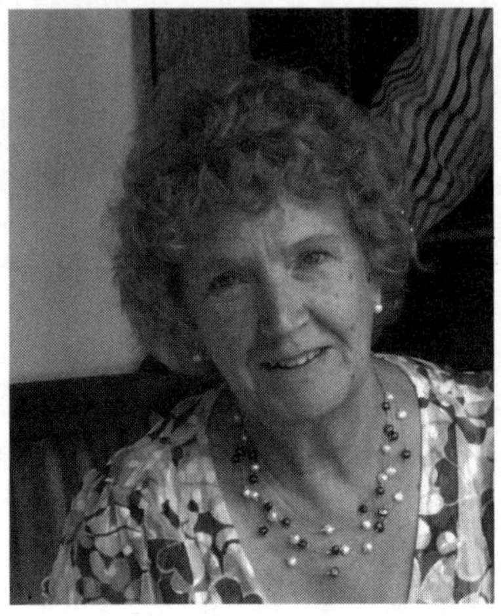

Lyn Lusi, cofounder of HEAL Africa, Democratic Republic of Congo

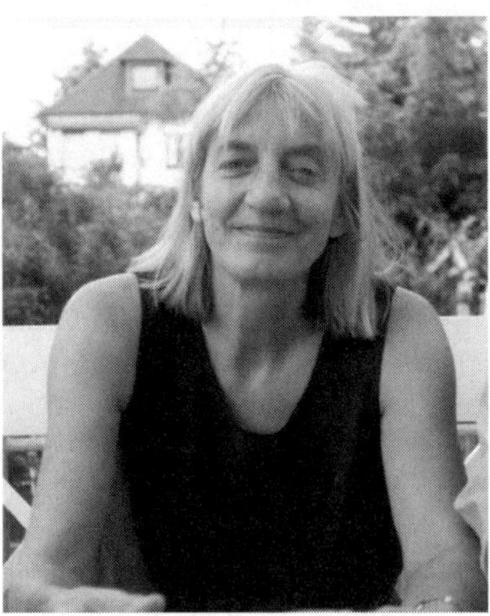

Christa Baatz, champion of CPHC in Guarjila, El Salvador

REVITALIZING HEALTH FOR ALL

Case Studies of the Struggle for
Comprehensive Primary Health Care

1 Introduction and Background

RONALD LABONTÉ, DAVID SANDERS,
CORINNE PACKER, AND NIKKI SCHAAY

Rationale

The ambitious goal of achieving "Health for All by the Year 2000" was first expressed in the Alma-Ata Declaration on Primary Health Care in 1978 (World Health Organization [WHO], 1978). The declaration's vision was for a broader, more inclusive approach to health across all care levels – one that emphasized the primary and community levels and that was sensitive to the social and economic conditions that impact both individual and community health.

Based upon the literature at the time of developing our research project, interest in and support for the revitalization of comprehensive primary health care (CPHC) resulted principally from three factors:

1 Despite impressive developments in biomedicine, progress in improving health has been moderate (Evans, Whitehead, Diderichsen, Bhuiya, & Wirth, 2001; WHO, 2004).
2 Inequities in both wealth and health have increased over the past decades, and, in some countries, health status has stagnated or even worsened. Action on social determinants of health (SDH) will contribute to reducing these health inequities (Adeyi, Chellaraj, Goldstein, Preker, & Ringold, 1997; Bates et al., 2004 May and June; Cornia, 2001; Cornia, Addison, & Kiiski, 2003; Farmer, 2003; Jenkins, 2004; Labonté, Schrecker, Sanders, & Meeus, 2004; Labonté, Schrecker, & Sen Gupta, 2005; People's Health Movement, 2005; Wade, 2004).
3 Despite reaffirmation of CPHC as the basis of their health policies by national governments and the WHO (National Primary Health

Care Conference: Celebrating the 25th Anniversary of the Alma-Ata, 2003; Sanders, 1998), emphasis on selective, vertical, and disease-centred approaches has led to an unsustainable patchwork of health interventions that is increasingly recognized as an impediment to achieving health equity in many parts of the world (Buse & Walt, 1997; Focus on the Global South, 2003; Magnussen, Ehiri, & Jolly, 2004; Pogge, 2004; UN Millennium Project, 2005; UN Millennium Project Task Force on Improving the Lives of Slum Dwellers, 2005; Wagstaff & Claeson, 2003; Widdus & White, 2004; SWEF, 2003).[1]

CPHC can be considered a sociopolitical philosophy as well as an implementation strategy for improved health equity. As a sociopolitical philosophy, it emphasizes equity in access to health care and to the SDH, while its implementation requires both sociopolitical processes and technological choices. Thus, the CPHC approach (in its earliest iteration in the Alma-Ata Declaration) embodied a set of five key principles, namely:

- universal accessibility and coverage on the basis of need: in other words support for the principle of equity;
- comprehensive care (which includes the integration of preventive, curative, rehabilitative, and promotive services);
- intersectoral collaboration and action to address the social and environmental determinants of ill health;
- active community participation in program and service planning; and
- appropriate care and use of technology.

The Alma-Ata Declaration also recognized that the possibility of attaining health equity through PHC was dependent on an equitable global economic system: that "economic and social development, based on a New International Economic Order, is of basic importance to the fullest attainment of health for all and to the reduction of the gap between the health status of the developing and developed countries" (WHO, 1978). We return to this point in our final chapter.

---

1   These concerns were also raised in the WHO 2008 World Report, *Primary Health Care: Now More Than Ever*, which was developed at the same time as our study, with input from several of our research team leads.

Key to operationalization of the CPHC approach are:

- an integrated referral system that facilitates the delivery of a continuum of care to clients across different levels and places of care in the health-care system without interruption; and
- multidisciplinary health teams, including community-based health care workers.

CPHC thus requires a "whole-of-health-system" approach. Intrinsic to CPHC is community empowerment as part of a strategy for better and more equitable health outcomes and improved health-system accountability. As such, it prioritizes community-based health care (Cueto, 2004). Different countries have implemented community-based care in different ways. For instance, some low- and middle-income countries (LMICs[2]) have made use of community health workers (CHWs). The massive expansion of rural health services in Communist China and (comparatively) low cost yet comprehensive health, education, and (in some cases) welfare programs in Tanzania, Cuba, Costa Rica, Nicaragua, and Sri Lanka (Halstead, Walsh, & Warren, 1985; Irwin & Scali, 2005; Rohde, Chatterjee, & Morley, 1993; Werner & Sanders, 1997) were examples that demonstrated the positive impact of such a strategy. The three essential features of these CPHC approaches were their recognition that promotion of health depends fundamentally on improving socioeconomic conditions and alleviating poverty and underdevelopment; that, in this process, people in their community or citizen roles should be both major activists and the main beneficiaries; and that health-care systems should be restructured to support priority activities at the community and primary levels because these respond to the most urgent health needs of the people (Magnussen, Ehiri, & Jolly, 2004; Werner & Sanders, 1997).

---

2 Previously, socioeconomic differences between countries were described by reference to First, Second, and Third World countries. More commonly, countries were referred to as developed (high income, industrialized), developing (low income, agricultural), and least developed (very low income). More recently, and given the imprecision of these categorizations, designation by per capita income levels (high, middle, and low incomes) is becoming the preferred choice. None is perfect, and all tend to ignore the historic political and economic forces that create conditions of chronic underdevelopment and inequality.

Building on the momentum of the Declaration of Alma-Ata, CPHC continued to inspire community health practitioners around the world, including the centrality of CPHC in the work of the People's Health Movement (PHM). PHM, an international network founded in 2000 with eight founding organizations and country circles throughout the world that comprises health researchers, policymakers, and civil-society activists, had two principal campaigns: 1) the renewal of CPHC; and 2) the strengthening of the right to health, with a focus on access to health care. It called for CPHC revitalization at both of its first two People's Health Assemblies (2000, 2005) and in the documents that were produced following these meetings – the People's Health Charter (People's Health Movement, 2000) and the Cuenca Declaration (People's Health Movement, 2005). The rapid rate at which the movement grew was testimony to both the desire for a revitalization of CPHC principles and strategies and to a strong civil-society movement backing these aims.

At the second People's Health Assembly in 2005, in anticipation of the thirtieth anniversary of the Alma-Ata Declaration in 2008,[3] a group of health researchers and activists formulated an innovative project entitled *Revitalizing Health for All: Towards Comprehensive Primary Health Care (RHFA)*. The project, which began in 2007 and ended in 2011, had approximately 50 collaborators from nearly 20 countries in Africa, Asia, Latin America, and Europe. It also included an Aboriginal component incorporating CPHC research from indigenous communities in Australia, New Zealand, and Canada. Although PHC from its beginnings has been a global strategy, its adoption and implementation have been predominantly in LMICs where the gains in terms of health outcomes, especially for mothers and children, have been perceived to be substantial where successful models have been developed. Equally, literature suggested that both health challenges and the potential impact of PHC were likely to be similar among (usually marginalized) indigenous minorities in high-income countries (Torzillo & Kerr, 1992).

Strategic leadership assistance was provided by the umbrella institutional partner, PHM, project co-leads located at the University of Ottawa (Canada) and the University of the Western Cape (South Africa), and a core team of representatives from Asia, Latin America, Europe, North

---

3 The importance of primary health care was reaffirmed upon the thirtieth anniversary of the declaration in the WHO World Health Report 2008 (WHO, 2008) and a special issue of *The Lancet* devoted to the theme (*The Lancet*, 2008).

America, and Australia. The project was carried out with support from the Global Health Research Initiative, a collaborative research-funding partnership of the Canadian Institutes of Health Research, the Canadian International Development Agency, Health Canada, the International Development Research Centre, and the Public Health Agency of Canada.

The principal goals of the *RHFA* project were threefold:

1 to renew the evidence base for the effectiveness of CPHC;
2 to enhance the capacities of researchers to generate and use new CPHC research knowledge for policy and program change in specific country contexts; and
3 to build regional and global networks of researchers and policy-makers to use research knowledge as one tool for advancing (and revitalizing) CPHC.

Distinctive Features of the Project

Synthesizing the existing evidence base: A review of CPHC literature

While there were documented CPHC experiences prior to the *RFHA* project, some of their weaknesses were also apparent. In some instances, for example, too little attention was given to the importance of the local sociopolitical context within which the CPHC effort took place. These contexts, in turn, both condition and constrain the full implementation of CPHC, leading to numerous partial implementations and a need to understand not only their accomplishments, but how those that have moved closer to an idealized CPHC have been able to do so (Brown & Fee, 2004; Kunitz, 2004; Sibthorpe, Glasgow, & Wells, 2005; Tatar & Tatar, 1997). The intention of our initiative was to fill this knowledge gap by conducting research on CPHC activities in the present and bringing together practitioners, researchers, and research-users to document more fully CPHC lessons from the past. Our goal was to increase our understanding of and support for CPHC as a basis for health-system revitalization. In short, we intended to renew, expand, and deepen the evidence base for CPHC, recognizing that no such systematic effort has occurred since the early 1990s.

One of the ways devised to *renew* the evidence base regarding the effectiveness of CPHC was to undertake a large global literature review. Seven bibliographic databases were consulted using an OVID interface: Medline (1966 to 2007), EMBASE (1980 to 2007), HealthStar (1966 to

1998), HealthStar (1999 to 2007), CINAHL (1982 to 2007), the Cochrane Central Register of Controlled Trials (2007), and Sociological Abstracts (1952 to 2007). As the literature was collected in mid-2007, only literature published through the first half of 2007 would have been captured. In addition, we called upon the 50-odd collaborators engaged in the *RHFA* project to search their own literature databanks for literature relevant to CPHC. The citations were entered into *Reference Manager* v11.0, and after removal of duplicates, a total of 95,845 citations remained. Other search strategies included internet Google searches, reference lists, and proceedings from key conferences for abstracts of unpublished data. Almost all of the database citations (notably those from high-income countries) used the term "primary health care" but were concerned only with primary medical or clinical care. Our inclusion criterion for the literature review required that the studies must address two or more of the Alma-Ata key principles (stated above) as we reconfigured them slightly for purposes of our study (described below). Based on rapid abstract reviews, most of the database citations were removed. A more deliberate search of grey literature supplemented the database search and led to a final list of 336 articles, reports, or papers.

This collection, which was divided into "grey" (nonpeer reviewed) and scientific (peer reviewed) literature, was distributed for analysis to geographically based teams. Review teams focused on "areas": Australia and New Zealand; Asia; Africa; Europe; South America; North America; and Indigenous Canada. An additional team reviewed the literature that discussed CPHC from a global perspective (i.e., not local or national CPHC initiatives).

The core project-management team developed a template for coding and analysing the global literature on CPHC experiences, with inter-rater reliability checks to ensure that the literature would be consistently reviewed. All teams conducting the literature review followed the established review protocol. The findings from this exercise are summarized in Chapter 2.

Research Triads

One of the ways devised to expand and deepen the evidence base regarding the effectiveness of CPHC was to select, fund, and train 20 research triads to carry out new research on CPHC experiences within their regions. The *RHFA* project leads recognized that to achieve this goal of generating new evidence, the capacities of researchers to generate and use new CPHC research knowledge also would have to be enhanced. To this end, the project sought to reduce the challenges that often arise between the researcher and the research-user in health systems studies by developing an innovative "research-to-action" model – a team that comprised three unique members:

1　An early-career researcher. He/she was typically located within an academic institution and was assigned to manage, facilitate, and implement the research project.
2　A research-user. This was a government official, health practitioner, manager, or policymaker in a mid- or senior-level position who was typically responsible for managing some aspect of the country's PHC policies or programs.
3　A mentor. He/she was a senior researcher with experience in research on CPHC or health-systems development. The role of the mentor was to help develop the research skills of the early-career researcher and nurture the collaboration between the early-career researcher and research-user.

With the guidance of the project's leads and trainers, the relationship between the team members was to be one of close collaboration, joint decision making, and mutual learning. Together, they would develop the research protocol, implement the study, and disseminate the findings. By establishing such mixed teams, it was anticipated that the research undertaken would better suit the needs and interests of the research-user, would find support throughout the data collection process, and would increase the likelihood of uptake or implementation of the research findings.[4] Throughout the course of the *RHFA* project, each of the research triads (located in Africa, Asia, Latin America, and those working with Indigenous/Aboriginal peoples in Canada, Australia, and New Zealand) worked collaboratively to a) design and implement

---

4　No explicit theory for the use of triads was used in this research study. Rather, the concept of triads was developed from the two coprincipal applicants' experiences in enhancing research capacities in low-resource settings (such as many low-income countries), in which the role of research mentors is important; and in the several community/university research partnerships undertaken by Labonté in the 1990s and early 2000s, in which engagement of research-users throughout all stages of research activity (including design of questions, methods, analyses, and final write-up and publication) proved successful in developing policy responsiveness to study findings.

a CPHC research project, and b) collectively advocate that the results (both in terms of outcome and process) be used to inform the development and/or implementation of health policy and practice in the local context. To this end, all three members of the team were expected to actively engage with local/zonal/district, regional/provincial, and national health policymakers in their respective countries. They would thus function as "knowledge brokers" or "policy entrepreneurs," engaging with peers locally, regionally, and nationally around the ability of health ministries to absorb such research findings and discussing with them what implications these results might have for policy and program development.

The "expression of interest" process

Fifteen members of the core project team, including those who had directed the regional CPHC literature reviews, met in Johannesburg, South Africa, in late 2007. With the initial regional results of the literature review in hand, the members finalized the project's "expressions of interest" (EOI) document. The EOI was essentially a call for research teams committed to developing important new knowledge and action on CPHC to apply for funding to support their proposed area of interest. The "Call for Expressions of Interest to Participate in New Research and Research Training in Comprehensive Primary Health Care" applied to four different areas/regions in which the *RHFA* project would focus, namely:

- India and South Asia;
- Africa;
- Latin America; and
- Indigenous/Aboriginal peoples in Canada and Australia.

Although PHC as codified in the Alma-Ata Declaration was intended to be the basis for health policy internationally, its adoption (as noted earlier) has been most enthusiastic in LMICs and especially in association with facilitative political or social movements (Alternative World Health Report, 2011). For this reason, and because of the limitations determined by the funding agency (which excludes high-income countries) and the scarcity of literature on CPHC emanating from high-income countries (where studies on primary *medical* care dominated), the call for EOIs was directed at the "Global South." This call nonetheless included Indigenous communities in high-income countries that were known to have developed efforts in CPHC under social and economic conditions similar to those in LMICs. However, it was intended that any general lessons learned would be communicated through publications, presentations, and via the People's Health Movement network to practitioners and PHC supporters in high-income countries.

The call for EOIs was widely circulated in English and Spanish through the project's network of collaborators and relevant listservs, notably that of the People's Health Movement. To submit an EOI, the team had already to be formed: an early-career researcher, research-user, and mentor had to be named, thus forming our triads. All members of the team (in a few cases teams had more than one mentor, or more than one research-user) had to submit a letter signed by their institutions stating that they would be given the time to commit to this project and participate in both the capacity-building and research processes over a three-year period. In circulating the call for EOIs, and based on extensive planning meetings for the overall project, we slightly amended the Alma-Ata principles to reflect the experiences of the core CPHC project team. In doing so, and in addition to the Alma-Ata principles, we described six ideal outcomes of CPHC. It should

1 increase equity in access to health care and other services/resources essential for health;
2 promote community empowerment and thereby reduce community vulnerabilities;
3 address the social and environmental determinants of health and thereby reduce exposure to risk;
4 improve community participation and political capabilities of marginalized groups;
5 increase intersectoral policy actions on social and economic determinants of health; and
6 improve population health outcomes and health equity.

We were clear at the outset of the project that we did not expect to see any examples of this fully idealized CPHC. The dominance of selective PHC since Alma-Ata, the role of international funders/donors in the health systems of many LMICs, and increasing pressures for privatization or creation of public-private partnerships in health-care delivery more globally were all seen as probable brakes on the comprehensiveness of PHC efforts. Rather, we anticipated that there would be pockets of innovation that were struggling to move beyond simply the first principle (equitable access) to incorporate different combinations of second through fifth principles, leading to some success in achieving the sixth. Thus, the EOIs were specific that not only was action in the first principle axiomatic (CPHC was grounded in health services), but also that the project to be studied must involve efforts in one or more of principles two through five, essentially following the same inclusion criteria as for the literature review.

Eighty-five applications were received. These were separated by region and given to regional teams of evaluators along with the *RHFA* project's "Protocol for Reviewing EOIs," which included a scoring chart. Twenty teams from 16 different countries were selected for participation and offered funding.[5]

Triad training and evaluations

As noted earlier, a principal goal of the *RHFA* project was "to enhance the capacities of researchers to generate and use new CPHC research." To this end, all members of selected teams were required to participate in capacity-enhancing workshops. The workshops, organized annually over a period of three years and together totalling more than four weeks of training, were conducted by the *RHFA* project faculty and mentors from each team and explored aspects of both research and policy development. The regional workshops were held in four parts of the world: Asia, Africa, Latin America, and Australia (for the Australian, New Zealand, and Canadian Indigenous teams). Regional meetings to bring together a larger number of interested groups, practitioners, and policymakers were organized alongside these workshops, in some cases involving several hundred attendees.

---

5 In addition to these 20 teams, one other team based in Nicaragua participated in the regional training sessions in Latin America at their own cost throughout the lifespan of the project. Another team in Asia (Gonoshasthaya Kendra in Bangladesh) also participated in the regional trainings in Asia, at their own cost, although extra funding was sought and received from IDRC to cover the costs of carrying out their studies. A team from Zimbabwe and another Kenyan team participated in the first Africa training workshop but not thereafter. A report on the separate Gonoshasthaya Kendra study is available on the project's website: Hassan, R. & Surur, H. "Study on GK's Comprehensive Primary Health Care (CPHC) Model: Social Capital, Community Participation, Gender Empowerment and Health Care Access for the Marginalized." http://www.globalhealthequity.ca/webfm_send/287

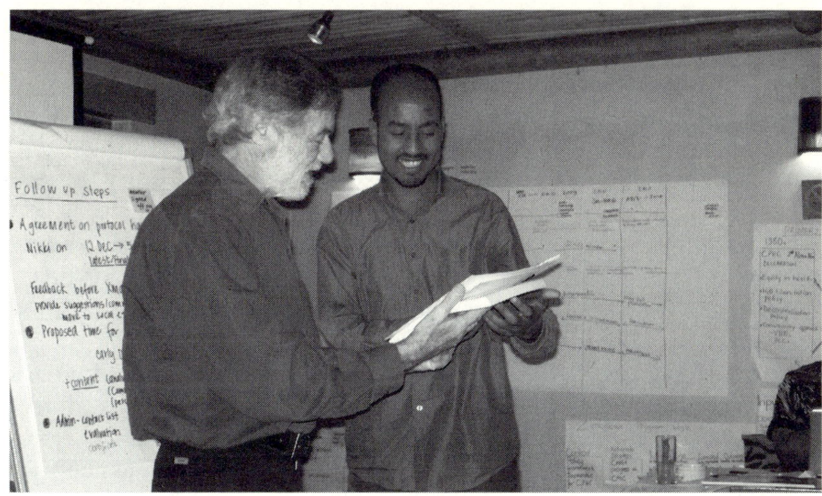

Project workshop for African research teams, Cape Town, South Africa

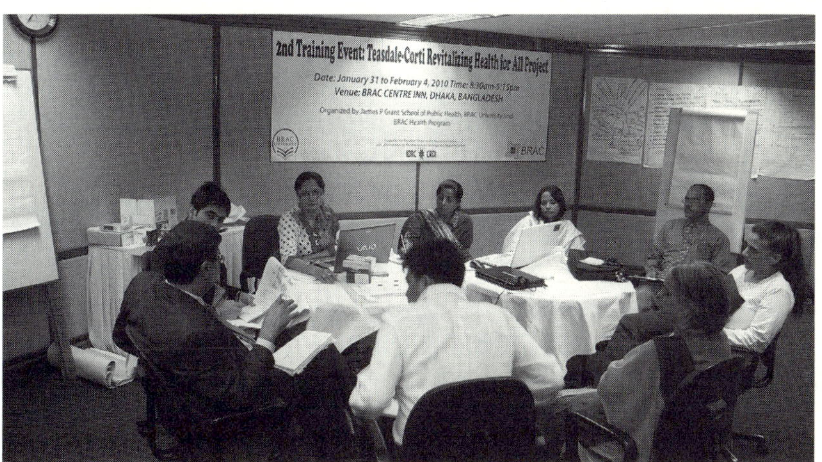

Project workshop for Asian research teams, Dhaka, Bangladesh

Curriculum at the first training included understanding the history, theory, and practice of CPHC; an overview of basic research and evaluation skills for proposed studies; and the revision and development of research protocols submitted with their original EOIs. By the end of the first training, teams were expected to have developed and finalized collaboratively robust research protocols ready to submit for ethics approval by local academic institutions or research councils. All teams received ethics clearances from their local institutions (a condition of funding transfer for their studies), and the overall project, including synopses of all of the individual studies, received ethics clearance through the Research Ethics Board at the University of Ottawa.

At the second workshop, teams reviewed and analysed preliminary results from their field research. Faculty members also worked to help them develop preliminary knowledge translation and exchange strategies. At the third and final training, teams presented the final analyses of their research findings and discussed their publication and dissemination strategies. Facilitators addressed how researchers could build their skills in relation to dissemination of the research results (e.g., through the media or in policy reviews).

Our teams conducted regular self-assessments of the effectiveness of their partnerships in order to advance their projects' potential to transform research into practice. This process began with a structured exercise during the second round of regional training sessions, which focused on some of the key elements of the "knowledge translation and exchange" process, adapting sections of the IDRC manual on outcome mapping (Earl, Carden, & Smutylo, 2001). During the final regional workshops, teams were asked to reflect on their triad experience.

The feedback from the teams on the triad experience was overwhelmingly positive. Most groups suggested that having individuals with different expertise enhanced the research relevance and usefulness as well as the ability to develop relationships and disseminate the research findings. The major constraining factor lay in communication challenges between triad group members due to differences in location and scheduling conflicts.

The involvement of the research-user was perceived as significantly increasing the opportunities and effectiveness of the program and improving relationships with both policy developers and local health workers. Many of the teams commented that the triad was a model that other researchers, government organizations, NGOs, and communities could use to strengthen their research-to-action and effectively bridge the worlds of people engaged in policy and program design and implementation and those involved in generating research and evaluation evidence.

One interesting and unexpected finding from the overall experience of the triads was that the distinction between researcher and research-user was often artificial and, in some cases, resented. "Research-users" (many of the teams included more than one) were often competent researchers themselves and not passive consumers of research knowledge or subordinate to the methodological expertise of researchers. Researchers, in turn, often had important insights into program and policy work. This in no way weakens the conceptual importance of establishing research triads but cautions that care and sensitivity are required when assigning the different labels.

Overview of the book

In the preceding sections of this chapter, we have provided some background on the project and how it set out to achieve its goals. Chapter 2 synthesizes the findings of reviews of the literature on CPHC on a regional basis, up to the year 2007 (when the review period ended). Table 1.1 provides a summary of all the different studies undertaken, identifying their authors, their methods, and which of the six ideal outcomes of CPHC they examined. Chapters 3 through 15 are the contributions from the funded triad teams that were able to make a full contribution to this book. Although all teams studied several aspects of CPHC, as Table 1.1 illustrates, their chapter contributions often spoke most strongly to one of four key themes that help to define PHC's "comprehensiveness." Each of these themes is introduced with a brief overview of the chapters in these sections.

The first section is on the theme of "Increasing Equitable Access to Health Care," of foundational importance in primary health care, comprehensive or otherwise. Three uniquely different contributions (in geography, history, and financing) are clustered here: a male-health program in Aboriginal Central Australia (Chapter 3), a safe-motherhood initiative in rural Democratic Republic of Congo (Chapter 4), and a more system-wide effort to implement CPHC reforms in Bogotá, Colombia (Chapter 5).

The second section is on the theme of "Community Engagement." Three more contributions are added to the book: a look at efforts to improve community participation in two provinces in South Africa

Table 1.1 CPHC *Revitalizing Health for All* research projects

Country and project title	Research team	Research focus and project publications	Key methods *	CPHC foci **
India (Bihar) The Contribution of the Accredited Social Health Activist (ASHA) under the National Rural Health Mission (NRHM) in the Implementation of Comprehensive Primary Health Care in East Champaran District, Bihar (State) India	Anil Cherian, Vandana Kanth, Jameela George	The role of community health workers (accredited social health activists, or ASHAs) in improving access to health services and advocacy on social determinants of health.	Survey of 299 households to measure knowledge, behaviour and practice changes attributable to ASHA interventions Structured key informant interviews of ASHAs (199), child-development workers (255), auxiliary nurse midwives (17), and village headmen/village committee members (27) Focus groups with village members	1, 2, 3, 4, 5
India (Arunachal Pradesh) Exploring Synergies between Empowerment and Gender and Comprehensive Primary Health Care in Three Tribal Districts of Arunachal Pradesh	Tage Kanno, Manjunath Shankar, Betsy Taylor, Hage Tam	The role of village health volunteers in promoting gender empowerment and community participation, and its impacts on comprehensiveness of and access to PHC services.	Key health indicators (control/gender empowerment intervention localities) Key informant interviews (n = 47) Participant observation (5 sites, multiple days) Focus group discussions (4 focus groups, total n = 60) Photovoice project/analysis (3 sites)	1, 2, 3, 4, 6
Iran The Contribution of Community Health Workers to the Implementation of Comprehensive Primary Health Care in Rural Settings	Sara Javanparast, Fran Baum, Gholamreza Heidari	The role of *behvarz* (Farsi term for community health workers) in enhancing all outputs of CPHC. (1) (2) (3)	Systematic literature review Document analysis including Iranian health ministry policy and unpublished reports Semistructured interviews with 91 *behvarz* in a representative sample of 18 Iranian provinces	1, 2, 3, 4, 5
Pakistan Perceptions about the Effectiveness of Three Models of Comprehensive Primary Health Care in Urban Squatter Settlements of Karachi	Parvez Nayani, Agha Ajmal, Yousuf Memon	Comparison of the comprehensiveness and sustainability of three models of PHC service development in poor communities supported by Agha Khan University: institution-led (externally financed, planned, and delivered), community-led (joint institution and community financed), community planned, copartnership (externally financed, community planned, and managed).	Document analysis Key informant interviews (n = 30) Focus-group discussions (12 focus groups, total n = 115)	1, 2, 3, 4, 5

Country and project title	Research team	Research focus and project publications	Key methods *	CPHC foci **
Bangladesh Revitalizing Health for All: Developing a Comprehensive Primary Health Care Model for Bangladesh	Taufique Joarder, Anwar Islam, Aftab Uddin	Identifying structural characteristics of CPHC through comparison of high- and low-performing health districts.	Document analysis and 4 key informant interviews (for history of PHC in Bangladesh) Index ranking of 10 urban and 10 rural health districts by health system performance using World Health Organization criteria from its 2000 report (for selection of high- and low-performing health districts) Ethnographic observations at 2 selected health districts; key informant interviews (n = 40); randomized household survey (n = 225 households) evaluating PHC services; participatory rapid appraisal (n = 30 participants) in each health district	1, 2, 3, 4, 5, 6
Uruguay Rural and Community Policlinics in Uruguay: Their Role in the New Integrated National Health System	Fernando Borgia, Ingrid Gabrielzyk, Jorge Soto, Marcela Azambuja, Alexis Gularte, Helena Giménez, Miguel Corneo, Marlene Arrarás, Sebastián González	The contribution and role of rural and community policlinics (health centres) in the country's new National System for Integrated Health.	Microdata from 4 waves of household survey (2007–9) Systematic document review and analyses Administrative data and historical narratives from 119 policlinics representing urban and rural settings Data from 5 regional policlinic meetings and from 11 local forums in 19 states (n = over 900 participants)	1, 3, 4, 5
El Salvador The Experience of Primary Health Care in El Salvador	Maria Argelia Dubón Abrego, Dagoberto Menjívar López, Eduardo Antonio Espinoza Fiallos, Christa Baatz	A detailed historical case study of the CPHC system developed in the village of Guarjila (1987–2007), now serving as a model of PHC development nationally.	In-depth interviews with community leaders, organized groups; and focus groups with community members Documentary and bibliographic analysis Participant observation	1, 2, 3, 4, 5, 6

Table 1.1 CPHC *Revitalizing Health for All* research projects (*Continued*)

Country and project title	Research team	Research focus and project publications	Key methods *	CPHC foci **
Colombia Learning From the Experience of Primary Health Care in Bogotá	Román Rafael Vega Romero, Paola Andrea Mosquera Méndez, Jinneth Hernández Torres, Jorge Martínez Collantes	The contribution of recent CPHC reforms in reducing health inequities through ecological analyses comparing high and low coverage in two disadvantaged localities, and pre- and post-implementation of PHC reforms on child health outcomes. (4) (5)	Data from 2 household surveys (2003 and 2007) and public health administrative databases; calculating concentration curves and indices, and regression analyses, related to child health outcomes and selected indicators of PHC coverage. Semistructured key informant interviews (n = 18) and 14 focus groups (n = 7–10/group) in district health localities, including decision makers, health staff, and community members	1, 2, 4, 6
Brazil Health-Care Coordination: Construction of Comprehensive Primary Health Care in Brazil	Patty Fidelis de Almeida, Lígia Giovanella, Berardo Augusto Nunan	Comparison of coordination mechanisms in four municipalities to integrate Brazil's CPHC model (family health teams) into secondary and tertiary levels of health care. (6) (7)	Health system administrative database. Key informant interviews with all level of health staff, including community health workers (n = 77)	1, 4, 6
Argentina The Political Dimension of Primary Health Care in Argentina: Repressed Components, Disordered Growth, and Models in Conflict: A Reconstruction from the Testimonies, Historical Footprints, and Clues in a Temporal-Spatial Exploration	Mario Rovere, Andrea Jait, Analía Bertolotto, Ana Fuks, Eugenia Bagnasco	Historical comparative study of different models of PHC programs targeting disadvantaged urban and rural populations. (8)	Bibliographic review and analyses. Key informant interviews (n = 35). Focus group discussions (3 focus groups, total n = 82). Discourse analysis	1, 2, 4, 5
Ethiopia (Jimma) Health Services Extension Program and Comprehensive Primary Health Care	Sudhakar Narayan Morankar, Mirkuzie Woldie Kerie, Abera Asefa Deressa	The role of community health workers and community participation in improving health outputs and outcomes. (9)	Representative household survey in 3 districts at early, mid and late implementation of program (n = 695). Key informant interviews (n = 4). Focus group discussions (5 focus groups, total n = 43)	1, 2, 4, 5

Country and project title	Research team	Research focus and project publications	Key methods *	CPHC foci **
Ethiopia (Tigray) The Contribution of the Health Extension Program in Promoting Comprehensive Primary Health Care in Tigray, Ethiopia: The Case of Maternal Health	Araya Abrha Medhanyie, Mark Spigt, Yohannes Tewelde Kifle, Yemane Berhane	The contribution of the Health Extension Program to the comprehensiveness of PHC services targeted to maternal health. (10)	Representative survey of women in areas served by program (n = 725) Key informant interviews (n = 15) Focus group discussions (8 focus groups, total n = 73)	1, 2, 4, 5
South Africa The Gauteng Province Community Health Worker Program: The Extent to Which It Contributes to the Provision of Comprehensive Primary Health Care	Nonhlanhla Nxumalo, Jane Goudge, Liz Thomas, Salamina Hlahane	A comparison of enablers and barriers to the effectiveness of community health workers in facilitating community participation, intersectoral action on social determinants of health, and access to formal health systems in three disadvantaged regions.	Key informant interviews (n = 24), including 4 focus group discussions Ethnographic participant/observation (74 household/CHW observations) Network mapping	1, 4, 5
Kenya Uptake and Contribution of a Community Strategy in the Renewal of Comprehensive Primary Health Care in Different Sociodemographic Contexts in Kenya	Jack Buong, Clementine Gwoswar, Dan Kaseje	An assessment of the contribution of the community health strategy (a model of CPHC now being generalized across the country) to the comprehensiveness of health system services in three socio-demographic contexts, and under three different modes of implementation.	Household survey (n = 3,694) Key informant interviews (n = 7) Focus group discussions (14 focus groups, total n = 134) Client exit interviews (n = 422)	1, 2, 3, 4, 5
Democratic Republic of Congo Exploring the Complex Contributions of a Community-based Safe Motherhood Program to Comprehensive Primary Health Care	Richard Bitwe Mihanda, Jean Robert Likofata, Gwendolyn J. Lusi	Evaluation of a maternal health program (Safe Motherhood) based upon local organization (solidarity groups, comprising microcredit/income generation, and pooled insurance) for its contribution to maternal health care and its potential as a model for health-systems reconstruction in a postconflict setting. (11)	Survey of solidarity groups (n = 174) and matched controls (n = 174) Key informant interviews (n = 6) 20 focus group discussions (solidarity group and control group members, traditional birth attendants, men in both solidarity group and control communities)	1, 2, 3, 4

Table 1.1 CPHC *Revitalizing Health for All* research projects (*Continued*)

Country and project title	Research team	Research focus and project publications	Key methods *	CPHC foci **
Australia (Alice Springs) Ingkintja: Learning from Comprehensive Primary Health Care Experiences	Clive Rosewarne, Gai Wilson, John Liddle	Evaluation of the comprehensiveness of an Aboriginal-controlled male-health program in a central Australian town. (12)	Document and program evaluation analyses Key informant interviews (n = 20) Community consultations (3 separate consultations, total n = 39) Service user consultation (1 consultation, total n = 12)	1, 2, 3, 4, 5
Australia (Utopia) Well-being at Utopia: The Role of Urapuntja Health Service	Sarah Doherty, Kevin Rowley, Ricky Tilmouth	Historical study of the comprehensiveness of an Aboriginal remote health service, serving medical and social health needs of 700 Aboriginal people spread over 250 square kilometres. (12)	Administrative data Census data (cross sectional analysis) Archival document analyses Key informant interviews (n = 11) Focus group discussions (2 focus groups, total n = 16) Participant/observation	1, 2, 3
Australia (Melbourne) Victorian Aboriginal Health Service: Revitalizing Health for All Project	Bronwyn Fredericks, Joanne Luke, Alan Brown	Historical study of the comprehensiveness of a community-run Aboriginal health service in an urban setting. (12)	Administrative data Archival document analyses Key informant interviews/oral histories Focus group discussion	1, 2, 3, 4, 5
Aotearoa/New Zealand Setting Up the Try! The Role of the Community Health Worker in a Māori Person's Health Journey	Tania Forrest, Pat Neuwelt, Rowena Gotty, Sue Crengle	The role of community health workers in improving access for Māori to culturally appropriate primary health care services.	Administrative data Archival document analyses Key informant interviews (n = 5) Focus group discussions (2 focus groups, total n = 10)	1, 2, 4
Canada Comprehensive Primary Health Care in the Island Lake Communities: What Does It Mean and How Does It Look?	Marcia Anderson DeCoteau, Grace McDougall, Carly Scramstad, Alex McDougall	Identification of Aboriginal health beliefs and values to inform a governance model for Aboriginal-run CPHC services. (13)	Literature review Focus group discussions (3 focus groups, total n = 23)	1, 3, 4

* The numbers appearing in the third column (Research focus and project publications) refer to publications from the studies, which are listed below.

** The numbers appearing in the fifth column (CPHC foci) refer to the output and outcome criteria of comprehensive primary health care used to guide the overall study, as follows: 1. increased equity in access to health care and other services/resources essential to health; 2. reduced vulnerabilities through increases in community empowerment; 3. reduced exposures to risk through improvements in social and environmental determinants of health; 4. improved participatory mechanisms and opportunities for, and increased political capabilities of, marginalized population groups; 5. increased intersectoral policy actions on the social and economic determinants of health; and 6. improved population health outcomes and health equity.

(1) Javanparast, S., Baum, F., Labonté, R. and Sanders, D. (2011). Community health workers' perspectives on their contribution to rural health and well-being in Iran. *American Journal of Public Health, 101*(12), e1–e6.

(2) Javanparast, S., Baum, F., Labonté, R., Sanders, D., Heidari, G., & Rezaie, S. (2011). A policy review of the community health worker programme in Iran. *Journal of Public Health Policy, 32*(2), 263–76. http://dx.doi.org/10.1057/jphp.2011.7

(3) Javanparast, S., Baum, F., Labonté, R., Sanders, D., Rajabi, Z., & Heidari, G. (2012). The experience of community health workers training in Iran: A qualitative study. *BMC Health Services Research, 12*, 291. http://dx.doi.org/10.1186/1472-6963-12-291

(4) Mosquera, P., Hernández, J., Vega, R., Martínez, J., Labonté, R. Sanders, D., & San Sebastián, M. (2012). The impact of primary healthcare in reducing inequalities in child health outcomes, Bogota - Colombia: An ecological analysis. *International Journal for Equity in Health, 11*, 66. http://dx.doi.org/10.1186/1475-9276-11-66

(5) Mosquera, P., Hernández, J., Vega, R., Martínez, J., Labonté, R., Sanders, D., & San Sebastián, M. (2012). Primary health care contribution to improve health outcomes in Bogota-Colombia: a longitudinal ecological analysis. *BMC Family Practice, 13*, 84. http://dx.doi.org/10.1186/1471-2296-13-84

(6) Almeida, P.F., Fausto, M.C.R., & Giovanella, L. (2011). Fortalecimento da atencao primaria a saude: estrategia para potencializar a coordenacao dos cuidados. *Revista Panamericana de Salud Pública, 29*(2), 84–95.

(7) Almeida, P.F., Giovanella, L., Mendonca, M., & Escorel, S. (2010). Desafios à coordenação dos cuidados em saúde: estratégias de integração entre níveis assistenciais em grandes centros urbanos. *Cadernos de Saúde Pública, 26*(2), 286–98.

(8) Rovere, M., & Laub, C. (2009). *Possibles: Una Publicacion Para Pensar Lo Local Junto A Lo Global*. Buenos Aires: Associación Civil El Agora.

(9) Woldie, M., Morankar, S., Feyissa, G.T., Labonté, R., & Sanders, D. (2015). Coverage of child health services in rural districts of Ethiopia with the Health Services Extension Program. *Journal of Public Health and Epidemiology, 7*(7), pp. 223–31. http://dx.doi.org/10.5897/JPHE2015.0733

(10) Medhanyie, A., Spigt, M., Kifle, Y., Schaay, N., Sanders, D., Blanco, R., Geertlan, D., & Berhane, Y. (2012) The role of health extension workers in improving utilization of maternal health services in rural areas in Ethiopia: A cross-sectional study. *BMC Health Services Research, 12*, 352. http://dx.doi.crg/10.1186/1472-6963-12-352

(11) Mihanda, R.B., Likofata, J.R., & Lusi, G.J. (2013). Contribution of safe motherhood solidarity groups in using and accessing maternity services during a period of armed conflict. *Health, 5*(7), 1085–91. http://dx.doi.org/10.4236/Health.2013.57146

(12) Fredericks, B., & Legge, D. (2012). Revitalizing health for all: International Indigenous representative group: Learning from the experience of comprehensive primary health care in Aboriginal Australia – A commentary on three project reports. Lowitja Institute. http://www.lowitja.org.au/sites/default/files/docs/Revitalising_Health_report.pdf

(13) Scramstad, C. (2012). Comprehensive primary health care in the Island Lake communities: What does it mean and how does it look? Department of Community Health Science, University of Manitoba.

(Chapter 6), a comparison of reforms based on a community PHC model in western Kenya (Chapter 7), and a comparison of different CPHC approaches in Bangladesh highlighting differences in "empowered" community engagement (Chapter 8).

Our third section focuses on the theme of "Community Health Workers": the *behvarz* CHW program in Iran (Chapter 9), the Accredited Social Health Activist (ASHA) program in North Bihar, India (Chapter 10), and the Health Extension Workers program in Ethiopia (focusing on two different regions in the country) (Chapter 11 and Chapter 12). All four contributions attempt to capture how CHWs contribute to service access and to actions on local SDH. In Iran and Ethiopia, the CHWs are paid employees of the formal health system; in India, they are volunteer village health workers.

Our final section is on the complex theme of "Governance and Intersectoral Action," and the three chapter contributions are all from Latin America. The first focuses on how CPHC services at a local level in Brazil became integrated with higher levels of care (Chapter 13), while a historical study of CPHC models in Argentina brings a more theory-driven exploration of sociopolitical barriers and enablers (Chapter 14). The small community of Guarjila, El Salvador, is the topic of the final case study chapter, which recounts how an entire community became a model of CPHC in action and an inspiration to national reform efforts (Chapter 15).

In reading these differing accounts, we want to emphasize three preliminary points:

1 Although we have organized the case studies into different thematic clusters, most teams explored several aspects of CPHC (Table 1.1). It was decided that to present the case studies in a somewhat (but not entirely) arbitrary thematic clustering would be more useful and interesting to readers, than, for example, organizing them by geographic region.
2 There are notable differences in the academic style and rigour displayed in the chapters. All contributors reported on their work using a standard outline provided by the editors, who in turn worked closely with the contributors on their individual chapters. As editors, however, we did not wish to impose a "standard" Western scientific voice on their work. The importance or implications of their findings thus remain expressed largely in the words of the research teams themselves. In a world of disparate means, resources, and experience, it should not be surprising that each chapter is unique in its presentation style.

3 The project was exceedingly ambitious in that the new studies were undertaken during a short period with minimal financial resources. Of necessity, this meant that their ability to empirically examine the broader comprehensiveness of many of their initiatives devolved to an emphasis on some components only.

We return to this last point in the book's final chapter (Chapter 16), in which we attempt a narrative synthesis across the different studies, linking their findings back to this introductory chapter and to some of the key findings from the literature review. More important, in the five years since this study came to an end the world has changed. We have a new set of post-2015 Sustainable Development Goals, a discourse on "universal health coverage" that has eclipsed much of the initial renewed attention to PHC after release of the 2008 World Health Report on the thirtieth anniversary of the Alma-Ata Declaration, simultaneous concerns over the rise of noncommunicable diseases globally in the midst of fears of new and emergent infectious pandemics, and a world still in a recessionary slump following a global financial crisis, the root causes of which remain to be addressed. These developments do not detract from the importance of some of the findings of our different studies but they do present a more challenging, if in some ways also enabling, global environment in which advances in CPHC might still proceed.

REFERENCES

Adeyi, O., Chellaraj, G., Goldstein, E., Preker, A., & Ringold, D. (1997, Jun). Health status during the transition in Central and Eastern Europe: Development in reverse? *Health Policy and Planning, 12*(2), 132–45. Medline:10168196

Bates, I., Fenton, C., Gruber, J., Lalloo, D., Medina Lara, A., Squire, S.B., …, & Tolhurst, R. (2004, May). Vulnerability to malaria, tuberculosis, and HIV/AIDS infection and disease. Part 1: Determinants operating at individual and household level. *Lancet Infectious Diseases, 4*(5), 267–77. Medline:15120343

Bates, I., Fenton, C., Gruber, J., Lalloo, D., Lara, A.M., Squire, S.B., …, & Tolhurst, R. (2004, Jun). Vulnerability to malaria, tuberculosis, and HIV/AIDS infection and disease. Part II: Determinants operating at environmental and institutional level. *Lancet Infectious Diseases, 4*(6), 368–75. Medline:15172345

Brown, T.M., & Fee, E. (2004, Nov). A role for public health history. *American Journal of Public Health*, 94(11), 1851–3. Medline:15514219

Buse, K., & Walt, G. (1997, Aug). An unruly mélange? Coordinating external resources to the health sector: A review. *Social Science & Medicine*, 45(3), 449–63. Medline:9232739

Cornia, G.A. (2001). Globalization and health: Results and options. *Bulletin of the World Health Organization*, 79(9), 834–41. Medline:11584731

Cornia, G.A., Addison, T., & Kiiski, S. (2003). Income distribution changes and their impact in the post- World War II period (Discussion Paper No. 2003/028). Helsinki: UNU-WIDER. Retrieved from UNU-Wider website: https://www.wider.unu.edu/publication/income-distribution -changes-and-their-impact-post-world-war-ii-period

Cueto, M. (2004, Nov). The origins of primary health care and selective primary health care. *American Journal of Public Health*, 94(11), 1864–74. https://www.ncbi.nlm.nih.gov/pmc/articles/PMC1448553/

Earl, S., Carden, F., & Smutylo, T. (2001). Outcome mapping: Building learning and reflection into development programs. Ottawa: IDRC. Retrieved from https://www.idrc.ca/en/book/outcome-mapping-building-learning-and -reflection-development-programs

Evans, T., Whitehead, M., Diderichsen, F., Bhuiya, A., & Wirth, M. (2001). *Challenging inequities in health: From ethics to action*. New York: Oxford University Press.

Farmer, P. (2003). *Pathologies of power: Health, human rights and the new war on the poor*. Berkeley: University of California Press.

Focus on the Global South. (2003, October). Anti poverty or anti poor? The Millennium Development Goals and the eradication of extreme poverty and hunger. Paper presented at the UNESCO Committee Meeting on Poverty Reduction, Bangkok, Thailand. Retrieved from http://www.focusweb.org /pdf/MDG-2003.pdf

Halstead, S.B., Walsh, J.A., & Warren, K.S. (1985). *Good health at low cost*. New York, NY: The Rockefeller Foundation.

Irwin, A., & Scali, E. (2005, March). Action on the social determinants of health: Learning from previous experiences. Paper prepared for the Commission on Social Determinants of Health, Chile.

Jenkins, R. (2004). Globalization, production, employment and poverty: Debates and evidence. *Journal of International Development*, 16(1), 1–12.

Kunitz, S.J. (2004, Nov). The making and breaking of Yugoslavia and its impact on health. *American Journal of Public Health*, 94(11), 1894–904. Medline:15514224

Labonté, R., Schrecker, T., Sanders, D., & Meeus, W. (2004). *Fatal indifference: The G8, Africa, and global health*. Cape Town: University of Cape Town Press/ IDRC.

Labonté, R., Schrecker, T., & Sen Gupta, A. (2005). *Health for some: Death, disease and disparity in a globalizing world*. Toronto: Centre for Social Justice.

Magnussen, L., Ehiri, J., & Jolly, P. (2004, May–Jun). Comprehensive versus selective primary health care: Lessons for global health policy. *Health Affairs, 23*(3), 167–76. Medline:15160814

National Primary Health Care Conference: Celebrating the 25th Anniversary of the Alma-Ata. (2003). Kopanong Declaration on Primary Health Care, Benoni, Gauteng. Retrieved from http://www.hst.org.za/news/national-primary-health-care-conference-celebrating-25th-anniversary-alma-ata

People's Health Movement (2000). The people's charter for health. Prepared for the First People's World Health Assembly, Dhaka, Bangladesh. Retrieved from http://www.phmovement.org/en/resources/charters /peopleshealth

People's Health Movement (2005). Cuenca Declaration. Presented at the Second People's Health Assembly, Cuenca, Ecuador. Retrieved from http:// www.phmovement.org/en/node/798

People's Health Movement. (2011). Primary health care: A review and critical appraisal of its revitalization. In *Global health watch 3: An alternative world health report*. London: Zed Books.

Pogge, T. (2004). The first United Nations millennium development goal: A cause for celebration? *Journal of Human Development, 5*, 377–97.

Rohde, J., Chatterjee, M., & Morley, D. (1993). *Reaching health for all*. Oxford: Oxford University Press.

Sanders, D. (1998). Primary health care 21: Everybody's business. Presented at WHO International Meeting to Celebrate 20 Years After Alma-Alta, Almaty, Kazakhstan. Retrieved from http://apps.who.int/iris/bitstream/10665 /66306/1/WHO_EIP_OSD_00.7.pdf

Sibthorpe, B.M., Glasgow, N.J., & Wells, R.W. (2005, Nov 21). Emergent themes in the sustainability of primary health care innovation. *Medical Journal of Australia, 183*(10 Suppl), S77–S80. Medline:16296958

SWEF Research Network. (2003). *Common research protocol*: Monitoring and evaluating the health system–wide effects of the Global Fund to Fight AIDS, Tuberculosis and Malaria. Bethesda: Partners for Health Reform*plus*, Abt Associates Inc.

Tatar, M., & Tatar, F. (1997, Sep). Primary health care in Turkey: A passing fashion? *Health Policy and Planning, 12*(3), 224–33. Medline:10173403

The Lancet. (2008). A renaissance in primary health care. *The Lancet, 372*(9642), 863.

Torzillo, P., & Kerr, C. (1991). Contemporary issues in Aboriginal public health. In J. Reid & P. Trompf (Eds.), *The Health of Aboriginal Australia* (pp. 326–80). Harcourt Brace Jovanovich Group [Australia] Pty Ltd.

UN Millennium Project. (2005). *Investing in development: A practical plan to achieve the Millennium Development Goals*. London: Earthscan.

UN Millennium Project Task Force on Improving the Lives of Slum Dwellers. (2005). *A home in the city*. London: Earthscan.

Wade, R.H. (2004). Is globalization reducing poverty and inequality? *World Development, 32*(4), 567–89.

Wagstaff, A., & Claeson, M. (2003). *The Millennium Development Goals for Health: Rising to the challenges*. Washington, DC: World Bank.

Werner, D., & Sanders, D. (1997). *Questioning the solution: The politics of primary health care and child survival, with an in-depth critique of oral rehydration therapy*. Palo Alto: HealthWrights.

Widdus, R., & White, K. (2004). Combating diseases associated with poverty: Financing strategies for product development and the potential role of public-private partnerships. Retrieved from: http://www.who.int /intellectualproperty/topics/ppp/en/CombatingDiseases-Abridged.pdf

World Health Organization. (1978). Declaration of Alma-Ata. International Conference on Primary Health Care, Alma Ata, former USSR.

World Health Organization. (2004). *Changing history*. Geneva: Author.

World Health Organization. (2008). *The world health report 2008. Primary health care: Now more than ever*. Geneva: WHO Press.

2 Summary of Comprehensive Primary Health Care Findings from the Structured Literature Review

RONALD LABONTÉ AND CORINNE PACKER

Our structured literature review took as its starting point the well-documented challenges to primary health care's abilities to fulfil its Alma-Ata vision:

- Its almost immediate eclipse by "selective" PHC, which privileged a few low-cost interventions, mostly directed to child survival, abetted by confusion over whether PHC was an "approach" or a level of care, and the equating in some rich countries of PHC with first-line or primary (medical) care provided by general practitioners (Tarimo & Webster, 1994).
- The globalization of market-driven models of health systems, coupled with the influence of the World Bank's 1993 *Investing in Health* report and its promotion of cost-effective "packages" that ignored the social determinants of health (SDH) and further disintegrated individual and collective health care (World Bank, 1993).
- The weakening and fragmentation of public health systems in many countries partly consequent to structural adjustment and the accompanying fiscal stringency, and the subsequent reliance of many low- and middle-income countries (LMICs) on a growing number of disease-specific global health partnerships for the financing of health services (Labonté & Schrecker, 2009).
- Political concern that PHC's emphasis on community participation could challenge elite group interests during a period marked by powerful left/right ideological struggles in many countries (Solar & Irwin, 2006).

Despite these challenges, the premise of our overall project was that considerable experience had been gained in implementing PHC as a

Table 2.1 Desired outcomes of comprehensive primary health care

- increased equity in access to health care and other services/resources essential to health
- reduced community vulnerabilities through increases in community empowerment (capacities)
- reduced community exposures to risk through improvements in social and environmental determinants of health
- improved community participation and political capabilities of marginalized population groups
- increased intersectoral policy actions on the social and economic determinants of health
- improved population health outcomes and health equity

more comprehensive approach, enriched by a subsequent rise in social models of health promotion (World Health Organization [WHO], 1986) and rights-based approaches to health and development. This knowledge had not (then) been systematically gathered and explored.[1]

Drawing on the experiences of our project's team and PHC commentaries, we created a list (Table 2.1) of the types of outcomes associated with idealized comprehensive PHC (CPHC), which also formed the basis of the call for expressions of interest described in Chapter 1.

We did not expect to find evidence of programs or health systems performing well on all of these outcomes; nor did we. Most of the literature concerned improving access to primary care only and occasionally also examined improvements in basic health knowledge/behaviours.

The approach to our structured literature review was described in Chapter 1. Our review covered literature that was current to mid-2007. The rise of "universal health coverage" as a WHO priority and target within the 2015 sustainable development goals has generated enormous discussion and commentaries in the intervening years. Our findings from the review nonetheless remain important insofar as they identify possibilities and challenges for CPHC that are no less relevant today in the global push to universal health coverage than they were when we first analysed them.

---

1 The descriptions of the challenges to primary health care are excerpts from Labonté, R., Sanders, D, Packer, C., and Schaay, N., (2014), "Is the Alma Ata Vision of Comprehensive Primary Health Care Viable? Findings from an International Project," *Global Health Action 2014*, 7: 24997. We thank the journal for allowing us to reproduce them.

There were notable differences in the findings across the regions; thus, we summarize key findings by region, focusing first on a group of high-income countries, followed by Latin America, South and East Asia, and Africa.

High-Income Countries: North America, Europe, Australia, and Aotearoa/New Zealand

Although our study focused on CPHC projects in LMICs and on Indigenous initiatives in high-income countries, our literature review was global in reach. Across all the high-income countries in this grouping, much of the literature centred on access to general practitioners or, in the case of uninsured Americans, provision of services through publicly funded community health centres (CHCs). Community involvement or empowerment was also a dominant theme, particularly with multidisciplinary CHCs (Franks & Fiscella, 1998; Yalnizyan, 2005). As with PHC experiences worldwide, such centres often began as ways to bring primary care services to rural/remote or disadvantaged populations but generally expanded to incorporate community participation and health promotion activities, very much in line with the Alma-Ata principles. In some countries, such as Canada and Australia, these centres became part of universally funded health systems serving a mix of population groups; while in others, such as Aotearoa/New Zealand, they remained largely independent and community controlled, albeit usually with government financial support. As community-initiated centres in Canada became more integrated within formal government health systems, the extent of their community control and the degree of their engagement in SDH and other facets of CPHC sometimes diminished, as access to clinical (primary medical) care came to predominate. This was more often the case when such centres lacked community governance structures and became services that were funded and delivered through central health departments (Laforest, 2006; O'Neill, 1992). Health services controlled by Indigenous organizations in Canada, the USA, Australia, and Aotearoa/New Zealand similarly implemented comprehensive forms of PHC, partly to deal with the poor health status of their communities. As with many CHC experiences, the community-governance structures of Indigenous health centres contributed to high responsiveness to local pressures and needs, notably in Australia (Hurley, Baum, Johns, & Labonté, 2010) (for a recent example, see Chapter 3 of this book).

While most of the studies described efforts to increase the comprehensiveness of PHC, few studies reported outcome or impact results. Those that did generally found that as PHC became more comprehensive (multidisciplinary teams, substantial community participation or governance), there were lower rates of lab tests, unnecessary hospitalizations, and prescriptions; greater equity in access to screening and other procedures, regardless of ethnicity, SES, or gender; and much greater emphasis on preventive programs and health-promotion activities (useful summaries of these studies can be found in the 2007 Final Report of the Health Systems Knowledge Network [Gilson, Doherty, Loewenson, & Francis, 2007]; as well as in the 2008 World Health Report on primary health care published just as our literature review was being completed [WHO, 2008]). Fewer studies estimated cost savings from CPHC (versus other forms of primary care provision), but there is some evidence that once patient volumes and needs are adjusted, CPHC shows lower costs (partly due to less medicalization), especially when there is a higher nonphysician to physician ratio of staff (Begley, Aday, & McCandless, 1989). Canadian studies that were completing at the time of our literature review further found that when compared to other primary care models (solo practitioners, group practices, fee-for-service/capitation payment systems), CPHC services with salaried physicians, large multidisciplinary teams, and community governance performed significantly better in community responsiveness, chronic-disease management, fewer prescriptions and hospital admissions, and socially oriented health-promotion activities (Dahrouge et al., 2009; Hogg et al., 2009; Liddy, Singh, Hogg, Dahrouge, & Taljaard, 2011; Muldoon et al., 2010). We also found several descriptive studies that reported on the creation and management of multidisciplinary teams and formative evaluations of intersectoral collaboration, both features considered aspects of CPHC; although relatively few included detailed evaluations, and some that did noted challenges related to training and power differentials in promoting multidisciplinary cooperation (Sicotte, D'Amour, & Moreault, 2002).

Similar to the North American literature, the bulk of the articles on PHC in Europe conflated the term with primary care, with little reference either to the Alma-Ata Declaration or information on efforts to engage community members on broader social health issues. A small number of the European studies did report on more comprehensive PHC projects. These included evaluations of a network of CHCs around Naples, the work of which was organized around issues of poverty, mental health, workplace hazards, and social exclusion (Füller, 1986); community and social-movement involvement in PHC centres in Madrid (Ruiz-Jimenez, 2007); and community-oriented primary care programs in Belgium that became triggers for intersectoral action on health determinants (De Maeseneer, De Roo, Art, Willems, & Van de Geuchte, 2007). In the UK, where PHC is often regarded as a "cornerstone" of health services, emphasis was placed on access to services, while the broader social vision of the Alma-Ata Declaration went largely unheeded (Green, Ross, & Mirzoev, 2007).

One reason for the small number of CPHC-relevant articles in our European findings: During the 1980s and into the 2000s, many European countries developed local "healthy cities" projects (in 2007 still numbering over 1,200), which emphasized community participation in broader public-health planning, intersectoral actions on SDH, and creation of "healthy public policies" following on from an invigorated social model of health articulated in the 1986 Ottawa Charter for Health Promotion (WHO, 1986). In the UK a number of government initiatives, such as "Health Action Zones," attempted to create a more "joined-up-government" approach to health inequalities, representing efforts at intersectoralism. In many of these instances, however, health services were absent or played only a minor part, effectively distancing health systems from actions on SDH. As with the North American literature, very little evidence was provided of actual health outcomes or changes in health inequities.

Some of the literature also discussed the political contexts that enabled or constrained CPHC. When local health centres or programs attempted to mobilize around the broader vision of CPHC, for example, they were sometimes met by opposition from medical associations, pharmaceutical firms, and conservative politicians (Labonté, 1998; Lefkowitz, 2007). This pattern was observed in other regions, underscoring the importance of progressive political support for efforts to sustain both the vision and the practice of CPHC. Several studies also identified the need for health workers in PHC services to be trained in the strategies essential to CPHC (e.g., community development, intersectoral processes, policy advocacy) and to be supported in applying these strategies in their work (Clendon, 2004; Si, Bailie, Togni, d'Abbs, & Robinson, 2006). Again, this was a finding common across many regions. There were a few studies that discussed the importance of "ring-fencing" funding for the comprehensive (nonclinical) aspects of PHC (e.g., community participation, community empowerment work, intersectoral initiatives) to prevent funds being redirected to primary care.

This last caution about funding reflects a major concern arising from reviews in North America, Australia, and Europe: the potential erosion of support for CPHC with the deepening of neoliberal and "new public management" models within public health systems. These models emphasize "core business" practices (i.e., clinical care), individualize risk and responsibility, and promote a "lifestyle drift" back to healthy behaviours and away from SDH. Much of the interest in Europe in PHC renewal, for example, was driven by its potential to reduce costs in secondary or tertiary care. A number of Australian papers based on a study in South Australia and the Northern Territory that followed the international one reported in this book provide extensive documentation of the "roll-back" of CPHC and its "lifestyle drift" away from the social model of health (see, e.g., Jolley et al., 2014; Baum et al., 2014; Baum et al., 2013).

Latin America

There is a rich, if episodic, history of CPHC programs across Latin America, many of which supported actions across most or all of the desired outcomes in Table 2.1. Unlike many of the localized initiatives found in our high-income group of countries, CPHC reforms in this region were often national in scope, notably in Cuba and Costa Rica, and more recently in countries such as Brazil, Venezuela, and Chile. The extent and sustainability of their comprehensiveness appears to have been significantly determined by the political climate, both national and international (Ramírez, Ruiz, Romero, & Labonté, 2011). There was a well-documented departure from comprehensiveness in PHC during the 1980s and 1990s, for example, when much of the region came under the sway of World Bank/International Monetary Fund structural-adjustment programs. These programs embodied neoliberal economic policies that emphasized privatization, cost-containment, and decentralization, with emphasis on the latter because it placed the onus for health care on local communities rather than on national policy and funding commitments, with the consequent need for redistributive programs. The result of these neoliberal policies was an increase in contracting out of basic services, a reliance on donor financing for specific (selective) PHC interventions, and the entrenchment of US-style social or private insurance, rather than tax-financed single-payer models (Ramírez et al., 2011). In some regions, notably Central America, CPHC programs became the sites of political struggle and repression.

This sometimes led to withdrawal of support for CPHC by governments who feared the citizen empowerment it emphasized and to CPHC's replacement by "safer" selective PHC programs. It also led to dangerous working environments for those still committed to CPHC, with CHWs sometimes targeted by paramilitary groups resisting democratic reform and citizen rights (Barten, Perez Montiel, Espinoza, & Morales, 2002; Muller, 1979). Although decentralization was often a feature of neoliberal health reforms, when both funding and power were transferred to local regions it often supported more comprehensive approaches to PHC, opening up space for advocacy for national-level programs (Ramírez et al., 2011).

Not all countries were as affected by the political and economic turmoil of the 1980s and 1990s, and an important finding from the Latin American experience was that more comprehensive approaches to PHC existed in countries with universal (or near universal) integrated health systems and strong civil-society movements. Other characteristics of these countries included a political (policy) commitment to improving health equity; a legal or constitutional right to health guaranteed by the state; and policies that clearly identified primary care, community participation, and intersectoral action as PHC components (for a recent example, see Chapter 13). A cautionary note expressed in several studies was that community participation was effective when generated "from below," but less effective when it was "top down" or mandated by funding programs (Ramírez et al., 2011). Selective PHC was associated with segmented and fragmented health systems reliant on multiple funding models (e.g., social insurance, public insurance, private insurance, out-of-pocket payment) and where more conservative politics and policy commitments prevailed (Ramírez et al., 2011).

By the early 2000s, following disenchantment with structural adjustment and the election of centre and centre-left governments in much of the region, health systems started becoming more progressive. Some of this progress was national in scope, although much of the regional shift towards comprehensiveness in PHC began with municipal efforts that arose as challenges to the selective PHC associated with structural adjustment (Ramírez et al., 2011). (For a discussion of the challenges faced in such local efforts, see Chapter 5 of this book.) One of the best-known examples of this national scaling up is the Brazilian *Programa Saúde da Família* (PSF), instituted nationally in 1994 but built on a social movement that began in one state (Ceará). It produced a threefold faster decline in infant mortality compared to the national average (Ramírez et al., 2011). At the time of our 2007 review, the PSF had expanded to cover more than 40% of the population; as of writing (January 2016), it now covers more than 90% and has changed its name to *Estratégia Saúde da Família* (ESF). While the PSF still tended towards clinical and selective interventions, albeit also emphasizing community development and intersectoral actions and supported by the large number of CHWs associated with each PHC team (Ramírez et al., 2011), the ESF is attempting to embody a fully comprehensive approach to PHC. (For a discussion of experiences of how the ESF is linking local CPHC to other care levels, see Chapter 13.)

The *Barrio Adentro* program in Venezuela is another national-scale program that is credited with shifting that country's approach to PHC from the privatized and selective interventions of the structural-adjustment era to one that is publicly financed and regulated. It rapidly increased access to a range of PHC services, with coverage extending to more than 73% of the population at the time of our review and now exceeding 80%. Its efforts at intersectoralism, however, have tended to emphasize health behaviours and individual risk factors, rather than those that are socially structured and determined (Ramírez et al., 2011).[2] It is not alone in this: while many PHC programs in the region enhanced their support for community development and participation, few have been successful in promoting intersectoral actions on health determinants. Those that have been somewhat successful were characterized by their intersectoral actions on concerns shared by both community groups (hence arising as part of their community development efforts) and government departments. The major impediment to such work, as in other regions studied in our review, was a lack of time to maintain the extensive networking required, especially when faced by frequent human resource shortages for primary care (Ramírez et al., 2011).

Similar to findings from high-income countries, PHC programs that were more comprehensive had better population health outcomes than those that were selective or targeted, the one exception being those (often donor-funded) selective programs targeting specific populations living in marginalized or impoverished conditions (Ramírez et al.,

---

2 Its reliance on Cuban doctors to deliver primary care has created some tension within the country (as it has also more recently in Brazil); and the rapid drop in oil prices in 2014, on which public-health financing in Venezuela is wholly reliant, may place its CPHC initiatives in some peril.

2011). In Costa Rica, for example, PHC reform was based on equitable access, multidisciplinary teams, comprehensiveness in terms of participation, actions on social determinants, and integration of care across levels. For every five years post PHC reform, child mortality dropped 13% and adult mortality by 4%, again controlling for other causes and health determinants (Pan-American Health Organization/World Health Organization, 2007). Echoing a similar caution emanating from the high-income nations, another Costa Rican study found that physicians paid on performance basis ("new public management") delivered poorer quality services that were less comprehensive and integrated, and which resulted in greater patient dissatisfaction (Gilson et al., 2007). Although it is not possible to generalize from a single study, studies from other countries have raised similar concerns about performance-based financing.

The "triple A-Q" (availability, accessibility, affordability, and quality) is considered axiomatic to ensuring an equitable health system. Most of the findings from the Latin American region showed positive results for the three A's when PHC was more comprehensive and publicly financed. While generally comprehensive PHC was also found to provide better (or at least similar) quality of care than other service modes (those offered under social or private insurance models), in some instances it was seen as providing lower quality care, stigmatizing the poor who were receiving it (Ramírez et al., 2011). This finding had less to do with PHC services per se than with the legacy of such services being underfunded and targeted only to the poor. Although hope remains for CPHC reforms in much of the region, some of the studies warned of opposition by elite groups in the medical community, as well as by private hospitals and insurers; the persisting dominance of the biomedical model; and limitations posed by a lack of appropriately trained and administratively supported health workers, whether they be doctors, nurses, allied health professionals, or community workers. (For a historical critique of how health-professional training can constrain CPHC, see Chapter 13.)

South and East Asia

Our approach to reviewing experiences in this vast region was undertaken in two waves: the first reviewed the indexed scientific literature. The second pursued a detailed search of so-called "grey literature," based on our understanding that much of the richness of CPHC experiences in this region, and notably in South Asia, was more likely to reside in detailed case-study reports than in journal articles.

The scientific literature, however, was not without insights into CPHC (Hurley et al., 2010). Most of the studies consisted of evaluations of donor-funded projects, which – common to such externally financed programs and their bias towards "selective" PHC – focused on specific health problems or population groups in the low-income countries in the region (Viswanatha & Narayan, 2008). Many of these PHC initiatives were rurally based, with an emphasis on improving access to basic care and reducing environmental hazards, such as lack of proper sanitation or potable water. Key elements ("packages") of these programs were maternal and child health and immunization, reproductive health, and health-worker training. A recurring theme was the problem of program sustainability in light of reliance on donor funding. Due to economic growth and urban migration, health-system reforms in wealthier nations in the region became more hospital centred, which increased pressure for greater privatization or user fees to offset reliance on full government funding. PHC studies in urban settings also became more concerned with "consumer satisfaction" and service effectiveness than with the broader dimensions of CPHC, although citizen participation in health services remained a central problem. Consistent with findings across all countries in the region, and all regions in our larger global study, such participation was cited as a key factor in improving PHC access and in contributing to actions on SDH. Such actions, however, were more commonly invoked in theory than found as a fact in practice. Several instances of successful intersectoralism were documented, often on specific diseases or environmental hazards in poorer, rural areas; or oriented to urban/town planning in cities and wealthier countries, many of which were part of the global Healthy Cities Network. In this respect, the findings were similar to those in Latin America: intersectoralism was more likely when there was pressure from below (community participation, activism) on issues that were simultaneously of concern to governments.

Historically, much of the inspiration for the original Alma-Ata conceptualization of PHC came from experiences in countries in this region, such as China (the "barefoot doctor" program as a model for basic rural health-care delivery), India (where large NGOs developed CPHC services in the absence of government programs, such as the Jamkhed Comprehensive Rural Health Project), and Bangladesh (where the Gonoshasthaya Kendra organization not only promoted access to

CPHC services but initiated several innovations aimed at gender empowerment[3]). (For a current review of CPHC issues in Bangladesh, see Chapter 8 of this book.) The work of these PHC innovators proved to be better captured in the "grey literature," which yielded more detailed and nuanced accounts of CPHC than those available in the scientific databases. Many of these accounts were also more rigorous in design and analysis (using quasi-experimental designs and mixed methods) than many of those in the peer-reviewed literature (Viswanatha & Narayan, 2008).

Many of the countries in the region, especially the low-income nations, had (and still have) very low levels of public health financing. This lack of public funding incentivized national nongovernmental organizations to attempt to fill the gaps in PHC. NGO-led PHC programs in the region were found to cluster into three different approaches. The first approach emphasized "bottom-up" community involvement, in which access to primary health-care services was the goal, but achieving it was seen as requiring inputs and coordination across local sectors, notably agriculture, education, and income generation. However, these programs neither featured an explicit focus on the process of political empowerment of communities nor questioned the existing local and larger power structures of society (Indian Council of Medical Research [ICMR], 1980a). The second approach viewed health-care services not as ends but as means to community empowerment that put citizens at the centre of decision making regarding development goals. An explicit concern with social justice and changing social power relations through health work were the driving forces for these CPHC programs (Arole & Arole, 1994; Chowdhury & Chowdhury, 2007; Haque, 2003; John & John, 1984). A third approach, falling somewhat between these two, built outwards from the Alma-Ata concept and pinpointed a range of essential primary care services while emphasizing community participation in identifying which services should be prioritized (ICMR, 1980b; Reynolds & Stinson, 1991). While NGO-led CPHC programs were primarily rural and targeted to the most marginalized populations (rarely adopting a whole-population approach), NGOs embracing the third approach saw themselves as models for national PHC efforts

---

3 A lengthy paper describing the history of this landmark organization was developed as part of the larger *Revitalization* study and is available at: http://www.globalhealthequity.ca/webfm_send/287.

which, although now expanding in many countries in the region, remain poorly financed or administered and focused almost exclusively on curative measures (Viswanatha & Narayan, 2008). A notable exception was Iran, which implemented a national PHC system in the 1980s built, in part, on having well-trained and publicly salaried CHWs stationed throughout the county's rural areas. This program is credited with contributing to a rapid decline in many key health measures and an elimination of the rural/urban health inequities that persist in many other countries in the region. (For a detailed study of this program, see Chapter 9 of this book.)

Several other large-scale NGO CPHC programs in Pakistan, India, and Bangladesh also showed dramatic improvements in infant and maternal health outcomes. Few were controlled studies, so it is difficult to attribute causality for the health improvements to the PHC elements alone, rather than to improvements in education, food security, employment, and other development sectors. One of the complicating factors is that the NGOs implementing these programs often simultaneously undertook development initiatives in agriculture, income generation, gender empowerment, and education. While embodying the principles of CPHC, this holistic approach to development (in which health plays a role but is not the totality) makes untangling the relative contributions of the different components challenging.

Across the South Asian region, the rhetoric of intersectoral action and community participation was strong in all reports of PHC, and both were associated with more successful PHC (in terms of health outcomes). Most of these programs, however, remained very localized (e.g., participation through village health committees rather than via political action) and focused primarily on the health-services elements of the Alma-Ata model without giving equal attention to intersectoral collaboration, political determination, and action on SDH. Among the reasons cited for this default to health services over empowerment processes were gross underfunding of public health care generally and the continued dominance of the hospital sector and the biomedical model within the public-health envelope. Intersectoral action, which perforce invokes a social model of health, was stronger in NGOs than in government programs, due not only to budgetary issues but also to competition among government sectors for control (i.e., bureaucratic, careerist obstacles). Only two countries in the region showed strong intersectoralism, at least at the time of our review (Sri Lanka and Oman) (Viswanatha & Narayan, 2008).

Africa

Africa, although helping to birth the concept of CPHC with the 1940s "community-oriented primary care" model developed in South Africa (Mullan & Epstein, 2002; Tollman & Pick, 2002), yielded the least amount of scientific literature on recent PHC innovations. As with the Asian and much of the Latin American literature, the focus of most African studies was on basic health care for the rural poor. This reflected need, but also often the more segmented or selective program approach favoured by donors. Most of the studies, and especially the better designed quasi-experimental ones, dealt only with specific health-care interventions. Those that attempted to capture a broader range of PHC activities were generally descriptive, lacking outcome data. One of only a few notable exceptions was the Ethiopian Health Services Extension Program. (For an update on this program, see Chapter 11 of this book.)

Historically, at the time of the Alma-Ata Declaration in 1978, the majority of African countries had attained their independence from the European colonial powers. PHC, in this new era of postcolonialism, was thus viewed by many as providing an opportunity for African countries to move away from the Eurocentric health systems they had inherited and embrace PHC as a guiding strategy for future health development (Chatora & Tumusime, 2004). However, the 1980s and early 1990s saw many African countries reduce their social-sector budgets, including health, as part of the economic structural-adjustment programs (Bassett, Bijlmakers, & Sanders, 1997; Schaay & Sanders, 2008). As a result of having to manage broader social and environmental issues such as armed conflict, civil war, political instability, and challenges related to food security, a large proportion of country resources were used to address resultant emergencies, ultimately serving as a detriment to the implementation of PHC (Chatora & Tumusime, 2004; World Health Organization [WHO] Regional Office for Africa [AFRO], 2008).

Along with the process of health-sector reform came the emergence in the 2000s of a plethora of global health initiatives or global health partnerships, such as Global Alliance for Vaccines and Immunization and United States President's Emergency Plan for AIDS Relief. These initiatives and partnerships privileged vertically implemented and managed programs and concentrated on a few selected elements of PHC, which has also been a factor contributing to the failure to promote a more comprehensive approach to PHC in the region (Schaay

& Sanders, 2008). Despite a number of regional declarations commit-ting to the PHC approach within the national health policies of most of the 46 WHO AFRO–member countries, progress towards PHC policy implementation has lagged behind, creating a discrepancy between the policy directives and their implementation in the region (WHO AFRO, 2008). In addition, stakeholders in the region have lacked a common understanding of PHC concepts and consensus on how PHC policies ought to evolve into strategies (WHO AFRO, 2008).

The reality of national politics had destabilizing effects on CPHC efforts in certain countries, such as in South Africa during apartheid (Andersson & Marks, 1988), Mozambique during the 1970s and 1980s (Cliff & Noormahomed, 1988), and Ethiopia during three different po-litical systems (Kloos, 1998). Others fared better. PHC principles were operationalized in Swaziland (Sukati, 1997) and Lesotho (Shonubi, Odusan, Oloruntoba, Agbahowe, & Siddique, 2005), and throughout the 1980s in the Dodoma region of Tanzania (Matomora, 1989), Kenya (Chaiken, 1998), The Gambia (Hill, MacLeod, Joof, Gomez, & Walraven, 2000), and Zimbabwe (Sanders, 1993).

The majority of the studies reviewed focused on rural populations, and, together with the urban studies, most were conducted in economi-cally disadvantaged communities that were experiencing limited access to health services. Although the PHC approach was not intended to be exclusively applied to the poor, especially in developing-country com-munities, this has been a common feature of PHC initiatives over the past 30 years. With the exception of the study by Albonico, Shamlaye, Shamlaye, & Savioli (1996) in the Seychelles, all of the studies included in the review concentrated on the local level (e.g., a village, a district, or a health facility) rather than the national level.

A large proportion of the 31 studies included in the final African re-view focused on assessing the possibilities and benefits of community participation and outreach and the inclusion of community-based or lay health workers within their interventions. Such studies, for example, described the positive impact a community-based health team, commu-nity or village health workers, traditional birth attendants, and commu-nity leaders had had on maternal and child health outcomes in villages in The Gambia, Zimbabwe, Benin, Ethiopia, and Tanzania (Hill et al., 2000; Jacobson, 1991; Velema, Alihonou, Gandaho, & Hounye, 1991; Ali, Asefaw, Byass, Beyene, & Pedersen, 2005; Ahluwalia, Schmid, Kouletio, & Kanenda, 2003;). Similarly, other studies (Ghebreyesus et al., 1996; Kidane & Morrow, 2000; Onwujekwe, Uzochukwu, Ojukwu, Dike, & Shu, 2007;

Pagnoni, Convelbo, Tiendrebeogo, Cousens, & Esposito, 1997) described how CHWs had assisted in increasing communities' access to malaria-treatment services in villages in Ethiopia, Nigeria, and Burkina Faso.

Combined with other strategies (such as increasing outreach services and health-educational campaigns), participatory mechanisms that were presented as making a positive contribution to the delivery of more accessible and responsive health services included the development of links with local community structures (Bedelu, Ford, Hilderbrand, & Reuter, 2007), the development of community health clubs (Waterkeyn & Cairncross, 2005), and the inclusion or representation of "community voice" in health-service activities (Báez and Barron, 2006). The importance of meeting client expectations as part of improving the quality of PHC health services also featured in studies by Haddad, Fournier, Machouf, & Yatara (1998) in Guinea and by Du Mortier & Arpagaus (2005) in the Democratic Republic of Congo.

Two Southern African studies (Bell, Ithindi, & Low, 2002; Scott, Stern, Sanders, Reagon, & Mathews, 2008) focused on operationalizing the PHC principle of equity by developing unique planning mechanisms to support a fairer distribution of health resources at a local primary care level.

Not surprisingly, the review did not find any studies of interventions that encompassed all four components of CPHC programming (promotive, preventive, curative, and rehabilitative) as described in the Alma-Ata Declaration. At best, interventions incorporated two components, generally some aspect of therapeutic (curative) care coupled with a preventive health education campaign – for example, the use of the SAFE strategy (surgery, antibiotics, facial cleanliness, and environmental improvement) to control trachoma in southern Sudan (Ngondi et al., 2006) and the implementation of simultaneous health education and deworming campaigns in schools in the Seychelles (Albonico et al.,1996) and in South Africa (Johnson & Chopra, 2002). The principle of intersectoral collaboration and its association with the SDH was rarely explored in the literature. One impressive example was a rural South Africa initiative called IMAGE (Intervention with Microfinance for AIDS and Gender Equity). Combining a "participatory gender and HIV training program, with poverty-focused group based microfinance" (International Planned Parenthood Federation, United Nations Population Fund, and Young Positives, 1997), the risk of past-year intimate-partner violence among IMAGE participants was reduced by 55% (Pronyk et al., 2006; Garcia-Moreno et al., 2006).

It is clear from our review that there remains a paucity of research that provides a solid evidence base of CPHC in the African region. Indeed, a possible limitation of this review was that some studies were likely "over-included" (i.e., included, even though they were not strictly about CPHC). Conversely, literature may also have been missed because it focused on a particular aspect of CPHC (e.g., community participation in health or health equity). Related to this is the (not unexpected) finding that the concept of PHC has been interpreted in several different ways in the regional literature: as a concept (Jelley & Madeley, 1984); a service (Haddad et al., 1998); an approach (Scott et al., 2008; Jelley & Madeley, 1984); a strategy (Bell et al., 2002); a system (Onwujekwe et al., 2007); a model (Norr, Norr, McElmurry, Tlou, & Moeti, 2004); and a program (Albonico et al., 1996). Both the complexity of the CPHC approach and the fact that there are multiple interpretations of the concept make it difficult to secure evidence for the effectiveness of CPHC and undermine support for its implementation, notwithstanding its persisting status in African health policies.

Conclusion

This chapter provides only a sketch of the evidence we analysed for our global study, and we encourage readers to review the published papers and draft reports generated by our review.[4] Our review highlighted a number of the limitations of the scientific literature on CPHC, including

- a large number of descriptive studies with limited ability to make causal attribution to population health outcomes;
- an emphasis on particular "slices" of a program rather than an examination of all of its elements, partly due to word-length constraints of the peer-reviewed literature;
- a preponderance of evaluations of selective interventions reflecting donor-funded priorities;
- an emphasis on health behaviour change over SDH;
- lack of a rigorous evidence base on intersectoral actions for health; and
- few studies examining CPHC as a national-level policy or approach, with most studying local initiatives.

---

4 Visit: http://www.globalhealthequity.ca/content/regional-literature-reviews.

Despite these limitations, some findings were fairly consistent across the regions, and the scientific and grey literature. These can be summarized as follows:

- CPHC remains rooted in improving access to health systems for marginalized groups, but with some evidence of actions on SDH, especially at the local level.
- Community governance matters in maintaining a comprehensive approach to PHC and in preventing it from being concerned primarily with primary (medical) care.
- Politics matters in sustaining funding and commitments to CPHC, with support for comprehensiveness generally associated with centre-left social-democratic politics and strong civil-society movements.
- CPHC shows some evidence of improving health outcomes and reducing health system costs, although much of the evidence is of low quality.
- Evidence of intersectoral actions remains weak, with some success apparent only when there is alignment between community pressure and government interests.
- In countries with weak public-health systems, NGOs have often initiated and sustained the most comprehensive forms of PHC.
- In countries with weak public-health financing, PHC services are often associated with lower quality care owing to poor staffing or resources.
- Across all countries in all regions, a focus on hospital care and the dominance of the biomedical model of health constrained support for CPHC.

In the conclusion of an article summarizing initial findings from our literature review, we reflected on another important concern captured in many of the studies: the threat of continued privatization of health-care delivery. Specifically, we cautioned that

perpaps the major future constraint to a revitalisation of PHC, and any deepening of its comprehensiveness, is the continued promotion of privately financed/provided health care in LMICs by the World Bank's International Financial Corporation and the "performance (results)-based" legacy of earlier health system market reforms. Health system financing, whether provided by states, donors or global public–private partnerships, is increasingly being evaluated by narrowly defined outcome measures that are largely unable to capture the long time-horizons of community empowerment strategies or advocacy and other work to bring about changes in public policies/determinants of health – two qualities distinguishing comprehensive PHC from its "selective" kin. ... How comprehensive PHC programs can manage the tension between the competing discourses of results-based efficiency and community-based empowerment, or can use selective PHC as a base for horizontal expansion into a more comprehensive approach, have emerged from our review as two key researchable questions for the future (Hurley et al., 2010).

ACKNOWLEDGMENTS

Numerous researchers contributed to the collection and analysis of literature for the regional literature reviews synthesized in this chapter. In alphabetical order they are: Naydú Acosta-Ramírez, Francoise Barten, Fran Baum, Emilie Efronson, Mikael Gebre-Mariam, Catherine Hurley, Julie Johns, Denise Laplante, Halli Manolakos, Suraya Mohamed, Thelma Narayan, Nacerdine Ouldzeidoune, Lillian Parsons, Lonneke Peperkamp, Jennifer Pollard, Ruth Stern, Hayat Tujuba Ali, Román Rafael Vega Romero, and Vinay Viswanatha.

REFERENCES

Ahluwalia, I.B., Schmid, T., Kouletio, M., & Kanenda, O. (2003, Aug). An evaluation of a community-based approach to safe motherhood in northwestern Tanzania. *International Journal of Gynaecology and Obstetrics: The Official Organ of the International Federation of Gynaecology and Obstetrics, 82*(2), 231–40. http://dx.doi.org/10.1016/S0020-7292(03)00081-X Medline:12873791

Albonico, M., Shamlaye, N., Shamlaye, C., & Savioli, L. (1996). Control of intestinal parasitic infections in Seychelles: A comprehensive and sustainable approach. *Bulletin of the World Health Organization, 74*(6), 577–86. Medline:9060217

Ali, M., Asefaw, T., Byass, P., Beyene, H., & Pedersen, F.K. (2005, Jan). Helping northern Ethiopian communities reduce childhood mortality: Population-based intervention trial. *Bulletin of the World Health Organization, 83*(1), 27–33. Medline:15682246

Andersson, N., & Marks, S. (1988). Apartheid and health in the 1980s. *Social Science & Medicine, 27*(7), 667–81. http://dx.doi.org/10.1016/0277-9536(87) 90327-3 Medline:3067361

Arole, M., & Arole, R. (1994). Jamkhed: *A comprehensive rural health project.* Hong Kong: The Macmillan Press Ltd.

Báez, C., & Barron, P. (2006). *Community voice and role in district health systems in East and Southern Africa: A literature review.* EQUINET Discussion Paper 39.

Barten, F., Perez Montiel, R., Espinoza, E., & Morales, C. (2002). Democratic governance: Fairytale or real perspective. Lessons from Central America. *Environment and Urbanization, 14*(1), 129–44.

Bassett, M.T., Bijlmakers, L., & Sanders, D.M. (1997, Dec). Professionalism, patient satisfaction and quality of health care: Experience during Zimbabwe's structural adjustment programme. *Social Science & Medicine, 45*(12), 1845–52. http://dx.doi.org/10.1016/S0277-9536(97)00122-6 Medline:9447633

Baum, F., Freeman, T., Jolley, G., Lawless, A., Bentley, M., Värttö, K., …, & Sanders, D. (2014, Dec). Health promotion in Australian multi-disciplinary primary health care services: Case studies from South Australia and the Northern Territory. *Health Promotion International, 29*(4), 705–19. http://dx.doi.org/10.1093/heapro/dat029 Medline:23656732

Baum, F.E., Legge, D.G., Freeman, T., Lawless, A., Labonté, R., & Jolley, G.M. (2013, May 10). The potential for multi-disciplinary primary health care services to take action on the social determinants of health: Actions and constraints. *BMC Public Health, 13,* 460. http://dx.doi.org/10.1186/1471-2458-13-460 Medline:23663304

Bedelu, M., Ford, N., Hilderbrand, K., & Reuter, H. (2007, Dec 1). Implementing antiretroviral therapy in rural communities: The Lusikisiki model of decentralized HIV/AIDS care. *Journal of Infectious Diseases, 196*(s3 Suppl 3), S464–S468. http://dx.doi.org/10.1086/521114 Medline:18181695

Begley, C.E., Aday, L.A., & McCandless, R. (1989, Summer). Evaluation of a primary health care program for the poor. *Journal of Community Health, 14*(2), 107–20. http://dx.doi.org/10.1007/BF01321541 Medline:2745740

Bell, R., Ithindi, T., & Low, A. (2002). Improving equity in the provision of primary health care: Lessons from decentralized planning and management in Namibia. *Bulletin of the World Health Organization, 80*(8), 675–81. Medline:12219160

Chaiken, M.S. (1998). Primary health care initiatives in colonial Kenya. *World Development, 26*(9), 1701–17. http://dx.doi.org/10.1016/S0305-750X(98)00067-9

Chatora, R.R., & Tumusime, P. (2004). Primary health care: A review of its implementation in sub-Saharan Africa. *Primary Health Care Research and Development, 5*(4), 296–306. http://dx.doi.org/10.1191/1463423604pc220oa

Chowdhury, R.H., & Chowdhury, Z. (2007). *Achieving the Millennium Development Goal on maternal mortality: Gonoshasthaya Kendra's experience in rural Bangladesh.* Dhaka, Bangladesh: Gonoprokashani Publishers.

Clendon, J. (2004, Dec). Demonstrating outcomes in a nurse-led clinic: How primary health care nurses make a difference to children and their families. *Contemporary Nurse, 18*(1–2), 164–76. http://dx.doi.org/10.5172/conu.18.1 -2.164 Medline:15729809

Cliff, J., & Noormahomed, A.R. (1988). Health as a target: South Africa's destabilization of Mozambique. *Social Science & Medicine, 27*(7), 717–22. http://dx.doi.org/10.1016/0277-9536(87)90331-5 Medline:3227373

Dahrouge, S., Hogg, W., Russell, G., Geneau, R., Kristjansson, E., Muldoon, L., & Johnston, S. (2009). The comparison of models of primary care in Ontario (COMP-PC) study: Methodology of a multifaceted cross-sectional practice-based study. *Open Medicine: A Peer-Reviewed, Independent, Open-Access Journal, 3*(3), e149–e164. Medline:21603051

De Maeseneer, J., De Roo, L., Art, B., Willems, S., & Van de Geuchte, I. (2007). *Equity, intersectoral action for health, primary health care and family medicine in Belgium.*

Du Mortier, S., & Arpagaus, M. (2005, Aug). Quality improvement programme on the frontline: An international committee of the Red Cross experience in the Democratic Republic of Congo. *International Journal for Quality in Health Care, 17*(4), 293–300. http://dx.doi.org/10.1093/intqhc/mzi042 Medline:15831544

Franks, P., & Fiscella, K. (1998, Aug). Primary care physicians and specialists as personal physicians. Health care expenditures and mortality experience. *Journal of Family Practice, 47*(2), 105–9. Medline:9722797

Füller, A. (1986). Health care and health promotion in southern Italian communities. *Health Promotion (Oxford, England), 1*(2), 225–31. http:// dx.doi.org/10.1093/heapro/1.2.225 Medline:10286860

Garcia-Moreno, C., Jansen, H.A., Ellsberg, M., Heise, L., Watts, C.H., & WHO Multi-country Study on Women's Health and Domestic Violence against Women Study Team. (2006, Oct 7). Prevalence of intimate partner violence: Findings from the WHO multi-country study on women's health and domestic violence. *The Lancet (London, England), 368*(9543), 1260–9.

Ghebreyesus, T.A., Alemayehu, T., Bosman, A., Witten, K.H., & Teklehaimanot, A. (1996, Apr). Community participation in malaria control in Tigray region Ethiopia. *Acta Tropica, 61*(2), 145–56. http://dx.doi.org /10.1016/0001-706X(95)00107-P Medline:8740892

Gilson, L., Doherty, J., Loewenson, R., & Francis, V. (2007). *Challenging inequity through health systems: Final report, Knowledge Network on Health Systems.* Geneva: WHO.

Green, A., Ross, D., & Mirzoev, T. (2007, Jan). Primary health care and England: The coming of age of Alma Ata? *Health Policy (Amsterdam), 80*(1), 11–31. http://dx.doi.org/10.1016/j.healthpol.2006.02.007 Medline:16545486

Haddad, S., Fournier, P., Machouf, N., & Yatara, F. (1998, Aug). What does quality mean to lay people? Community perceptions of primary health care services in Guinea. *Social Science & Medicine*, 47(3), 381–94. http://dx.doi.org /10.1016/S0277-9536(98)00075-6 Medline:9681908

Haque, T. (2003). *With the people, for the people: Gonoshasthaya Kendra, Bangladesh.* The People's Health Centre. London: One World Action.

Hill, A.G., MacLeod, W.B., Joof, D., Gomez, P., & Walraven, G. (2000, Feb). Decline of mortality in children in rural Gambia: The influence of village-level primary health care. *Tropical Medicine & International Health*, 5(2), 107–18. http://dx.doi.org/10.1046/j.1365-3156.2000.00528.x Medline:10747270

Hogg, W., Dahrouge, S., Russell, G., Tuna, M., Geneau, R., Muldoon, L., Krissjansson, E, & Johnston, S. (2009). Health promotion activity in primary care: Performance of models and associated factors. *Open Medicine: A Peer-Reviewed, Independent, Open-Access Journal*, 3(3), e165–e173. Medline:21603049

Hurley, C., Baum, F., Johns, J., & Labonté, R. (2010). Comprehensive primary health care in Australia: Findings from a narrative review of the literature. *Australasian Medical Journal*, 1(2), 147–52.

Indian Council of Medical Research (Ed.) (1980a). *Community participation: A problem in a semi-urban community health programme.* National conference on evaluation of primary health care programmes; 80; New Delhi: ICMR.

Indian Council of Medical Research (Ed.) (1980b). *Comprehensive health project, Rangabelia.* National conference on evaluation of primary health care programmes; 80; New Delhi: ICMR.

International Planned Parenthood Federation, United Nations Population Fund, and Young Positives. (1997). *Change, choice and power: Young women, livelihoods and HIV prevention: Literature review and case study analysis.* London: International Planned Parenthood Federation.

Jacobson, J.L. (1991, Jul–Sep). Maternal mortality and morbidity. Zimbabwe's birth force. *Newsletter (Women's Global Network on Reproductive Rights)*, 36, 16–17. Medline:12284525

Jelley, D., & Madeley, R.J. (1984). Primary health care in practice: A study in Mozambique. *Social Science & Medicine*, 19(8), 773–82. http://dx.doi.org /10.1016/0277-9536(84)90392-7 Medline:6505746

John, J.C., & John, H.C. (1984). We learn through our failures: The evolution of a community based programme in Deenabandhu. *Contact*, 82, 1–9.

Johnson, B., & Chopra, M. (2002). *Evaluation of a primary education programme to combat worm infestation in Khayelitsha, Cape Town: A research report.* Cape Town: University of the Western Cape and South African Medical Research Council, on behalf of the Khayelitsha Task Team.

Jolley, G., Freeman, T., Baum, F., Hurley, C., Lawless, A., Bentley, M., Labonté, R., & Sanders, D. (2014, Aug). Health policy in South Australia 2003–10:

Primary health care workforce perceptions of the impact of policy change on health promotion. *Health Promotion Journal of Australia*, 25(2), 116–24. http://dx.doi.org/10.1071/HE13088 Medline:25169802

Kidane, G., & Morrow, R.H. (2000, Aug 12). Teaching mothers to provide home treatment of malaria in Tigray, Ethiopia: A randomised trial. *Lancet*, 356(9229), 550–5. http://dx.doi.org/10.1016/S0140-6736(00)02580-0 Medline:10950232

Kloos, H. (1998, Feb–Mar). Primary health care in Ethiopia under three political systems: Community participation in a war-torn society. *Social Science & Medicine*, 46(4–5), 505–22. http://dx.doi.org/10.1016/S0277 -9536(97)00194-9 Medline:9460830

Labonté, R. (1998). *A community development approach to health promotion*. Edinburgh: Health Education Board of Scotland/Research Unit in Health and Behaviour Change.

Labonté, R., & Schrecker, T. (2009). Rights, redistribution, and regulation. In R. Labonté, T. Schrecker, C. Packer, & V. Runnels (Eds.), *Globalization and health* (pp. 317–33). New York: Routledge.

Laforest, R. (2006). State and community sector relations: Crisis and challenges in Quebec. *Philanthropist*, 20(3), 171–84.

Lefkowitz, B. (2007). *Community health centers: A movement and the people who made it happen*. New Brunswick, N.J.: Rutgers University Press.

Liddy, C., Singh, J., Hogg, W., Dahrouge, S., & Taljaard, M. (2011, Oct 18). Comparison of primary care models in the prevention of cardiovascular disease: A cross sectional study. *BMC Family Practice*, 12(1), 114–24. http:// dx.doi.org/10.1186/1471-2296-12-114 Medline:22008366

Matomora, M.K.S. (1989). A people-centered approach to primary health care implementation in Mvumi, Tanzania. *Social Science & Medicine*, 28(10), 1031–7. http://dx.doi.org/10.1016/0277-9536(89)90385-7 Medline:2717967

Muldoon, L., Dahrouge, S., Hogg, W., Geneau, R., Russell, G., & Shortt, M. (2010, Jul). Community orientation in primary care practices: Results from the Comparison of Models of Primary Health Care in Ontario Study. *Canadian Family Physician/Medecin de Famille Canadien*, 56(7), 676–83. Medline:20631283

Mullan, F., & Epstein, L. (2002, Nov). Community-oriented primary care: New relevance in a changing world. *American Journal of Public Health*, 92(11), 1748–55. http://dx.doi.org/10.2105/AJPH.92.11.1748 Medline:12406800

Muller, F. (1979). *Participacion popular en programas de atencion sanitaria en America Latina*. Universidad de Antioquia: Facultad Nacional de Salud Publica/ Katholieke Universiteit Nijmegen.

Ngondi, J., Onsarigo, A., Matthews, F., Reacher, M., Brayne, C., Baba, S., …, & Emerson, P.M. (2006, Aug 12). Effect of 3 years of SAFE (surgery, antibiotics, facial cleanliness, and environmental change) strategy for trachoma control in southern Sudan: A cross-sectional study. *Lancet, 368*(9535), 589–95. http://dx.doi.org/10.1016/S0140-6736(06)69202-7 Medline:16905023

Norr, K.F., Norr, J.L., McElmurry, B.J., Tlou, S., & Moeti, M.R. (2004, Mar). Impact of peer group education on HIV prevention among women in Botswana. *Health Care for Women International, 25*(3), 210–26. http://dx.doi .org/10.1080/07399330490272723 Medline:15195767

O'Neill, M. (1992). Community participation in Quebec's health system: A strategy to curtail community empowerment? *International Journal of Health Services, 22*(2), 287–301. http://dx.doi.org/10.2190/AKBE-UN31-6QEF -VG15 Medline:1601547

Onwujekwe, O., Uzochukwu, B., Ojukwu, J., Dike, N., & Shu, E. (2007, Feb). Feasibility of a community health worker strategy for providing near and appropriate treatment of malaria in southeast Nigeria: An analysis of activities, costs and outcomes. *Acta Tropica, 101*(2), 95–105. http://dx.doi.org /10.1016/j.actatropica.2006.07.013 Medline:17270139

Pagnoni, F., Convelbo, N., Tiendrebeogo, J., Cousens, S., & Esposito, F. (1997, Sep–Oct). A community-based programme to provide prompt and adequate treatment of presumptive malaria in children. *Transactions of the Royal Society of Tropical Medicine and Hygiene, 91*(5), 512–17. http://dx.doi.org /10.1016/S0035-9203(97)90006-7 Medline:9463653

Pan-American Health Organization/World Health Organization. (2007). *Renewing primary health care in the Americas: A position paper of the Pan-American Health Organization/World Health Organization.* Washington, DC: Author.

Pronyk, P.M., Hargreaves, J.R., Kim, J.C., Morison, L.A., Phetla, G., Watts, C., …, & Porter, J.D. (2006, Dec 2). Effect of a structural intervention for the prevention of intimate-partner violence and HIV in rural South Africa: A cluster randomised trial. *Lancet, 368*(9551), 1973–83. http://dx.doi.org /10.1016/S0140-6736(06)69744-4 Medline:17141704

Ramírez, N.A., Ruiz, J.P., Romero, R.V., & Labonté, R. (2011, Oct). Comprehensive primary health care in South America: Contexts, achievements and policy implications. *Cadernos de Saúde Pública, 27*(10), 1875–90. http://dx.doi.org/10.1590/S0102-311X2011001000002 Medline:22031193

Reynolds, J., & Stinson, W. (1991). *Lessons learned from primary health care programmes funded by the Aga Khan Foundation.* Geneva: Aga Khan Foundation.

Ruiz-Jimenez, J.L. (2007). *Experiencia en España sobre APS con enfoque comunitario.* Estrategia de promoción de la salud en el área 1 del SERMAS de Madrid. Paper presented at ALCUEH workshop in El Salvador.

Sanders, D. (1993). The potential and limits of health sector reforms in Zimbabwe. In Rohde, J., Chatterjee, M., & Morley, D. (Eds.), *Reaching health for all* (pp. 239–66). Oxford University Press.

Schaay, N., & Sanders, D. (2008). *International perspectives on primary health care over the past 30 years. South African health review 2008*. Durban: Health Systems Trust.

Scott, V., Stern, R., Sanders, D., Reagon, G., & Mathews, V. (2008, Feb 04). Research to action to address inequities: The experience of the Cape Town Equity Gauge. *International Journal for Equity in Health, 7*(6), 6. http://dx.doi.org/10.1186/1475-9276-7-6 Medline:18248666

Shonubi, A.M.O., Odusan, O., Oloruntoba, D.O., Agbahowe, S.A., & Siddique, M.A. (2005, Jul). "Health for all" in a least-developed country. *Journal of the National Medical Association, 97*(7), 1020–6. Medline:16080673

Si, D., Bailie, R.S., Togni, S.J., d'Abbs, P.H.N., & Robinson, G.W. (2006, Jul 3). Aboriginal health workers and diabetes care in remote community health centres: A mixed method analysis. *Medical Journal of Australia, 185*(1), 40–5. Medline:16813550

Sicotte, C., D'Amour, D., & Moreault, M.-P. (2002, Sep). Interdisciplinary collaboration within Quebec community health care centres. *Social Science & Medicine, 55*(6), 991–1003. http://dx.doi.org/10.1016/S0277-9536(01)00232-5 Medline:12220099

Solar, O., & Irwin, A. (2006, Dec). Social determinants, political contexts and civil society action: A historical perspective on the Commission on Social Determinants of Health. *Health Promotion Journal of Australia, 17*(3), 180–5. Medline:17176231

Sukati, N.A. (1997, Apr). Primary health care in Swaziland: Is it working? *Journal of Advanced Nursing, 25*(4), 760–6. http://dx.doi.org/10.1046/j.1365 -2648.1997.1997025760.x Medline:9104672

Tarimo, E., & Webster, E.G. (1994). Alma-Ata recommendations: A critical review I: Strategic approaches. In *Primary health care concepts and challenges in a changing world: Alma-Ata revisited* (pp. 10–26). World Health Organisation Division of Strengthening of Health Services. Geneva: World Health Organization.

Tollman, S.M., & Pick, W.M. (2002, Nov). Roots, shoots, but too little fruit: Assessing the contribution of COPC in South Africa. *American Journal of Public Health, 92*(11), 1725–8. http://dx.doi.org/10.2105/AJPH.92.11 .1725 Medline:12406793

Velema, J.P., Alihonou, E.M., Gandaho, T., & Hounye, F.H. (1991, Jun). Childhood mortality among users and non-users of primary health care in a rural West African community. *International Journal of Epidemiology, 20*(2), 474–9. http://dx.doi.org/10.1093/ije/20.2.474 Medline:1917252

Viswanatha, V., & Narayan, T. (2008). *Synthesis of grey literature from select Asian countries about comprehensive primary health care experiences.* Available at: http://www.globalhealthequity.ca/sites/default/files/imce/Vinay%20Asia%20Final%20Report%203%20Sept%20with%20some%20concls.pdf

Waterkeyn, J., & Cairncross, S. (2005). Creating demand for sanitation and hygiene through Community Health Clubs: A cost-effective intervention in two districts in Zimbabwe. *Social Science & Medicine, 61*, 1958–70.

World Bank. (1993). *World development report 1993: Investing in health.* New York: Oxford University Press.

World Health Organization. (1986). *Ottawa charter for health promotion.* Ottawa: World Health Organization, Health and Welfare Canada, Canadian Public Health Association.

World Health Organization. (2008). *The world health report 2008. Primary health care: Now more than ever.* Geneva: WHO Press.

World Health Organization Regional Office for Africa. (2008). *Report on the review of primary health care in the African region.* Brazzaville, Republic of Congo: Author.

Yalnizyan, A. (2005). *Canada's commitment to equality: A gender analysis of the last ten federal budgets (1995–2004).* Ottawa: The Canadian Feminist Alliance for International Action.

SECTION ONE

Increasing Equitable Access
to Health Care

Our research program considered equitable access to health care as the baseline for CPHC: necessary, but insufficient without actions specifically related to the other desired outputs (see Table 2.1). Ultimately, all of the health systems studied in the *Revitalizing Health for All* (*RHFA*) project had as a fundamental goal improved equitable access to health services. Although few of the projects specifically analysed the equity dimension (i.e., did access disproportionately increase for those in greatest need?), all of the PHC services being studied were targeted at areas or population groups experiencing both need and relative disadvantage. Findings generally noted that the PHC services studied were successful in improving access. Two *RHFA* projects in particular (one based in Australia and the other in the Democratic Republic of Congo) illustrate unique ways in which equitable access to health care was increased for targeted populations: Aboriginal males and women, respectively. In Colombia, arguments based on national human rights obligations also proved useful in improving equitable access to health systems that were more comprehensive in treating and preventing disease.

Specifically, one of our Aboriginal teams, based in Alice Springs, **Australia**, sought to examine how the Male Health Program run through the Central Australian Aboriginal Congress (Congress) would be able to address equitable access to health care and the social determinants of health (SDH) affecting Aboriginal men. Aboriginal men in this part of Australia experience high levels of social disadvantage compared to Aboriginal men in other regions of Australia, Aboriginal women in general, and the broader non-Aboriginal population. They also experience poorer health outcomes overall. In addition, Aboriginal males in the region suffer from high levels of depression and other mental-health conditions. After extensive community consultation, the existing Male Health Program, which was largely stigmatized from being originally branded as a sexually transmitted infections program and therefore severely underused, was transformed into a program addressing the larger SDH affecting Aboriginal men. In short order, the program gained credibility and acceptance by the community, and visits by Aboriginal men for clinic-based services increased 13-fold while visits for counselling services increased 10-fold. This was achieved largely by employing a strong peer educator and Aboriginal liaison officer, employing a multidisciplinary workforce, and reconceptualizing the health program to address both the health needs and social conditions faced by the Aboriginal males in the region. Other aspects of the program (such as shower and washing-machine facilities for men who may be "sleeping rough," and the involvement of male elders in running speaking sessions) reflected the efforts of Congress to ensure the comprehensiveness of this program. Congress itself is an Aboriginal-run comprehensive health- and human-service organization, with community leadership and the capacity to advocate for all people who access its programs.

Developing primary health-care services (comprehensive or otherwise) in remote and postconflict areas of poorer countries is seen as one of the most challenging tasks in ensuring equitable access to health care. This led our study to work with the team in the **Democratic Republic of Congo** (DRC), which explored the effectiveness of an NGO-supported program using community insurance and microcredit to improve pre- and post-natal care, and safe delivery. While the range of services and limited form of financing do not represent "comprehensive" PHC, the approach taken in this "Safe Motherhood" program often forms the base from which more comprehensive approaches develop. Our DRC team found that where women participated in "solidarity" groups (the "Safe Motherhood" intervention), maternal and child health outcomes dramatically improved. These groups also included income-generating activities for women, regarded as foundational to greater health and gender empowerment, as well as to identifying new roles for men in the program. The microcredit and community-insurance schemes used by the NGO in this study have become viewed as a panacea for improving health-care access in many low-income settings. What our DRC study found, however, is that the viability and expansion of this program relied upon, and will continue to rely upon, ongoing financial resource transfers from the NGO to the communities. The team also concluded that the concept of community self-sufficiency or self-reliance needs to be discarded and replaced by one that emphasizes community self-determination in a context of local, regional, and even global interdependencies. A number of *RHFA* projects simultaneously noted strengths and weaknesses in CPHC contributions. In the case of DRC, for instance, husbands of members of the women's solidarity groups in DRC still expressed concern over their wives giving birth in a health centre, partly because of the possibility of a male health worker seeing their wives unclothed. These concerns were being addressed, in part, through the program's partnerships with strong community and religious leaders and tribal chiefs, encouraging their support for safe, facility-based childbirth.

Our third contribution in this section highlights the political complexities of moving from a CPHC policy vision to one implemented in actual practice. In 2004, the Government of the City of Bogotá in **Colombia** adopted a CPHC policy to secure the right to health and reduce inequalities in health and access to health care. The Colombian team analysed the policy's implementation from 2004 to 2008 with the aim of examining where and how improvements were made in terms of impacts on health and health equity. Although the policy sought to deliver a complete CPHC package, the tensions between the content of the policy and the realities at the district level resulted in a hybrid CPHC model: comprehensive in efforts to support community participation and intersectoral collaboration, but selective in providing "cost-effective" and vertical program interventions associated more with traditional primary care models. The program, while intended to implement the more visionary CPHC policy, has been reduced to a strategy in which community health managers' main objectives are to induce demand for services and to promote community participation in identifying needs, although without having the ability to act upon these needs. Although advances have been identified in the access to and expansion of services, these are still insufficient when measured against the intent of CPHC reforms. The study attributes these shortcoming to tensions between differing levels of government and the fragmentation of the country's health-care system, which divides health into public goods (public health) and private goods (market-oriented insurance for individual medical care). Despite these limitations, the CPHC initiative in the City of Bogotá managed to contribute to improving health indicators and health equity.

3 Ingkintja: The Congress Male Health Program, Alice Springs, Australia

CLIVE ROSEWARNE, GAI WILSON,
AND JOHN LIDDLE

Background

Central Australian Aboriginal Congress (Congress), an Aboriginal community-controlled comprehensive primary health service, was chosen as one of the Indigenous/Aboriginal sites to participate in the *Revitalizing Health for All* (*RHFA*) project. The Congress cabinet nominated the Ingkintja,[1] previously the Male Health Program, as the focus.

Congress was established in 1973 as an advocacy body for central Australian Aboriginal[2] people and has contributed to the comprehensive primary health care (CPHC) movement in Australia (Rosewarne, Vaarzon-Morel, Bell, Carter, Liddle, & Liddle, 2007). It provides a range of health services to Aboriginal people within the town, and immediate surrounding areas, of Alice Springs, in the Northern Territory (NT), Australia. Alice Springs has a population of approximately 27,500 people, of which 5,700 are Aboriginal, and is located 200 kilometres south of the centre of Australia. The Central Arrernte people are the traditional custodians of the town area; however, people from roughly 15 different language groups live in or regularly visit the town to utilize services.

---

1 The name "Ingkintja" was formally adopted by the service in 2009. Ingkintja is a central Australian Aboriginal word that means a meeting place for males.

2 In this report, the term Aboriginal people will be used when referring to Indigenous people in the region. The term Aboriginal and Torres Strait Islander will be used if reference is being made to all Indigenous people in Australia or data that cannot be disaggregated. It is also the preferred term used by Aboriginal people from the community-controlled health service, the Central Australian Aboriginal Congress, which is the location of this research.

Table 3.1 Life-expectancy comparison: Northern Territory (NT)
Aboriginal males and other populations

Population	Life expectancy (years)
NT Aboriginal male	61.5
NT Aboriginal female	69.2
NT non-Aboriginal male	75.7
National Aboriginal male	67.2
National non-Aboriginal males	78.7

The expansion of European settlement, based on Alice Springs, occurred after 1880, relatively later than in most other areas of Australia. As of mid-2011, the Aboriginal and Torres Strait Islander population of Australia was estimated at 669,900, or 3% of the total Australian population (Australian Bureau of Statistics [ABS], 2013).

The poorer health status of Australian Aboriginal and Torres Strait Islander peoples in comparison to non-Aboriginal and Torres Strait Islander Australians is well documented (ABS & Australian Institute of Health and Welfare [AIHW], 2008). Aboriginal male[3] health status, as measured by a number of indices, is poor compared with non-Aboriginal males and women. Life expectancy at birth over the period 2005–7 for NT Aboriginal and Torres Strait Islander males was estimated at 61.5 years, which represented a life-expectancy gap of 17.2 years compared to non-Aboriginal and Torres Strait Islander males nationally (ABS, 2009; AIHW, 2008).

Aboriginal males in the NT have a shorter life expectancy than the region's Aboriginal female residents (7.7 years). This is larger than the disparity between Aboriginal males and females nationally (5.7 years) or between non-Aboriginal males and females in the NT (5.5 years) or nationally (3.9 years). (See Table 3.1.) Aboriginal males are also over-represented in mortality statistics in almost every age group (except 65 years and over) and have age specific death rates at least twice that of non- Aboriginal and Torres Strait Islander people. For the age groups 35 to 44 and 45 to 54, the age-specific death rates for Aboriginal males

---

3 The term male is used throughout this report, as the terms men and man have particular cultural meaning in central Australian Aboriginal communities, denoting a male who has certain status related to cultural practices and knowledge.

are around 5 times that of non-Aboriginal males (ABS & AIHW, 2008). For cardiovascular disease in Aboriginal 25 to 54 year olds, the rate is 7 to 12 times that of non-Aboriginal people (Brown & Blashki, 2005). These health status indices indicate that there is an urgent need to address Aboriginal male health in this region.

Most Aboriginal organizations are directly funded from the Commonwealth (the federal Australian government), including the Aboriginal Community Controlled Health Organisations, funded since 1995 through the Commonwealth Department of Health's Office of Aboriginal and Torres Strait Islander Health. Over the previous decade, the Commonwealth government under the conservative Liberal-National Party Coalition moved away from the bilateral policy of Aboriginal self-determination to a policy of mainstreaming Aboriginal programs and dismantling a rights-based approach to Aboriginal affairs.

Until recently, most of the literature concerning the social determinants of health (SDH) has not been framed from an Indigenous point of view and has omitted some important facets that could be termed "Indigenous social determinants" of health. However, there is a growing literature articulating the discourse about the SDH from an Indigenous framework (Anderson, Baum, & Bentley, 2007; Calma, 2006; Carson, Dunbar, & Chenhall, 2007; Nettleton, Napolitano, & Stephens, 2007; World Health Organization [WHO], 2007). In addition to those themes encapsulated in the broader literature, the Indigenous social-determinants framework highlights a number of other themes. These include colonization and diversity of Indigenous experiences; human rights and self-determination; poverty reduction; marginalization; education opportunities; data invisibility; culture, cultural security, cultural competence, and Indigenous world views; institutional reform; control of land; racism; family and community health; control over health; incarceration and the justice system; and family separation and reconciliation (Carson, Dunbar, & Chenhall, 2007; Dick, 2007; Houston, 2004; Houston, 2006; McCoy, 2008; Paradies, 2006; WHO, 2007).

There is also an increasing body of work that specifically considers gender and the SDH within an Aboriginal-male context (McCoy, 2008; Wenitong, 2002; Wenitong, 2006). Indigenous participants in the WHO Adelaide Symposium highlighted the need for a gender perspective (WHO, 2007). Within the Aboriginal population of the region serviced by Ingkintja, there are marked disparities in social disadvantage between Aboriginal males and Aboriginal women. Using the

Gender-Related Index for Indigenous Australians (GRIFIA)[4] as a tool to create a ranking of relative disadvantage, Yap and Biddle (2009) have shown that central Australian Aboriginal males are more socially disadvantaged than Aboriginal women and most other Aboriginal males.

CPHC services have the potential to address Aboriginal male health issues because they encapsulate a range of principles and practices that recognize that health care must address both individual and social dimensions of health. The Australian National Strategic Framework for Aboriginal and Torres Strait Islander Health states that CPHC includes at least the following elements: clinical services, illness-prevention services; specific programs for health gain; access to secondary and tertiary services and related community services; and client/community assistance and advocacy (National Aboriginal and Torres Strait Islander Health Council [NATSIHC], 2003).

That access to CPHC services can make a significant contribution to redressing health-care disadvantage has been noted in the Australian context (Commonwealth Grants Commission, 2001; Robert Griew Consulting & Office of Aboriginal and Torres Strait Islander Health [OATSIH], 2008), and Aboriginal community controlled health services (which reflect many attributes of the CPHC approach and model) were found to have an essential role in addressing Indigenous disadvantage (Dwyer, Siburn, & Wilson, 2004). However, it is also noted that there is a shortage of robust evaluation and documentation of the effectiveness of CPHC programs, especially regarding Australian Aboriginal CPHC services (Burns, Thomson, Brooks, Burrow, Kirov, McGougan & Valenti, 2002; Dwyer, Siburn, & Wilson, 2004).

Concern over low access rates of Aboriginal males to health services in central Australia was the main reason for the establishment of the Congress Male Health Program (MHP) in 1994. Aboriginal males had

---

4 Variables used to construct the GRIFIA were employment to population percentage; year 12 as highest level of schooling; did not attend school; managerial or professional occupation; degree as nonschool qualification; individual income less than $250 per week; and income more than $1,000 per week. These variables are based on 2006 census data available at the gender disaggregated level of Indigenous regions. Two variables, "children engaged in preschool" and "core activity restriction" (as a proxy for health – this variable relates to people who need assistance because of self-care, mobility, and communication issues) were not included as their loading in absolute value was less than 0.3 and was therefore statistically not significant. The GRIFIA model does not include dimensions such as culture, direct health, and development and justice issues, which were not available at this regional level.

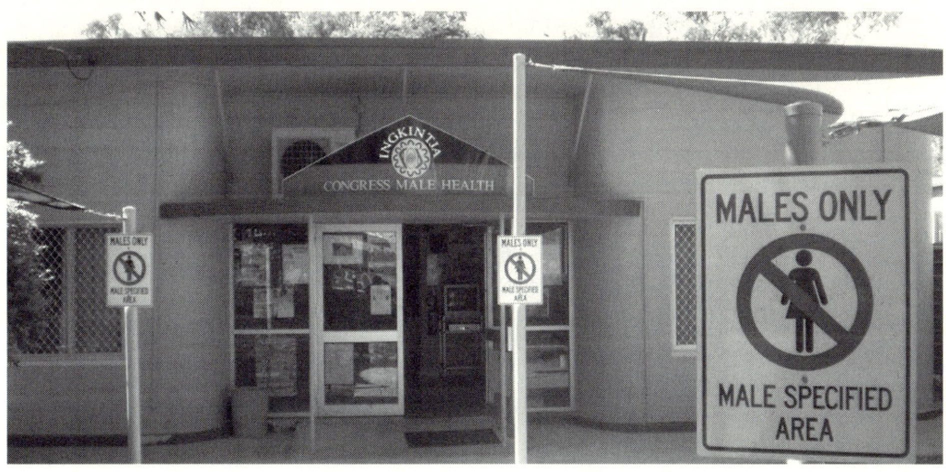

Aboriginal, male-only health clinic in Alice Springs, Australia

raised the issue of cultural safety in accessing health services. Clinics were often perceived as "women's places" by Aboriginal males who, despite their high levels of chronic and communicable disease, avoided attaining care until conditions were advanced. In its first 10 years, the MHP was funded through the National Indigenous Australians' Sexual Health Strategy. As a consequence, it struggled to balance a desire to offer a CPHC service that addressed the SDH with a funding model designed to prioritize outcomes aimed at dealing with sexually transmitted infection (STI) rates. There was a broad agreement that early versions of the MHP did not reflect the health needs of Aboriginal males in the region very well.

Congress established a male-only health centre in 2003 that was predicated on a CPHC approach and supported by the NATSIHC. Agitation by Aboriginal male staff and cabinet members, as well as growing community pressure, prompted the Congress cabinet to undertake a Community Consultation and Program Planning Project (in 2004) to identify the health-service needs of Aboriginal males in the region. The findings of this project provided a clear direction for service development, which has guided the program's growth. There was general agreement that it was not until the program began to expand during and after the community consultation that Aboriginal male health issues were more adequately addressed.

From two staff members at its inception in 2003, the program (at the time of this study) came to employ nine staff. Moreover, in addition to Aboriginal male health checks, it was enlarged to offer general practitioner (GP) clinics, a range of counselling services, a drop-in centre, and twice weekly health-education sessions. There were outreach services to remote communities and town camps. In 2008, the MHP hosted the Central Australian Aboriginal Male Health Summit, attended by 300 mainly central Australian Aboriginal males. Another smaller summit that focused on violence issues was held in 2010. It was in 2009 that the name Ingkintja was adopted by the service.

It is in this context that The Congress Male Health Program – Revitalising Health for All: Learning from Comprehensive Primary Health Care Experiences project was developed. This study was undertaken in 2009–2010.

Research Questions and Methods

The main research question for this project was, how does the Central Australian Aboriginal Congress MHP reflect the SDH affecting Aboriginal male health, as articulated by Aboriginal males, in the Alice Springs region?

The following set of more in-depth questions was developed to interrogate the data and investigate the main question in more detail:

1 Why was the Congress MHP developed?
2 How has the history of the MHP reflected the health needs of Aboriginal males?
   a How has health status, health needs, and their causes been defined from the perspective of Aboriginal males using the service?
   b What are the theoretical understandings of male social, emotional, and physical health that informed the MHP service's development?
3 How have social and political issues shaped the capacity of the program to address Aboriginal males' health needs, including their SDH?
4 What are the key principles guiding the MHP?
5 How have the SDH been understood by Congress and its program staff?
6 What have been some of the more notable CPHC efforts of this program aimed at influencing the SDH of Aboriginal male health?

7 What have been enablers/barriers to offering a comprehensive approach to PHC that incorporates actions on the SDH of Aboriginal male health?
8 How effectively is the MHP carrying out its functions and implementing its principles?
9 Are the principles and functions around which the MHP has been constructed the right ones?
10 What are the next steps to further the program's capacity to address the SDH needs of Aboriginal males in this context?

This research employed a narrative case-study approach, incorporating lay knowledge perspectives. Qualitative methods included a literature review, document analysis, key-informant interviews, and community and service-user consultations. The quantitative data collected consisted of de-identified service-use data from the patient information recall system *Communicare*, service data sourced from program records, program evaluation and funding reports, and Australian Bureau of Statistics (ABS) population data. Capacity development was envisaged to occur through a formal training strategy, an informal transfer process during the research between researchers and program staff, and mentoring. A steering committee of Aboriginal people guided the project's implementation.

Results and Analysis

Central Australian Aboriginal males interviewed as part of this study conceptualized their health status and health needs using social, emotional, and mental health frameworks.

A profound sense of disempowerment, caused in part by the changing nature of male roles in Aboriginal society since colonization and in contemporary society, leading to loss of self-esteem was a commonly described experience. Aboriginal males interviewed described being unable to cope with these changing roles in society, which also led to frustration, anger, alienation, and worry. Most of the males commented on this, as in the following example:

I tell you what if you really worried, what that what cause, what it leads you to, worry suicide, you'll kill yourself. It leads you to suicide. A lot of people done it. You see a lot of people dying suicide. I got problem. Same problem you mob got but it just got bigger and you can't handle anymore.

This loss of self-esteem, often manifesting in depression, was linked to negative social behaviours and outcomes. For many, drinking was identified as a means of escaping these feelings, leading in turn to further problems, such as fighting; getting caught in drinking circles that entrap people into further drinking; and poverty, marital breakdown, and promiscuous sexual behaviour. As some males explained,

> And a lot of men out there are just sitting down and numbing themselves because they can't see their kids, can't have access to their kids or that other thing about when they do go and see, there's bail conditions in that and they can't go near a partner when they're intoxicated or drugs and so it's dividing.
>
> That stuck in a cycle thing, that'll be just like, if you get out, who's going have, everyone else is just drinking, well what are you going to do? You're going to come back and drink too, Mate.

People became unable to deal with issues such as getting a job, supporting their families, and being strong emotional partners for their wives. One male noted that "when you're a healthy bloke you can do exercise, you can shower, you can take a walk with your wife."

Difficulties in relationships and being unable to express emotions often led to problems involving anger and violence. These males were isolated, depressed, and struggling. This process was then compounded by a deep sense of the social censure of Aboriginal males, as well as negativity apparent in representations of Aboriginal males, particularly in relation to child abuse and domestic violence. As these men stated,

> Aboriginal males were no longer just, there are some bad guys there, it was now getting to the point of Aboriginal blokes being all sex abusers and paedophiles and hiding behind their culture and all this stuff. So the plan became much more aggressive, an anti-Aboriginal agenda I reckon, that's in my perception.
>
> And then from that then came the intervention. And then it became almost open warfare on an Aboriginal identity and an Aboriginal ability to determine their own future, I think that's changed. When that happened, we were getting ... all these blokes and they were ringing me or coming into me at work and saying, I'm frightened to walk down the street with my kids, people are looking at me funny.

Strong individuals who respected themselves and their families were seen as being people who avoided problems in life. The images evoked of a healthy Aboriginal male were described as someone who was working, who took their responsibilities seriously, who was a happy family man who got exercise, had health checks, and regularly went out to the bush to escape town pressures and reconnect with the land:

I'm telling you ... you stop drinking you see a whole new life. Your work, you can buy anything you want, you can buy merne (food), you can help people with problems them got now, right now, you want to talk about problems, I've been through that, I've been worse. Worse problem. Drink every day. Morning, sundown, during weekend. This bloke can tell you. He can tell you how I was, drinker. I used to go look for fight. I got proof of violence. Like I'm not frightened of anyone. I stopped that. I did like, "No that's not the way to go." All these people, my family; I could help them to help their self.

Like I said if you want to learn culture you've got (to have) a clear mind. You can't learn when you've got alcohol.

Many Aboriginal males interviewed believed that the first step in addressing these issues required the individual to decide that he wanted to change his life. For some, this was a highly individualized journey:

Just myself. I was thinking, "I got kids now. My kids growing up, I'm going to be a grandparent." That stopped me. You don't want to be blind all your life. You've got to open your mind, see what's out there.

Well I wanted to make a change because you know, I didn't want my kids growing older have to look at me like, "Dad's a drunk." That embarrassed me and I'm not that type of guy, I'm educated, I'm a smart person …

However, most felt that the individual needed support. There were many potential sources identified for this support; the family, community, or an external agency. It was seen as a legitimate role of agencies like Congress to create a sense of empowerment within individual males to assist them to take control over their lives and to realize their image of a healthy male. It was commonly stated that agencies needed to be flexible in their approach so that they could respond to an individual's need whenever they presented:

The principles are to be responsible to the wishes of senior Aboriginal men and to be sensitive to cultural practices. There are two good ones for which there is a little bit of tension between them. One is to be a compassionate gentle respite, place for respite from some of the pressures on the street. The second principle is that clients won't be mollycoddled and treated too softly, this is perceived as being one of the reasons that some of the problems have occurred in the past. So both those principles are kind of acted on. It also works under the principle that we need new ideas; so it's open, very open to creative solutions.

Equally important was that agencies, in working with people, did not create dependency on their services but rather empowered people to take action for themselves. With this positive approach, some respondents felt that change could be affected at the individual level fairly quickly, assisting people to break out of a destructive cycle. Significantly, affecting change at the individual level with its consequent effects on the family, and hence on the community, was seen by many males as being a strategy whereby the broader health determinants, such as employment, education, social cohesion, empowerment, and alcohol abuse could be addressed:

> I think that a lot of men they need to, these fellas coming in here they need to sit down and sort their thinking first, what are their priorities, what do they want to do with their life and with their families and then go from there I guess.
>
> I mean, you have to work within reality and the reality of some people is pretty grim. And that's why people ask me, "Oh, do you think you're doing any good?" and I think, "Yes, I am, but it's one at a time." I'm not changing the world, I'm not even changing a town camp, but if I can change a household by changing one person within that household, well that's a good outcome. That's as good as I can hope to do. Changing the world, no. Haven't got my cape yet.

While positive benefits could be felt almost immediately within the family, these benefits would flow into the local community, creating community capacity to deal with social issues. Thus, collective action at the community level was usually seen as a concurrent pathway to individual agency to address the SDH.

Increasing equity in access to services

The MHP/Ingkintja saw a dramatic and sustained increase in service access and usage after the implementation of the 2004 community

Figure 3.1 Contacts by financial year by type of service at MHP/Ingkintja

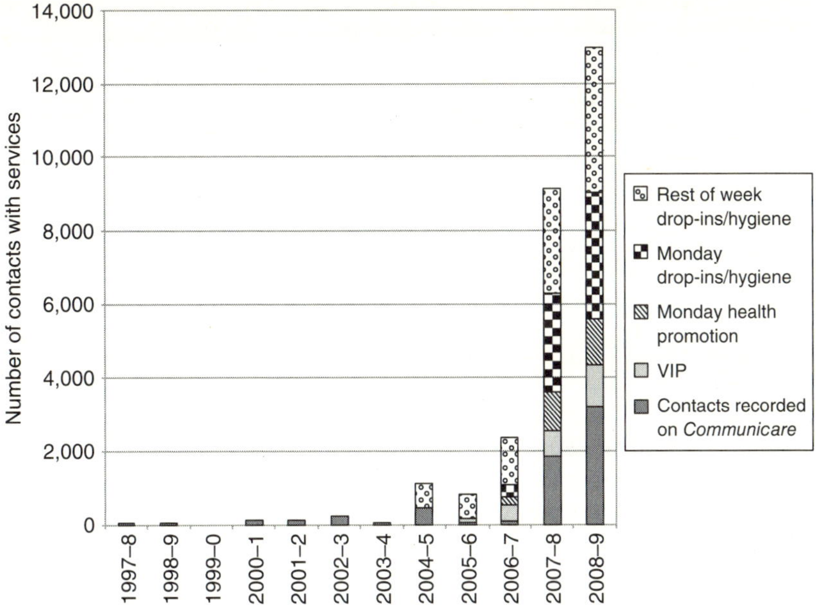

Note: The patient information recall system *Communicare* had no data available for 1999–2000.

consultation. From a previous yearly high of 235 contacts, the program grew to 12,981 contacts in the year 2008–9 (Figure 3.1). This growth was reflected in all services provided by the program; it also reflected the greater diversity of programs being offered and a much higher level of staffing.

For the year prior to 2002, Aboriginal health worker (AHW) or GP contacts (as recorded on the patient information recall system *Communicare*) numbered 60 to 70, reflecting a service that was struggling to meet its screening performance indicators for STIs. Contact rates remained variable for a number of years as the program worked through appropriate service-delivery issues and dealt with difficulties in maintaining staff. After 2007–8, with a full complement of staff and other activities in the centre (a male-only centre established in 2003), there was exceptional growth in the number of contacts with GPs and nurses/AHWs. In 2008–9, there were 3,214 contacts. The Violence Intervention Program

(VIP) established in April 2006, which employed a second psychologist in 2008, grew significantly from 428 contacts to 1,142 contacts during 2008–9. The continued dramatic increases in contacts in those services that required professional positions suggest that at the period studied, the service was still not meeting the level of demand for these types of services in the community.

The health education/promotion sessions quickly passed 1,000 contacts per year. The number of contacts of people using the service in 2008–9 was almost as high on Mondays and Tuesdays (3,452) as on the following three days (3,951). This indicates that access to the GP service and (or possibly coupled with) the health discussion sessions offered only on Mondays and Tuesdays were important services, drawing participants beyond what was available on the other days. An alternative explanation or additional contributing factor could have been that demand was higher for the other drop-in services after the weekend, when the centre had been shut for two days.

The largest number of contacts occurred through the drop-in centre. Combining the Monday and Tuesday contacts with the rest of the week, there were 7,403 drop-in contacts, representing 57% of all contacts for 2008–9, the final years of data collection for this study. These figures include people accessing the program for a variety of reasons, including using the hygiene program, stopping in to talk informally with staff and other Aboriginal males present, and using the centre as a respite site.

Contacts for both Aboriginal males and females at Congress had steadily grown over the last 20 years. However, the gap in access by Aboriginal males compared to females had also grown.

This disparity in contacts is graphically illustrated in Figure 3.2, which shows these contacts as recorded on *Communicare*. However, if services that were not amenable to being recorded on *Communicare* are included, the gap in the access rates is noticeably reduced. Figure 3.3 shows the same *Communicare* data with contacts added from the MHP VIP and the drop-in centre.

While there may be other programs for which contacts were not recorded on *Communicare*, none of these were female only, so their exclusion from this graph would not significantly distort the result.

At the time of this study, it was possible only to consider some potential factors or interplays between factors that may explain the gap in contact rates. Negative views of Aboriginal male behaviour became especially apparent after the revelation on national television that child sexual abuse occurred in some NT Aboriginal communities. This and the subsequent description of the situation as a national crisis by the

Figure 3.2 Contacts at Congress by gender,[5] from *Communicare* by financial year

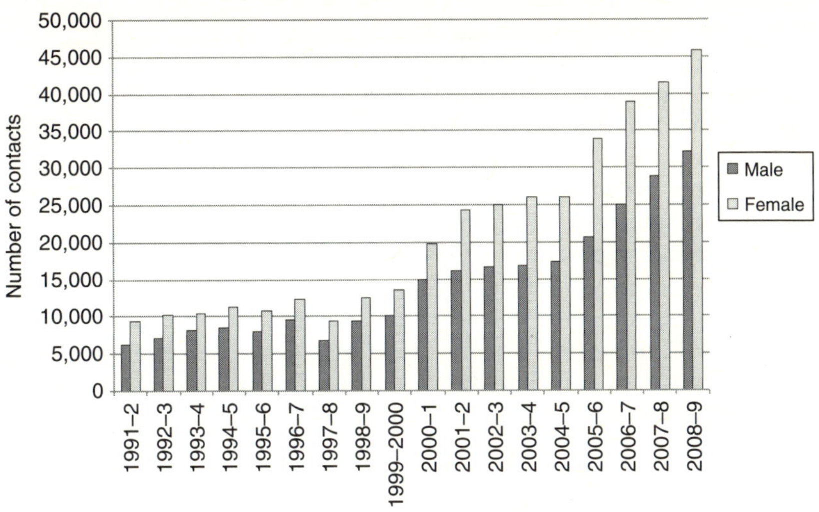

Figure 3.3 Contacts at Congress by gender, from *Communicare* plus MHP drop-in centre and VIP by financial year

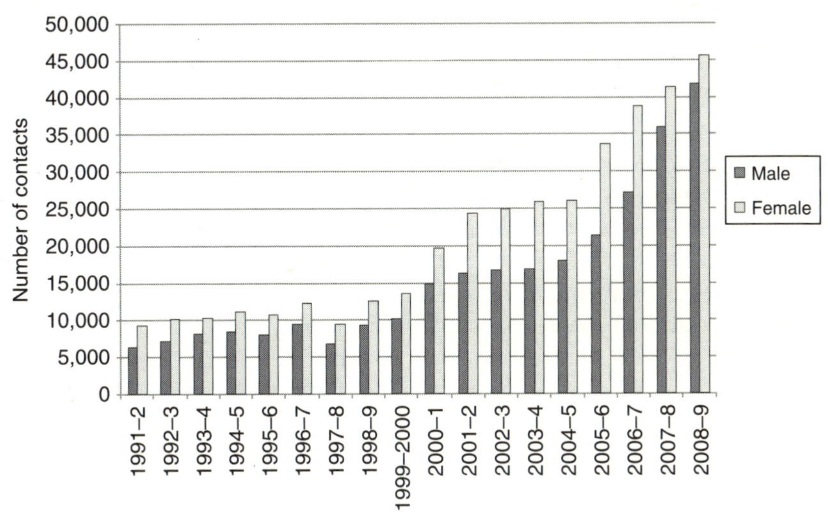

5 In the patient information recall system, only male and female gender options were being used during the project period.

Commonwealth government, which then permeated all aspects of Aboriginal affairs in the NT,[6] may have created a sense of shame and kept Aboriginal males from accessing services, thus counteracting to some degree the work of the MHP to improve access. Over the same period, Congress saw substantial growth in both the number of services offered and the number of staff. This increased capacity could have contributed to the greater rates of access by Aboriginal women. First, the increase in service access by Aboriginal women could have occurred by magnifying an existing trend in the disparity, making it more apparent because of increased levels of usage. Second, if the increase in capacity occurred at a time when Aboriginal males were avoiding using services due to perceived stigmatization, then the increased capacity would more likely be absorbed by women, as capacity would most likely still be less than demand in a population with high levels of chronic disease and poor health. Third, the greater rate of service access by Aboriginal women could have occurred if some of the new or expanded programs specifically targeted Aboriginal women or were perceived as targeting Aboriginal women, such as the expansion of the home-visitation service under the Nurse-Family Partnership Program (2007). What is apparent from the access data is that while the MHP had contributed to a substantial increase in Aboriginal male access to health services, there was still a gap in access rates between males and females to Congress services as whole. This gap would close significantly if the drop-in centre access data was added to the overall Congress data, showing that this approach can assist in bridging this gap.

Factors that contributed to increased equity of access to health services also reduced vulnerabilities through changes in community empowerment starting at the individual level

The open drop-in centre approach of the MHP was recognized as being an effective strategy in increasing Aboriginal male health-service access rates. The drop-in centre provided a culturally safe and welcoming place that was responsive to the needs of the people on any given day.

---

6 For more information regarding this policy, see the full project report at http://www .globalhealthequity.ca/electronic%20library/Australia%20Final%20Project%20 Report.pdf and also the *Submission of the Human Rights and Equal Opportunity Commission (HREOC) to the Senate Legal and Constitutional Committee on the NT National Emergency Response Legislation*, Australian Human Rights Commission, 2007.

It was important that people were able to come to the service when they needed to and when they were ready to seek information. The safe and welcoming atmosphere was achieved through an informal process of staff taking the time to talk with people when they came in, checking on their moods, and spending time with them straight away, if needed.

Having senior Aboriginal men involved in the program contributed significantly to the cultural safety practices of the place. The men employed at the time of the study had a profound knowledge and understanding of cultural matters, spoke a number of Aboriginal languages, and had an extensive awareness of the local and nearby communities. The males accessing the service felt the activities were undertaken in a culturally respectful manner. At the same time, these activities also provided a reference point for information and guidance to non-Aboriginal staff. This culturally safe environment contributed to improved health outcomes in a number of ways. The provision of a service that is perceived to be culturally safe contributes to acceptance of that service by Aboriginal people, and therefore improves access. When a service publicly recognizes the importance of cultural values, it reinforces to the community not only the priority of cultural diversity, but also that Aboriginal culture is respected. This perception in turn contributes to building cultural pride and helps strengthen cultural identity.

The provision of showers and washing machines through the Hygiene Program was recognized as a valuable and innovative service that addressed core issues around self-esteem and personal dignity. This service was particularly appreciated by Town Camp residents and those living rough or coming in from bush communities. Being able to access the showers and washing machines gave these Aboriginal males the opportunity to feel better about themselves and to feel confident in seeking other services. Consequently, this strategy also contributed to improving access to other services and helped develop individuals' capacity to take greater control over their lives.

Having access to medical services, screening, health checks, and treatments in the Male Health Centre setting was valued by Aboriginal males. This strategy seems to have been effective because they could access the medical service while using some other aspects of the service at the same time: attending the health promotion and education sessions, using the showers and washing machines, or just sitting around talking with other people present. This informal setting had a friendly and casual feel, very different from the more formal setting of the main Congress clinic. Aboriginal males attending the Male Health Centre also had more contact with staff, which contributed to feelings of ownership about the facility and comfort with the staff. Having senior Aboriginal workers on hand greatly enhanced this program, as they were able to explain some procedures in the person's first Aboriginal language or discuss issues involving cultural matters with clients and staff.

Known as the Monday or Tuesday morning sessions, the education or health-promotion sessions were recognized as providing an important opportunity for Aboriginal males to access a broad range of information regarding such matters as employment, education and training, legal rights, and health education on such topics as chronic-disease management, STI prevention, nutrition, environmental health matters, family and fathering programs, and personal-development issues around anger management or other behavioural concerns. In this way, these sessions explicitly addressed CPHC principles and some of the SDH. These sessions also played an important role in acting as a front door to the other services. This occurred in a number of ways. The sessions allowed people to come to the service without immediately having to ask for help or to see someone, so that clients could become comfortable with the place and staff. The sessions also gave people something to do while waiting to access health staff. Matters raised in these sessions acted as the trigger for some males to then seek professional assistance from staff for issues confronting them; for example, accessing counselling services or referrals to other sections of the organization.

Significantly, this setting also provided opportunities for Aboriginal males to provide assistance to each other and develop a sense of mutual support and strength. Participants noted how new friendships developed through attending these sessions. The outcomes of these discussions were fed back into the planning for future sessions and were the recognized basis for discussion topics at the 2008 Aboriginal Male Health Summit. In this way, participants saw immediate and tangible results of their involvement, which contributed to a sense of being valued. It is an important form of community consultation that helped the program reflect some of the contemporary community needs and it represented one form of community participation in, and control of, the program.

The counselling service offered through the VIP, which addressed a range of issues including depression, family support, empowerment, and anger management or other violence-related matters, was noted as an important strategy that addressed the social determinants of Aboriginal male health. The need for this type of service had been recognized for some time. The community consultation (2004) articulated these needs and identified the issues the counselling service could most effectively address. Based on this information, funding was pursued. While at the time of the study the program could take on clients only if violence was a factor, we believe that locating the counselling service contextually in the findings of the community consultation, and physically and structurally within the MHP, contributed to its successful uptake by Aboriginal males. In addition, the qualities of the staff involved were also recognized as contributing to the counselling service's success. Through a focus on violence, the counselling service addressed many broader issues. The building of individuals' capacity to manage their own lives was recognized as having positive effects on their family and partners, as well as on their ability to engage with employment, education, and access to other services, such as health services. The ability to engage in public life without fear or shame should not be underestimated in its impact on an individual's ability to deal with social issues.

The Central Australian Aboriginal Male Health Summit (2008) was held as a community response to the destructive political atmosphere and negative portrayals of Aboriginal males that were caused by recent federal government policy changes. It was widely recognized as being a pivotal event in challenging negative stereotypes of Aboriginal males and providing (symbolic and practical) support to Aboriginal males in the region. There were varying views as to its impact at a policy level. Locally, a view was expressed that the message from the summit fell on deaf ears in government because it did not fit with government policy. It was also felt that it was only because Aboriginal males apologized to women that the summit received any attention at the political level. Nevertheless, Congress management argued that after the summit, access to funding for programs for Aboriginal male health became easier and that Ingkintja was recognized at a government level as a program to be consulted on male health issues. Nationally, it has been recognized by both Aboriginal and non-Aboriginal commentators and political leaders as a key moment in political advocacy in that it presented Aboriginal males in a positive manner at a crucial time in the policy debate regarding Aboriginal affairs. Most notably, this recognition included being cited in the then prime minister's Indigenous Affairs Statement (Rudd, 2009).

The 2004 community consultation was identified as an important process in establishing what the Aboriginal male community defined as their needs and in renewing the dialogue with Aboriginal males about the direction of the service. It helped to establish the MHP's legitimacy with the local community and gave Aboriginal males and agencies with an interest in Aboriginal male health a chance to share their views. Most importantly, the documented evidence gathered during this 18-month process was used immediately to shape the program and it has guided the direction and style of the MHP since that time. Community consultation, if it is seen to lead to change that is in line with the community's views, is an important empowering process. Since changes in the program's design and delivery occurred quickly, and those changes reflected the views being expressed through the consultation, they contributed positively to both the program's acceptance in the community and to building a sense of personal value for those who were interviewed and consulted.

Finding appropriate ways to engage with Aboriginal male health around important cultural ceremonial practices has been a long-term aim of the MHP. Two issues were involved: first, establishing a community understanding of the difference between men's (male) health and *men's business* (cultural ceremony and law), which is seen as an important part of the spiritual health of a person; and second, establishing a way to have medical support available at ceremony time to minimize the potential spread of blood-borne viruses.

It is recognized that through the efforts of Congress MHP staff, a community understanding has been established regarding the difference between *men's business* and what is commonly being discussed when people talk about male health. Aboriginal men's cultural ceremony is an essential component of Aboriginal cultural practice and is open only to those males participating. Concerns that *men's business* was what was to be discussed when talking about "men's health" had caused concern and, for some, profound distress in early discussion about establishing "men's" health programs. Congress MHP work in this area helped to resolve confusion and allay concerns when talking about the need for Aboriginal males to access health services and look after their health. This process is another important example of the program's activity being located within a cultural safety framework, which has helped build acceptance of the service and could potentially lead to better access to health services for some Aboriginal (particularly senior) males.

Discussion and Conclusion

The Congress MHP, as it was known until 2009, was poorly resourced in its early years, inappropriately located, and suffered from the social stigma related to being funded as an STI program. The decision, driven by a variety of reasons, of the Congress cabinet in 2004 to undertake an extensive community consultation and program-planning project led to a number of positive outcomes, including improved community credibility and acceptance. A clear programmatic vision based on need, as defined by the local community, was identified. Since then, the program has been better resourced, has moved into larger premises, and has broadened its funding and range of services.

Ingkintja adopted a drop-in centre service model, which incorporated a community-development approach based on individual capacity building and CPHC frameworks that successfully addressed both the physical and emotional health needs of Aboriginal males in the region. Key to creating an appropriate environment for Aboriginal males to access health care and support was the cultural sensitivity of the program and its cultural safety aspects. These included Ingkintja being a male-only space, the Aboriginal staff, and most importantly, the active participation of senior Aboriginal men in the program. Because of these approaches, there was a significant increase in access rates by Aboriginal males, which included a 13-fold increase in the number of contacts per year for the MHP's clinic-based services. Also notable was the number of contacts with the counselling services through the VIP, which grew 10-fold after its establishment. By far the greatest numbers of contacts occurred with the hygiene facilities and attendance at the health-promotion and education sessions, achieving more 8,600 contacts in 2008–9.

Aboriginal males interviewed as part of this study located their health in an emotional and social well-being framework. Using this framework, they recognized the impacts of colonization, changing male roles in contemporary society, social alienation, and exclusion from access to employment opportunities as key contributing factors to their states of health. These Aboriginal males identified the need for individuals to take responsibility for their own lives and actions; they also recognized that people may need support and that there were a number of factors that contributed to triggering an individual to decide to take action. Such triggers included responsibility to and support from family, their own sense of self-esteem, and their understanding of their community obligations. Of significance was the recognition of the need for the individual to take action, with an understanding that change can then occur at a family and then community level, enabling some people to engage with those structural issues that contribute to a community's health.

This awareness represented a sophisticated understanding of the pathways to address the individual structural divide, often discussed in SDH and social-change literature. Empowerment was understood as a process. Disempowerment, through structural action without community participation and empowerment, was acknowledged as leading to further alienation. One senior manager stated,

> That's what I mean, that's the risk of institutionalising resources and empowering the institution to provide these things doesn't translate to empowerment in the community and if you think about all the things that are going on in our communities, that's, we've really got to get back to that, because we've got to empower people to make the change within the environment.

This study found Congress Ingkintja recognized and worked towards empowering Aboriginal males in the region, boosting self-esteem and creating community capacity to address and take action on social issues.

The literature review of Aboriginal male health programs and documents reviewed as part of this study verified Ingkintja's approach and the range of services as consistent with models of health services developed for Aboriginal males elsewhere, and with the expectations of central Australian Aboriginal males. This finding was confirmed during the interviews.

The identified strengths of Ingkintja at the time of the study included a high degree of cultural safety; the mix of preventive, health promotion, and treatment and rehabilitation services; the drop-in centre approach; multidiscipline staffing; advocacy on SDH; and the flexibility and responsiveness in approach and service delivery.

There was a complex and multilayered interrelationship between the provision of medical services and other comprehensive primary health care approaches at play within Ingkintja. The provision of GP services at Ingkintja was recognized as being a key element in attracting some people to the service. At the same time, it was recognized that many people came for the other drop-in centre functions and then, over time, having become more comfortable, decided to utilize the GP service. Many staff believed that to have credibility in the local community as "a fair dinkum health service," they needed to have a GP on site. However, it was the mixture of services, the fact that people could attend when they were in the mood or ready, the physical layout of the centre, and it being a welcoming and safe male-only environment that were recognized by most people interviewed as being the reasons for success in achieving good access rates.

At the time of this study, the Congress Ingkintja successfully modelled a number of key elements of CPHC:

- It employed a multidisciplinary workforce in programs that had health promoting, preventive, curative, and rehabilitative foci.
- It took a broad definition of health and well-being that addressed the immediate health needs and concerns of individuals and their social conditions.
- Through a broad range of programs, it had both a medical and SDH agenda.
- It placed great emphasis on the active involvement of Aboriginal males in service delivery, program development, and governance.
- It had a strong ethos of seeking the views of Aboriginal males on their health needs and on the development of the programs to meet those needs.
- It maintained strong emphasis on health-service access as a determinant of health, and developed a number of innovative approaches and programs to support that aim.

By contributing to Congress advocacy on such things as the Commonwealth Aboriginal affairs, alcohol, and child-protection policies, Ingkintja's perspective contributed to creating policy frameworks and programs of action that could support and address Aboriginal peoples' needs and perspectives. Its impact on policy was most recognized when Ingkintja took direct action on issues coupled with advocacy and capacity building, such as with the summit.

The study identified a number of often interrelated issues that may have acted as barriers to the work of the program. These factors included problems in accessing adequate and flexible funding to develop and deliver appropriate services in the region, male-health policy being too narrowly focused on reproductive and sexual health, and government policies that vilified Aboriginal males and undermined their dignity and roles within their communities. While policy continues to accept the dominance of a medical model of health, rather than recognizing the essential SDH that influence Aboriginal male health, Ingkintja will continue to struggle with health-program funding parameters that do not adequately reflect local health needs.

Despite these quite substantial barriers, this study found that Congress Ingkintja provided a very successful health service program for Aboriginal males in the central Australian region. Using community development and comprehensive primary health care principles, Ingkintja staff worked sympathetically and effectively with Aboriginal males to empower them to take action to address the SDH affecting the quality of life of the local Aboriginal community. At the same time, Ingkintja has worked as an advocacy body at a structural and policy level. The provision of medical services occurred within a social-health framework. There was a high level of community support for the program's services and approach, reflected in the impressive rates of the various services.

Since this project, Congress has continued to undertake research with the aims of identifying and being responsive to community health needs, ensuring reflexive health practices, and strengthening the evidence base of its CPHC approach. Current research with this focus includes participating as one of six Australia primary health service sites in Evaluating the Effectiveness of Comprehensive Primary Health Care in Local Communities, a collaborative research project with Flinders University. The project specifically aims to extend the evidence base and work of the *Revitalizing Health for All: Learning from Comprehensive Primary Health Care Experiences* collaboration by evaluating CPHC as a system. There are other smaller projects describing the impacts of specific Congress programs, such as the Lowitja Institute–funded Learning from Central Australian Aboriginal Women's Experiences: Reflections on Participation in the CAAC Family Partnership Program in Alice Springs.

ACKNOWLEDGMENTS

We gratefully acknowledge the contributions of the many Aboriginal males who participated in this research project. Their generosity in sharing their experiences provided a rich and honest description of their lives and feelings. We also would like to thank Congress staff and cabinet members for their involvement, noting in particular the work of past CEO Stephanie Bell, who was instrumental in the development and implementation of the project; Baydon Williams and David Blue, for their time, humour, and patience; and Korey Summers, trainee Aboriginal research officer. The Congress cabinet directive that Congress undertake this type of research reflects an important commitment on behalf of the organization to ensure that the evidence base for quality comprehensive primary health care is broadly available. We also note and appreciate the additional funding provided by the Australian Cooperative Research Centre for Aboriginal Health (Lowitja Institute) and the considerable financial contribution of Congress to the project.

REFERENCES

Anderson, I., Baum, F., & Bentley, M. (2007). *Beyond Bandaids: Exploring the underlying social determinants of Aboriginal health.* Darwin: Cooperative Research Centre for Aboriginal Health.

Australian Bureau of Statistics. (2009). *Experimental life tables for Aboriginal and Torres Strait Islander Australians, 2005–2007 (3302.0.55.00).* Canberra: Author.

Australian Bureau of Statistics. (2013). *Aboriginal and Torres Strait Islander population nearing 700,000.* Canberra: Author.

Australian Bureau of Statistics & Australian Institute of Health and Welfare. (2008). *The health and welfare of Australia's Aboriginal and Torres Strait Islander peoples* (Cat. no. IHW 21). Canberra: Australian Institute of Health and Welfare.

Australian Human Rights Commission. (2007). *Submission of the Human Rights and Equal Opportunity Commission (HREOC) to the Senate Legal and Constitutional Committee on the NT National Emergency Response Legislation.* Canberra: Author. Retrieved from http://www.hreoc.gov.au/legal/submissions/2007/NTNER_Measures20070810.html

Australian Institute of Health and Welfare. (2008). *Aboriginal and Torres Strait Islander Health Performance Framework 2008 report: Detailed analyses (Cat no. IHW 22).* Canberra: Author.

Brown, A., & Blashki, G. (2005, Oct). Indigenous male health disadvantage: Linking the heart and mind. *Australian Family Physician, 34*(10), 813–19. Medline:16217564

Burns, J., Thomson, N., Brooks, J., Burrow, S., Kirov, E., McGougan, B., & Valenti, A. (2002). *Describing an iceberg from a glimpse of its tip: A summary of the literature on achievements in Aboriginal and Torres Strait Islander health.* Perth, Australia: Australian Indigenous Health Info Net.

Calma, T. (2006). *Creating futures: Influencing social determinants of mental health and well-being in rural, Indigenous and Island peoples.* Sydney: Australian Human Rights Commission; Retrieved from https://www.humanrights.gov.au/news/speeches/site-navigation-26.

Carson, B., Dunbar, T., & Chenhall, R. (Eds.). (2007). *Social determinants of Indigenous health.* Sydney: Allen & Unwin.

Commonwealth Grants Commission (CGC). (2001). *Report on Indigenous funding 2001*. Canberra: Commonwealth of Australia.

Dick, D. (2007). Working paper presented to the International Symposium on the Social Determinants of Indigenous Health: *Social determinants and the health of Indigenous peoples in Australia: A human rights based approach*. Adelaide, Australia. Retrieved from https://www.humanrights.gov.au /news/speeches/social-determinants-and-health-indigenous-peoples -australia-human-rights-based.

Dwyer, J., Siburn, K., & Wilson, G. (2004). *National strategies for improving Indigenous health and health care* (Aboriginal and Torres Strait Islander Primary Health Care Review: Consultant Report No. 1). Canberra: Commonwealth of Australia.

Houston, S. (2004). Cultural security as a determinant of Aboriginal health. In H. Keleher & C. MacDougall (Eds.), *Understanding health: A determinants approach* (pp.101–111). South Melbourne: Oxford University Press.

Houston, S. (2006, Dec). Equity, by what measure? *Health Promotion Journal of Australia, 17*(3), 206–10. Medline:17176236

McCoy, B. (2008). *Holding men*. Canberra: Aboriginal Studies Press.

National Aboriginal and Torres Strait Islander Health Council. (2003). *The National Strategic Framework for Aboriginal and Torres Strait Islander Health: Framework for action by governments*. Canberra: Author.

Nettleton, C., Napolitano, D., & Stephens, C. (2007). *An overview of current knowledge of the social determinants of Indigenous health*. Adelaide: World Health Organization.

Paradies, Y. (2006). *Race, racism, stress and Indigenous health*. (Submitted PhD thesis, Department of Health, University of Melbourne, Melbourne, Australia).

Robert Griew Consulting & Office of Aboriginal and Torres Strait Islander Health. (2008). *The link between primary health care and health outcomes for Aboriginal and Torres Strait Islander Australians*. Canberra: Office of Aboriginal and Torres Strait Islander Health, Department of Health and Ageing.

Rosewarne, C., Vaarzon-Morel, P., Bell, S., Carter, E., Liddle, M., & Liddle, J. (2007). The historical context of developing an Aboriginal community-controlled health service: A social history of the first ten years of the Central Australian Aboriginal Congress. *Health and History, 9*(2), 114–43. http:// dx.doi.org/10.2307/40111578

Rudd, K. (2009). *Ministerial statement Indigenous Affairs* (Commonwealth of Australia Parliamentary Debates House of Representatives Official Hansard No. 3). Canberra: Commonwealth of Australia.

Wenitong, M. (2002). *Indigenous male health*. Canberra: The Office for Aboriginal and Torres Strait Islander Health Commonwealth Department of Health and

Ageing. Retrieved from http://health.gov.au/internet/main/publishing.nsf /Content/health-oatsih-pubs-malehealth.htm1.

Wenitong, M. (2006, Oct 16). Aboriginal and Torres Strait Islander male health, wellbeing and leadership. *The Medical Journal of Australia, 185*(8), 466–7. Medline:17137444

World Health Organization. (2007). Presented to the International Symposium on the Social Determinants of Indigenous Health: *Social determinants of Indigenous health: The international experience and its policy implications.* Adelaide: Flinders University.

Yap, M., & Biddle, N. (2009). *Towards a gender-related index for Indigenous Australians* (CAEPR Working Paper No. 52). Canberra: Centre for Aboriginal Economic Policy Research, Australian National University.

4 Exploring the Complex Contributions of the Community-based Safe Motherhood Program to Comprehensive Primary Health Care in the Democratic Republic of Congo

RICHARD BITWE MIHANDA, JEAN ROBERT LIKOFATA, AND GWENDOLYN J. LUSI

Background

This chapter presents the results of a study on safe motherhood carried out in North Kivu, Democratic Republic of Congo (DRC). It was conducted by HEAL (Healthcare, Education, community Action, and Leadership development) Africa, in partnership with the DRC's Provincial Division of Health. Although a complex web of possible factors impact on maternal mortality and morbidity, the study described here attempted to ascertain the added value of the community-based Safe Motherhood Prenatal Care and Micro-insurance Program being carried out in North Kivu.

Maternal mortality remains very high in sub-Saharan Africa, with rural areas having the highest rates. This is a result of numerous factors, the most important of which include maternal undernutrition (including anaemia) and short stature – which are both influenced by dietary intake during childhood and adolescence, as well as the presence of HIV infection and the frequency and severity of such communicable diseases as malaria and diarrhea, and access to safe assisted delivery – which is affected by physical and financial accessibility and the availability of maternity services of sufficient quality. The failure of the great majority of African countries to achieve the UN's Millennium Development Goal 5 – reduce maternal mortality by three-quarters of its 1990 level – serves to underline the above challenges (World Health Organization [WHO], 2010). The DRC starkly exemplifies this challenge: official statistics – which are almost certainly an underestimate – put the national maternal mortality ratio in 2005 at 1,100 per 100,000 live births (WHO, 2010). North Kivu is acknowledged to be one of the most underdeveloped regions of the DRC, and its development has been further compromised by persistent and widespread conflict. In 2007, national data revealed that only 21% of women accessed family planning services, 85% attended prenatal care at least once, and 74% had a skilled attendant at delivery (WHO, 2010). Data for the territory of Masisi in North Kivu confirm very low levels of service utilization along the continuum of care.

The study was conducted in the rural health zones of Birambizo and Kayna, where maternal health indicators are poorer than in urban areas (Ministère du Plan et Macro International, 2008), and focused on one specific aspect of maternal health: safe delivery care.

Policy context and health-service provision

Since 1985, the DRC has implemented a health system based on the principles of primary health care as codified in the Declaration of Alma-Ata, with significant sustained funding from the United States Agency for International Development (USAID) (1981–2006), the World Bank, and other donors. The coverage is based on health zones, ideally serving a population of 150,000, and subdivided into 15 *airès de santé*. Each *aire de santé* has a general referral hospital capable of emergency surgery and a health centre that is staffed and equipped to minimal standards and able to provide preventive and curative health care. A comprehensive package of health services is offered in each zone.

Despite the policy framework, the package fails to address the social determinants of ill- health. For example, in the areas of maternal and child health – and in particular, safe motherhood in rural areas – the government has targeted specific problems that contribute to risky delivery and identified solutions. The solutions include family planning through health centres, delivery in health centres, prevention of post-partum hemorrhage, and the use of partograms. But the barriers that prevent women from using health centres at the time of delivery have been left unaddressed; inequities in access to and availability of health centres able to provide maternity care have not been explored.

Impact of war

Eastern DRC has experienced uninterrupted war since 1992. The effects of the war on CPHC and maternal health are significant and affect several social determinants and important components of the health system. These effects include the destruction and looting of health infrastructure; the flight of trained personnel; the continual displacement of populations, with ensuing poverty; illness; malnutrition; war injuries; the disruption of immunization programs; and the unchecked spread of communicable diseases, especially sexually transmitted infections and HIV, often related to sexual violence in war time.

These intersecting factors and barriers have resulted in the DRC having some of the worst maternal mortality statistics in the world, despite theoretical coverage in 515 health zones. Maternal mortality rates (MMRs) worldwide are between 140 and 200 per 100,000, whereas in the DRC the MMR is 1,298 per 100,000. The under-5 mortality rate in the DRC is 205 per 1,000 live births. Both the high under-5 mortality rate and MMR are the results of poor access to health care, as well as the quality of health care and CPHC in the country (World Bank, 2007).

HEAL Africa's Safe Motherhood Program

It is within this context that HEAL Africa's Safe Motherhood Prenatal Care and Micro-insurance Program works to address the social and structural factors that undermine maternal health and safe birth practices. The program has a two-pronged approach: strengthening health-care structures and encouraging community change. In terms of health care, this program works with structures such as health centres and general-referral hospitals. Activities include capacity building of health personnel, equipping health facilities with supplies, and revitalizing maternity centres. The community aspect includes training traditional birth attendants (TBAs) in the techniques of safe birth and reducing risky practices, training officers who conduct awareness-raising sessions in the community, and training local religious and tribal leaders.

There are a number of barriers to safe motherhood in North Kivu's four health zones, notably

- technical barriers, including
  destruction of infrastructure,
  looting of equipment,
  lack of lighting for surgery and delivery,
  lack of trained personnel,
  poor training of surgeons on safe surgical procedures for a Caesarean section (C-Section), and
  lack of medicines;

- policy barriers, including
  "selective" interventions instead of a comprehensive set of activities, and
  neglect of the importance of TBAs, despite the reality that more than half of all deliveries are conducted by TBAs;
- economic barriers, including
  cost of delivery in a health centre ($5 cash; instead of a chicken to the TBA),
  cost of a C-Section ($35 minimum),
  cost of absence from the farm while awaiting delivery at the hospital,
  cost of transport from home to health centre, or health centre to hospital, in case of emergency obstetric care, and
  men's control over money and decision making; and finally
- social barriers, including
  traditional beliefs about women and maternity,
  wishes and values of husbands and mothers-in-law,
  role and influence of TBAs,
  question of who will provide care for children and husband if the woman is absent from home,
  early marriage,
  multiparity, and
  gender inequities.

Given the challenging barriers to safe motherhood in North Kivu, HEAL Africa had to determine how its Safe Motherhood Program could build on the foundation of existing community structures to effectively address some key social determinants of maternal health. An intervention devised by HEAL Africa was to create "Safe Motherhood Solidarity Groups," intended to organize maternity insurance through a rotating credit scheme to mitigate the poverty of their members' households.

The maternity microinsurance scheme is extremely innovative and increases health-care access for prenatal mothers. Women of reproductive age pay into maternity microinsurance programs that ensure that they can receive proper health care during pregnancy, delivery, and the neonatal period. The insurance programs are locally managed, with each member paying into the program to receive the needed support from an appropriate health facility when she becomes pregnant. The appropriate level of care might be provided by a retrained TBA, the local health centre, or a local hospital. Early screening and prenatal care are essential to identifying high-risk deliveries and assessing the appropriate level of care for pregnant women.

Each maternity microinsurance program starts with eight to10 members and a small grant of money for them to manage for their own childbirth costs. They receive training in family planning, managing a small business, and understanding the concept of a "solidarity group." They meet weekly, get to know each other, and develop trust. Their husbands become involved in the classes on family planning. They arrange to work together to transport their wives to the clinic to deliver, thus avoiding the alternative: a two-day walk. Ultimately, the multipronged approach of the Safe Motherhood Program attempts to address all the factors that prevent women from seeking maternity care in an established clinic or health institution.

Research Questions and Methods

The objectives of the study were as follows:

- to measure the contribution made by the safe-motherhood solidarity groups in improving the utilization of maternity services in Kayna and Birambizo health zones;
- to identify the experiences and perceptions of project stakeholders regarding the value of the safe-motherhood solidarity groups; and
- to identify the constraining and facilitating factors in the operation of the Safe Motherhood Program as reported by the project stakeholders.

Two of the four rural areas in which the Safe Motherhood Program has been initiated were chosen for the study that was carried out in 2009. The first was the health zone of Birambizo, where the Safe Motherhood Program had been operational for three years, and the second was Kayna, where the program was just being implemented. The Birambizo health zone has 32 *aires de santé*, each with its own health centre, and 356 villages. In addition, the zone has 39 public health centres, three mission-related health centres, 18 health posts, a general-referral hospital, and a mission-related hospital. Kayna's health zone, by contrast, has 20 *aires de santé*, each with its health centre, and 107 villages. This zone has 16 state health centres, four referral health centres, and 42 health posts.

The necessary sample size to demonstrate significant differences in key indicators of improved utilization of maternity services was calculated using *Epi Info* 6.04. In each of the two zones, our target was to interview 87 women who were members of solidarity groups and 87 women who were not. We did not quite meet our target of an even split between both groups. In the end, we had fewer participants who were nonmembers of solidarity groups: 60% of respondents were members of solidarity groups and 40% were nonmembers. Four additional women participated, rendering a total of 352 respondents. Of the women surveyed, 48% lived in Birambizo and 52% in Kayna.

In addition, semistructured interviews were conducted in focus-group format involving

- two heads-of-zone doctors;
- four supervising nurses;
- women of childbearing age, members of safe-motherhood solidarity groups;
- women of childbearing age, nonmembers of safe-motherhood solidarity groups;
- TBAs who were members of safe-motherhood solidarity groups; and
- TBAs who were not members of safe-motherhood solidarity groups.

Results and Analysis

The large majority of female respondents were of childbearing age. Most women who were from areas where the Safe Motherhood Program was operating recognized the positive impact of the program on maternal health and on knowledge and access to information about reproductive health. Most respondents also agreed that information from the program on family planning had a positive impact. There was a strong association between belonging to a solidarity group and utilization of maternity services (Table 4.1).

In describing the impact of the program on access and utilization, focus-group participants from the solidarity groups made the following statements and testimonies: "the program has abolished the bad habit of women giving birth at their homes"; "thanks to the program, women work together and pay maternity fees for members of the

Table 4.1 Utilization of maternity services by solidarity group members and nonmembers

Comparison indicators	Solidarity group members	Solidarity group nonmembers	RR	P
Utilization				
Yes	168	31	3.71	0.0001
No	3	86	1	

solidarity groups"; "our wives have learned a variety of skills; they have been educated in giving birth at the hospital and seeking health care earlier on"; "new mothers have been educated to pursue care in the hospital even after they have delivered"; and "it reduces the ratio of women who deliver at home."

Doctors, nurses, and other health workers also reported changes in health behaviours related to access and utilization. Regarding members of the solidarity groups, one stakeholder from the Birambizo health zone reported that

> …women, especially with teachings from the Safe Motherhood Program, have discovered that they must not wait until they have problems to come to the hospital. It is necessary to come to the health centre from conception so that we can daily keep an eye on her pregnancy and find out what problems can occur.

Another explained that

> they now know that for every pregnancy, you must go to the health centre even if they have gone to see a TBA. These days, even TBAs are sending pregnant women to the health centre. Another thing they are informed about is cleanliness, breast feeding, and family planning.

Project stakeholders also reported nurses' and doctors' positive attitudes towards the Safe Motherhood Program. Stakeholders in Kayna health zone reported on the opinions of nurses, stating that nurses would like to see the program last a long time, as they are taught new material and are also reminded of knowledge and skills they learned in nursing school. A similar response was noted from TBAs, who appreciate the program and the knowledge they gain from it.

In terms of availability of medicines and staff, cost reduction, information knowledge, and financial barriers, all stakeholders reported appreciating the value of solidarity groups. The following statements from both solidarity-group members and nonmembers who participated in the focus-group discussions demonstrate also the positive social and environmental impact the program has had on whole communities: "it brings change in the way of thinking of people"; "it contributes to the fraternity of people here"; "the number of members is only growing and they are working more and more"; "from the Safe Motherhood Program, people are learning how to live together in union and fraternity"; "thanks to the program, there is change within families: There are now dialogues within families concerning family planning"; and "the Safe Motherhood Program has helped our community with advice on preventing maternal mortality."

Discussion

Improving access to maternity services

It is evident that the Safe Motherhood Program has been effective in addressing the factors that affect access to maternity services, while at the same time encouraging utilization and confronting barriers that deter utilization.

Solidarity group members receive financial support through the rotating credit allowances and income-generating activities. This financial support provides the means for women to afford maternity care. Women reported that they were able to afford prenatal care, delivery fees, and postnatal care due to the support of the solidarity groups. The groups have enabled women from all social classes to access quality maternity services and pay for them. Pregnant women are commencing prenatal visits much earlier than they had previously. Members of solidarity groups who give birth in hospital have enough money to pay their bills. The Safe Motherhood Program has therefore contributed to reducing inequities of access to maternity services through overcoming economic barriers.

Contributions to social and environmental change

The Safe Motherhood Program has succeeded in reducing financial, physical, and technical obstacles that hinder access and utilization. This success, in turn, has enabled communities to address the social and cultural factors that influence decisions to seek maternity health care.

It is evident that study participants and community members perceive the program as beneficial: they have seen changes in their families, communities, and health status. The program's ability, and that of its solidarity groups, to work with all members of society, rather than just targeting women of childbearing age, is a key factor in its success.

Solidarity, team work, and the involvement of leaders are all integral to the Safe Motherhood Program, as they give individuals a sense of having a stake in how the project unfolds. Fostering connections and relationships with community leaders assists in achieving full community buy-in, thereby laying the groundwork for change in habits, health beliefs, and behaviours. Members of the Safe Motherhood solidarity groups reported various incentives for joining, including the training women receive regarding income-generating activities; access to rotating credit allowances; information on family planning, and HIV, and gender; literacy classes; and access to social support. These benefits encourage membership and also address the gamut of social aspects that contribute to poor health.

The program catalyses a number of environmental changes as well. For instance, TBAs who were called to home births in the past now often work within health structures. TBAs who are members of solidarity groups are also referring women to clinics to give birth. The training of health personnel (including midwives and TBAs) is also a remarkable change brought about by the program.

The participatory mechanism of the solidarity groups and their political capacity have been improved due to close partnerships with strong community leaders, such as religious leaders and tribal chiefs. The voice of vulnerable groups is promoted and heard through the weight of these leaders and their specific power to influence the whole community and effect change.

In communities where the Safe Motherhood Program operates, women's access to solidarity groups greatly reduces the risk of maternal mortality and improves maternal and infant health. The reinforcing effects of community mobilization, education, solidarity-group membership, rotating credit, and support for TBAs and health centres have successfully reduced factors that lead to women giving birth at home. Members of the solidarity groups use maternity services more than nonmembers. They prefer to give birth within health structures and clinics – and with trained health personnel – where the detection and treatment of complications are available.

Finally, solidarity groups encourage equitable access to medical care. Because there is no discrimination within the group-membership system, the program is open to all ethnic groups and all generations. As the maternity-insurance aspect of the program enables the women to pay for health care, the women also send an encouraging signal to employees of clinics and hospitals who, in turn, are more motivated to provide quality care.

The importance of women's empowerment and social mobilization

To reduce maternal mortality, women must be involved in matters that concern their fate. A good relationship between women and health-care services is essential so that women seek out access knowing they will receive quality care and be supported by the community. Such a goal is not easy to achieve in Africa, because a high percentage of women are illiterate, and specialized services are inaccessible both geographically and financially.

Women should be trained in and informed about prevention and promotion of maternal health care. Any activity in favour of mothers and newborn babies depends on social mobilization; otherwise, it is doomed. The Safe Motherhood Program enables women's empowerment and social mobilization in the context of CPHC and maternal mortality.

The impact of this initiative in North Kivu is similar to that recorded in recent large community-intervention trials in Nepal and Malawi in which facilitation of women's groups by community-level "animators" has resulted in significant increases in utilization of maternity services and a sharp and significant reduction in newborn deaths, as well as some improvement in maternal mortality, albeit just short of statistical significance (Manandhar et al., 2004; Lewycka et al., 2013). As noted by Rosato et al.,

> Women's groups in Malawi and Nepal are increasing the important capacities within communities, such as the ability to identify maternal and neonatal health problems and their root causes; the ability to mobilise resources necessary for improving the health of mothers and newborn infants; the internal and external social networks they can draw on when needed; and the development of strong local leaders who have the motivation and drive to improve maternal and neonatal health in the community.

A large proportion of this effect is thought to be due to community mobilization bringing about changes in socio environmental risk factors by developing the capacities of communities, the choices they make, and their ultimate empowerment. (Rosato et al., 2008)

Limitations

The limitations of this research study relate mainly to the fact that the selection of groups (members and nonmembers) for study was not randomized. This could have created bias in the results since it is possible, although unlikely in these universally poor zones with poor health infrastructure and staffing, that there were other important differences between the comparison groups that could have influenced utilization of services and thus maternity outcomes.

Conclusion

A sustainable reduction in maternal morbidity and mortality will require not only improved access to relevant services but also improved quality of basic and comprehensive emergency obstetric care at health centres and referral hospitals respectively (Souza et al., 2013). Moreover, it will be necessary over the longer term to address the key social determinants of poor maternal health to ultimately have a positive impact on the tragedy of maternal mortality. Expanding the use of Safe Motherhood solidarity groups throughout the DRC would be an excellent tool for reducing maternal mortality and high-risk childbirth. The poor infrastructure, instability, and conflicts that to this day erupt in Eastern Congo make a community-based approach the most sustainable option. HEAL Africa continued to expand its Safe Motherhood Program in 2012, expanding into six new health zones in Maniema Province. The goal is to create 240 solidarity groups among these zones, training 480 group leaders over the course of three years. In addition, HEAL Africa is attempting to extend the solidarity group approach for women of childbearing age and incorporate children and eventually the whole community in developing health insurance to cover all health needs that may arise. The project in Maniema will start this expansion, including mothers and their children below the age of 1 year in the solidarity group health-insurance scheme. Future research will examine the success of this project and the feasibility of providing health insurance to an entire community to achieve universal coverage.

The Safe Motherhood Program has partnered with other community-development programs that HEAL operates throughout Eastern Congo, evolving into a powerful tool to improve CPHC. This coexistence with other programs involving women's empowerment, leadership, and conflict resolution, as well as gender and justice, can assist in reducing the barriers that inhibit access to, and utilization of, maternal health services. The goal is to address all the factors that influence poor CPHC, as it is well known that the social, cultural, and structural factors in any given context are just as integral to health as its health systems. This approach can only support and enhance the progress that the Safe Motherhood Program is already making.

ACKNOWLEDGMENT

Some material in this chapter previously appeared in Mihanda, R.B., Likofata, J.R., and Lusi, G.J. (2013), Contribution of safe motherhood solidarity groups in using and accessing maternity services during a period of armed conflict. *Health*, 5(7), 1085–91. http://dx.doi.org/10.4236/Health.2013.57146

REFERENCES

Lewycka, S., Mwansambo, C., Rosato, M., Kazembe, P., Phiri, T., Mganga, A., …, & Costello, A. (2013, May 18). Effect of women's groups and volunteer peer counselling on rates of mortality, morbidity, and health behaviours in mothers and children in rural Malawi (MaiMwana): A factorial, cluster-randomised controlled trial. *Lancet*, *381*(9879), 1721–35. http://dx.doi.org/10.1016/S0140-6736(12)61959-X Medline:23683639

Manandhar, D.S., Osrin, D., Shrestha, B.P., Mesko, N., Morrison, J., Tumbahangphe, K.M., … de L Costello, A.M., & Members of the MIRA Makwanpur trial team. (2004, Sep 11–17). Effect of a participatory intervention with women's groups on birth outcomes in Nepal: Cluster-randomised controlled trial. *Lancet*, *364*(9438), 970–9. http://dx.doi.org/10.1016/S0140-6736(04)17021-9 Medline:15364188

Ministère du Plan et Macro International (2008). *Enquête Démographique et de Santé, République Démocratique du Congo 2007*. Calverton, Maryland, U.S.A.: Author. Retrieved from http://www.measuredhs.com/pubs/pdf/FR208/FR208.pdf

Rosato, M., Laverack, G., Grabman, L.H., Tripathy, P., Nair, N., Mwansambo, C., …, & Costello, A. (2008, Sep 13). Community participation: Lessons for maternal, newborn, and child health. *Lancet, 372*(9642), 962–71. http:// dx.doi.org/10.1016/S0140-6736(08)61406-3 Medline:18790319

Souza, J.P., Gülmezoglu, A.M., Vogel, J., Carroli, G., Lumbiganon, P., Qureshi, Z., …, & Say, L. (2013, May 18). Moving beyond essential interventions for reduction of maternal mortality (the WHO Multicountry Survey on Maternal and Newborn Health): A cross-sectional study. *Lancet, 381*(9879), 1747–55. http://dx.doi.org/10.1016/S0140-6736(13)60686-8 Medline:23683641

World Bank (2007). *The World Bank annual report.* Retrieved from https:// openknowledge.worldbank.org/handle/10986/7534

World Health Organization. (2010). *Trends in maternal mortality: 1990 to 2008.* Geneva: Author.

5 Implementing a Primary Health Care Program in Bogotá, Colombia

ROMÁN RAFAEL VEGA ROMERO, PAOLA ANDREA
MOSQUERA MÉNDEZ, JINNETH HERNÁNDEZ
TORRES, AND JORGE MARTÍNEZ COLLANTES

Background

Colombia is an Andean country located in northwestern South America and is considered an upper-middle income country. According to 2014 figures, it has an estimated population of 47.8 million inhabitants, 76% of whom live in the capital city of Bogotá (World Bank, 2016). Despite the fact that the country has a presidential system of government, it has a certain degree of government decentralization in its departments, municipalities, and districts. Bogotá is subdivided into 20 localities, one of which, Sumapaz, is rural. It is a socially and spatially segregated city and is divided into social strata zones that range from level one to level six, with level one being the poorest and level six the wealthiest, according to the income of the residents and the living conditions of the locality and homes. Approximately 50% of the population lives in stratas one and two (DANE-SDP, 2011), and the primary health care program that was implemented in these strata is the focus of this study.

In Colombia, PHC was implemented after the Declaration of Alma-Ata (Organización Panamericana de la Salud/Organización Mundial de la Salud [OPS/OMS], 1978) under the old National Health System and was organized along four main approaches (Hernández, Obregón, & Miranda, 2002; Vega, Hernández, & Mosquera, 2012). The first approach was one of "primitive" PHC (Testa, 1983) that sought to make low-complexity public health services provided by assistant health personnel accessible, particularly in rural areas. The second consisted of a selective approach to PHC (Cueto, 2006; Hernández et al., 2002), promoted by organizations such as UNICEF and the World Bank, and prioritized certain cost-effective interventions such as vaccination, oral rehydration, family planning, and nutritional supplements, among others, that helped reduce the rates of morbidity and mortality in prioritized populations. The third approach was one of traditional basic care based on medical attention provided by general practitioners and nurses (Hernández et al., 2002; Vega, 2009). Finally, the fourth approach was a combination of local health systems (OPS/OMS, 1989) and health promotion (Pan American Health Organization, 1986; Restrepo, 1992) advocated by the Pan American Health Organization and the Colombian government (Ministerio de Salud, 1989, 1990, 1992) in order to strengthen the local and national health systems within a context of state decentralization. Under the previous National Health System, a combination of selective and basic PHC had prevailed (Vega, 2009).

Thus, for instance, few health-care programs were developed that focused on PHC such as the one promoted at Alma-Ata, which, beyond treatment and prevention of diseases, included a significant component of community participation and intersectoral coordination under local health systems that were created with the decentralization of the health-sector starting at the end of the 1980s (Hernández et al., 2002). However, these experiences with PHC did not refocus the predominantly curative care model of a fragmented and segmented health system in which access to services was tied to employment or poverty, which is what happened with social security for state and private-sector workers, or with public assistance for those who did not have social security or any means to pay for private health-care services (Hernández et al., 2002; Vega, 2009).

Law 100 of 1993 reformed the health-care system and created the General System of Social Security in Health (*Sistema General de Seguridad Social en Salud*, SGSSS), which was based on a model of managed competition that opened up contributory and subsidized insurance and the provision of services to the market. Subsequently, with this law, individual services were separated from public or collective ones, and PHC disappeared from the national health policy (Vega, 2009). Under the SGSSS, insurance companies manage payments from individual enrolment, contract out the provision of health services, and enrol individuals into the two different insurance schemes: a contributory scheme for those who contribute a portion of their wages, and a subsidized scheme for those who receive a total or partial subsidy from the state, depending on their level of poverty. The two schemes had different benefits packages and capitation payment units for individual services according to the individual's ability to pay, with greater coverage for the contributory scheme and less for the subsidized one. Only in 2010 did the two schemes begin to equalize for certain age brackets, and they are now in the process of becoming completely identical, although the values of the capitation-payment units are still different. With regard to public health services, those covered under a different benefits package – the Collective Intervention Plan (*Plan de Intervenciones Colectivas*, PIC) – are the responsibility of the public health authorities at the local level (Colombia, 1993; Hernández, 2002).

Under the current fragmented, segmented, and market-oriented health-care system, the last two centre-left district governments in Bogotá decided to embrace PHC as one of their policies and strategies for improving access to health services as well as the quality of life and living standards of the population. As the result of this policy and within the context of a segmented and fragmented health system, a new approach to PHC emerged that combined selective, basic, and comprehensive[1] elements of PHC and that we named a hybrid and segmented primary health-care model in the city of Bogotá (Vega et al., 2012).

Starting in 2004, PHC began to be integrated into the network of first-level public hospitals operating under the District Health Secretariat (DHS, *Secretaría Distrital de Salud*) through the program *Salud a su Hogar*, subsequently renamed *Salud a su Casa* (SASC, Home Health). Two of the program's main objectives were to improve health outcomes and reduce health inequities. Therefore, the program was created with a focus on rights and included community participation, the empowerment of social groups, and intersectoral collaboration as key elements for its development (Vega, Acosta, Mosquera, & Restrepo, 2008; Secretaría Distrital de Salud de Bogotá, 2004).

The primary functional characteristics that were proposed to guide the implementation of the PHC strategy in Bogotá and improve the health status of the population were

- the organization of basic health-care teams (two full-time community health workers [CHWs], one full-time environmental technician, and a part-time nurse and physician for each microterritory) that attend to 1,200 families and are supported by a supplemental team in each locality (consisting of an oral hygienist, dentist, physiotherapist, psychologist, and environmental engineer);

---

1 We understand CPHC as an "approach aimed at reducing health inequities that is based on meaningful community participation, multidisciplinary teams, and action across sectors" (Labonté et al., 2008, p. 58).

- the division of the population into microterritories, prioritizing the poorest and most vulnerable (strata one and two) with access to the basic health-care teams;
- the coordination of the two types of interventions covered under the SGSSS (individual medical services provided by the Compulsory Health Plan (*Plan Obligatorio de Salud*, POS) for the insurer-run contributory and subsidized schemes, and the public health services covered under the PIC) under the claim of a family and community orientation of PHC (Vega, Acosta, & Mosquera, 2009);
- the integration of public health services into the daily lives of the population (in settings such as the family, neighbourhood, school, kindergarten, and workplace) as different gateways to PHC;
- the coordination of intersectoral responses aimed at satisfying the needs of the community; and
- the promotion of social participation, which recognizes the community as a legal entity and creates opportunities for social organization and mobilization to enable the community to demand its rights (Secretaría Distrital de Salud de Bogotá, 2008).

Various studies have been conducted in Colombia on the subject of PHC, with the majority of them concerned with analysing the evolution of national health policies and their implementation before the creation of the SGSSS. These studies have revealed that a CPHC approach had never been completely attempted (Apraez, 2010; Vega, 2009). The first studies and assessments of the PHC strategy developed in Bogotá in 2004, which included the first phase of this study, were conducted four years after the strategy's implementation (Centro de Estudios, 2008). These first studies analysed the functional management model designed at the district level. In the first phase of the study, a case study was conducted on the implementation of PHC in the locality of Suba, in which a performance analysis was conducted on the characteristics of PHC, following Macinko and Almeida's methodology (2007). The study revealed that the locality had performed poorly in terms of having a family- and community-based approach and access to the public network in charge of implementing PHC (Vega, Martínez, & Acosta 2009). This same study analysed the association of PHC implementation with certain child health indicators sensitive to PHC and its possible contribution to reducing inequalities. It was found that in the localities with high coverage, infant, postneonatal and under-5 mortality rates due to pneumonia declined and had a greater percentage reduction during the SASC implementation period compared with the rates in localities where the strategy had been less developed. Moreover, these rates tended to decline faster during this period among the localities with lower income per capita compared with the rates for the higher-income localities, suggesting an inequality in reduction related to the SASC implementation (Mosquera, Granados, & Vega, 2008).

Research Questions and Methods

In this context, six years after the implementation of PHC in Bogotá, the second phase of this study set out to analyse in greater detail PHC's functional management model designed at the district level. The study also assessed the model that was implemented by the public network of first-level services in certain localities. This was done by assessing PHC's impact on certain health outcomes and the extent to which PHC's values, principles, and characteristics had been met.

To this end, two types of analyses were conducted: a multicase study using qualitative methodology, and an analysis of PHC's impact on the health outcomes of the population. The multicase study was carried out in six localities in Bogotá (Bosa, Ciudad Bolívar, San Cristóbal, Tunjuelito, Usme, and Kennedy) where the PHC strategy had been implemented through the SASC program. Data collection for this study consisted of a documentary analysis, 18 semistructured interviews (with SASC senior managers and operational personnel at district and local level) and 14 workshops (with employees from different local institutions and with the community). Documents reviewed consisted of health policies, guidelines, and tools used at the district and local level to support the PHC implementation process; working documents and internal reports were also reviewed since those allowed identification of the characteristics of the management models that were implemented. The interviewees were selected using snowball sampling. Using *ATLAS.ti* software, the material was transcribed and codified. PHC principles, characteristics, and components, as well as other emerging categories, were used as the categories of analysis. Triangulation of data was used in each case and among the cases.

To determine PHC's impact on the population's health outcomes, an ecological analysis that included a comparison of two periods (one before and one after the implementation of the SASC program) was conducted. Based on this analysis, the associations and possible effects of the implementation of the program started in 2004 were assessed using different selected child health indicators and controlling for socioeconomic variables. This study used the city of Bogotá as the unit of analysis. Of the 20 localities into which Bogotá is administratively and politically divided, 16 were included as subunits of observation. Four localities were excluded because three did not have strata one and two populations (the target population of the strategy), and, for the other, the socioeconomic information necessary for the analysis was not available.

Three types of variables were used for analysis of the associations of health outcomes: 1) health outcome/status indicators (dependent variables); 2) PHC coverage intensity (PHCI, independent variable); and 3) socioeconomic or control variables (covariables). The following indicators were selected as health outcome/status variables and were identified in the literature review as sensitive to PHC implementation (Macinko, Almeida, & de Sá, 2007; Shi, Starfield, Kennedy, & Kawachi, 1999: infant mortality rate; under-5 mortality rate; infant mortality rate due to acute diarrheal disease and pneumonia; postneonatal mortality rate due to acute diarrheal disease and pneumonia; prevalence of acute malnutrition in children under 5 years of age; diphtheria, pertussis, and tetanus vaccination coverage in infants under 1 year of age; and prevalence of exclusive breastfeeding in infants under 6 months. The information sources for the above indicators were the DHS's and the Vital Statistics databases of the National Administrative Department of Statistics (*Departamento Administrativo Nacional de Estadísticas*), the Feeding and Nutrition Epidemiological Surveillance System (*Sistema de Vigilancia Epidemiológica de Alimentación y Nutrición*), and DHS's registry for rapid monitoring of immunization coverage.

The PHCI variables were characterization[2] coverage of the SASC program and the ratio of physicians, nurses, and CHWs per target population of the program. The ratio of physicians and nurses was calculated in full-time equivalents, and the estimates of the program's target population (strata one and two) were calculated using past figures from the 2002, 2009, and 2010 stratification data from the Secretariat of District Planning and census data from 2005. The following socioeconomic

---

2 Characterization is the first activity carried out by a SASC basic health-care team to enrol families in the program and consists of a household survey that is applied to identify the structure and dynamics of the family and its socioeconomic and health status. This information is then used to design an action plan and a family follow-up plan for the team.

indicators were used as control variables: the Quality of Life Index (QLI),[3] the population living under the poverty line, the percentage of households with high economic dependence, the percentage of the population with reduced food consumption due to lack of money, sewerage coverage, contributory insurance coverage, and subsidized insurance coverage. These indicators were taken from the District Quality of Life surveys of 2003 and 2007, publicly available sources of the National Administrative Department of Statistics.

In order to conduct the analysis, the PHCI was first created through a statistical process known as a principal component analysis. The PHCI was standardized and assigned values on a scale of 0–100; this variable summarizes the behaviour of the four original variables of coverage over time. Using the behaviour of the PHCI, the localities were classified into two groups for the quasi-experimental multivariate analysis: one group showed a consistent increase in the PHCI (high coverage) and the other group showed a declining or stagnant PHCI behaviour (low coverage) during the period studied.

To assess the relationship between SASC coverage according to high- or low-coverage groups and the different health outcomes, correlation analyses were conducted prior to a principal component analysis of the different variables and the PHCI in each of the groups. This process identified the correlation structure of the variables to be included in the multivariate regression models. The health and socioeconomic variables according to group were included in the models, and the years 2003 (one year prior to the implementation of the SASC program) and 2007 (three years after the implementation of the program) were used as cut-off points in the analysis, due to the availability of information on the covariables in the Quality of Life survey. The analyses were conducted using Poisson regressions, creating a separate model for each year through which the incidence rates attributable to PHC were calculated and adjusted for the socioeconomic variables. Lastly, to precisely

---

3 The QLI combines 12 variables measuring material well-being, organized into four categories: 1) education and human capital: the education attained by the head of household; average education of the members 12 years of age or older; youth between 12 and 18 years of age who attend secondary school or university; children between 5 and 11 years of age who attend school; 2) housing quality: materials of walls and floors; 3) access and quality of services: sanitation, water supply, kitchen appliances, waste collection; and 4) household size and composition: children 6 years of age or younger in the home; number of people per room.

measure the changes in the health outcomes among the groups and years, a panel Poisson regression model was used in which each of the years in the analysis was included as a panel and the difference among the groups was compared. The analyses were conducted using the *Stata 11 Data Analysis and Statistical Software* package. A more detailed explanation can be found in Mosquera et al. (2012).

Results and Analysis

PHC implementation in Bogotá was assessed based on the cases of the six first-level hospitals in the public network. The district government had set out to refocus the provision of health-care services in the city under the PHC strategy and the Quality of Life and Health Promotion Strategy (*Estrategia Promocional de Calidad de Vida y Salud*) (D'Elia, 2002; Secretaría de Salud de Bogotá, 2008) in order to improve access to health services and health equity. Despite the city's efforts, the study showed limited progress on that front.

Initially, the DHS began by organizing a working task force at the undersecretariat level, with the participation of different departments, to guide health policy, implement the CPHC model, and involve all SGSSS actors. However, from the beginning, Law 100 of 1993 limited the scope of the proposed PHC model. Law 100 had brought about a neoliberal reform of the health sector in Colombia and subsequently prevented the DHS from obligating the Health-Promoting Enterprises (*Empresas Promotoras de Salud*, EPSs) to fund certain key components of the PHC strategy. The EPSs, including those that participated in the subsidized scheme and contracted locally by DHS, were not obligated to provide funds for the provision of individual health services rendered through basic health-care teams. Likewise, the EPSs were not legally bound to comply with certain elements of the PHC model related to access to services, coordination, and continuity and comprehensiveness of care, among others. Therefore, it was neither possible to integrate POS services (i.e., services foreseen in the Compulsory Health Plan) with those of the PIC (Collective Intervention Plan), nor to ensure that the basic health-care teams were truly multidisciplinary (Vega, Acosta, Mosquera, & Restrepo, 2009).

Thus, the PHC strategy was implemented primarily under the SASC program and within the functional organization of the PIC teams in different areas of daily life (family, community, school, and work), with a family-centred approach. These services, delivered at the family and community level, are provided by CHWs (later renamed "health managers") whose background as nursing assistants allow them to carry out the characterization of the families and their surroundings using standardized forms. Using this information, a plan is designed with the family that induces demand for individual services not provided by the basic health-care teams. The health information, education, and communication intervention then takes place during the initial home visit, and if the family is prioritized, more frequent follow-ups are made. The health managers also lead activities to promote community participation and intersectoral health efforts with community groups and leaders to search for solutions to health needs and to improve quality of life. The health managers work under the supervision of the physician and nurse, who accompany them on some of their activities on the ground (Secretaría de Salud Dirección de Salud Pública, 2010a). However, depending on the needs of the assigned population, the manager does not have health-care duties as part of the basic health-care team.

Moreover, the work of the health managers is strengthened by other professionals from a supplemental team who work in each locality and attend to problems relating to mental health, nutrition, oral health, community-based rehabilitation, and environmental sanitation, and by other PIC teams that work in schools, workplaces, and with community groups and organizations. The basic health-care teams and the supplemental teams coordinated with the PIC teams until 2011 by channelling or directing families to the services provided by the PIC teams. In some cases, the supplementary teams were also assigned to a group of several microterritories so that they established ties with the population (Secretaría de Salud Dirección de Salud Pública, 2010a).

In some of the public hospitals, the physicians and nurses on the basic health-care teams were organized to provide services at the intramural as well as extramural level to guarantee closer ties with the population. However, the intention that each microterritory have a complete team of professionals was never fulfilled because hospitals claimed they did not have the financial resources necessary to incorporate the basic-care team into their services. This happened because the EPSs, in accordance with national law, are obligated to contract out only 60% of POS spending on health services to public hospitals and can provide the remainder of the services through their own network or other private institutions.

The State Social Enterprises (*Empresas Sociales del Estado*) made significant efforts to develop or improve PHC features with the support of the district government on a number of fronts, such as improved access through the creation of new health centres and mobile care units; a diversified offering of outpatient services in a greater number of care centres; improved organizational aspects of care (such as extended service hours and improved systems for making appointments, including on the ground by the health managers of the basic-care teams and even online); provision of transportation to prioritized groups to facilitate access within the different points of care of a single State Social Enterprise and to different levels of care within the network of services; and with a policy of free health care, elimination of sliding scale fees, and copayments for prioritized groups that others must pay in other parts of the country. Despite these advances, in the performance evaluation undertaken in another section of this study that is not described in this chapter, the State Social Enterprises were given low scores by users in the categories of "access" and "family- and community-centred approaches."

Regarding the continuity of care, mechanisms were created that helped organize the work of the basic health-care teams in following up with families who did not attend health-promotion or prevention programs and in monitoring cases of families identified during the delivery of services. Although the characterization and monitoring records filled out by the basic health-care teams are systematized in an online database known as *APS en línea* (PHC online), information is not reviewed by professionals during intramural care, given that, on the one hand, not all institutions use systematized medical-history registries, and, on the other hand, in the institutions that have it at the district level, *APS en línea* is not linked to its registries or to its search functions. The continuity of care at other levels of care is maintained under a single reference and counter-reference system for emergency care and hospitalization, but there are difficulties in managing the flow of information, particularly with counter-references. This system does not guarantee complete coordination and management, from the first level of access to specialized outpatient services at other levels of care, given that those aspects depend on an EPS's contracts with the local enterprise affiliated with the population and, for certain services, on the EPS's previous authorization of the service.

Community participation in health was promoted by basic health-care teams through the formation of management centres in each microterritory, in which community plans were defined through a process of joint identification of health needs. Although some interesting intersectoral responses were developed at the start of the PHC implementation, in general, the response of the health sector to the plans resulting from this process was limited to hospitals' capacity to provide services, including those of the PIC. The problem lay in the fact that the implementation plans were not clearly anticipated in the design or in the allocation of budget resources and were confined to whatever the health sector could advocate for with other sectors and district institutions. Moreover, another difficulty was that, in some microterritories, the management centres served as merely another space that other institutions promoted for community participation. Because of this, in certain localities, these spaces were exclusively functional and used to carry out health information, education, and communication interventions at the community level. Furthermore, in each locality, intersectoral management became the responsibility of PIC teams that were different from the PHC teams and were dedicated solely to this task. Although the PIC teams did not participate in the management centres, by identifying management needs in different areas, they fulfilled advocacy roles in each of the different settings of intersectoral coordination and community participation at the local and microterritorial level. The management centres, although they allowed the different institutions to get closer to the communities in order to identify their needs and prioritize them, also came up short when it was time to respond to those same needs.

During its six years of implementation, the SASC program covered 1,497,750 people in the lowest socioeconomic strata in the city, corresponding to 41% of the target population (Secretaría de Salud Dirección de Salud Pública, 2010b). Between 2004 and 2007, the SASC program showed a pronounced increase in PHCI in the study, although it was followed by a period of lesser growth between 2007 and 2009 (Figure 5.1), with differential behaviour among the localities. This is explained by the fact that some localities had greater priority in the allocation of resources that was not always linked to the number of people to be covered, but rather to criteria such as the way in which the resources were used and, in some cases, to political criteria.

Thus, the analysis identified two groups of localities: the first had a sustained trend towards growth in program coverage, which included 10 of the 16 localities in the study, and the second showed stagnation or a decline in program coverage, which included the remaining six localities (Figures 5.2 and 5.3).

In the analysis of the socioeconomic and health-status characteristics of the localities included in the study between 2003 and 2007, the period when the program was implemented, an increase in the QLI was noted, as well as a slight increase in sewerage coverage and a significant decline

Figure 5.1 Behavioural trend of PHC program coverage in Bogotá, 2004–9

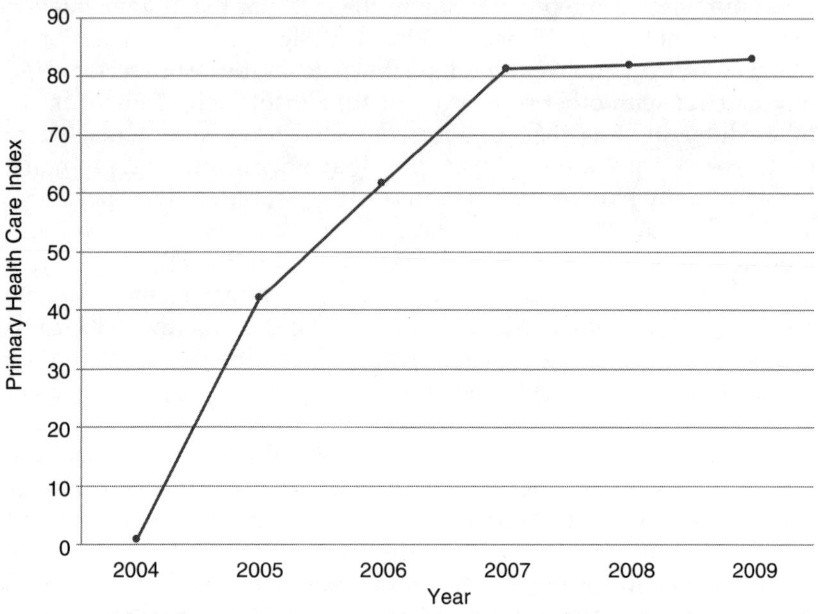

Figure 5.2 Behaviour of PHC program coverage in group 1 localities

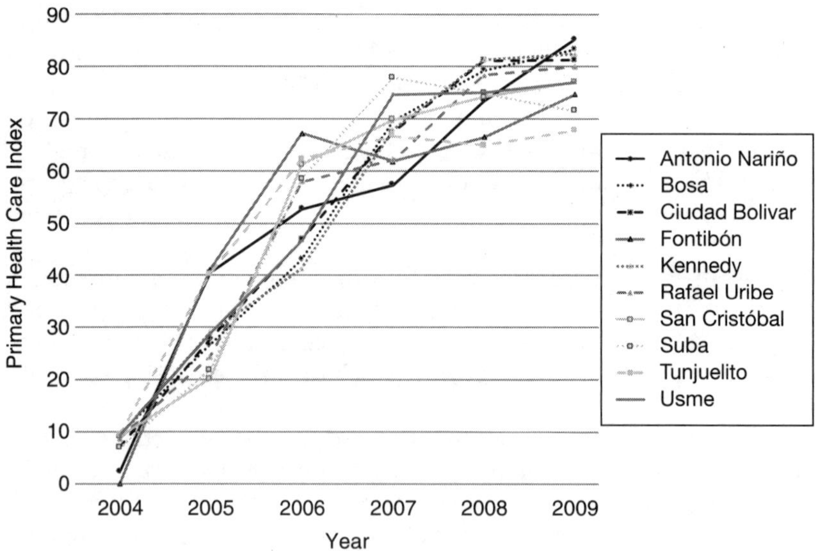

Figure 5.3 Behaviour of PHC program coverage in group 2 localities

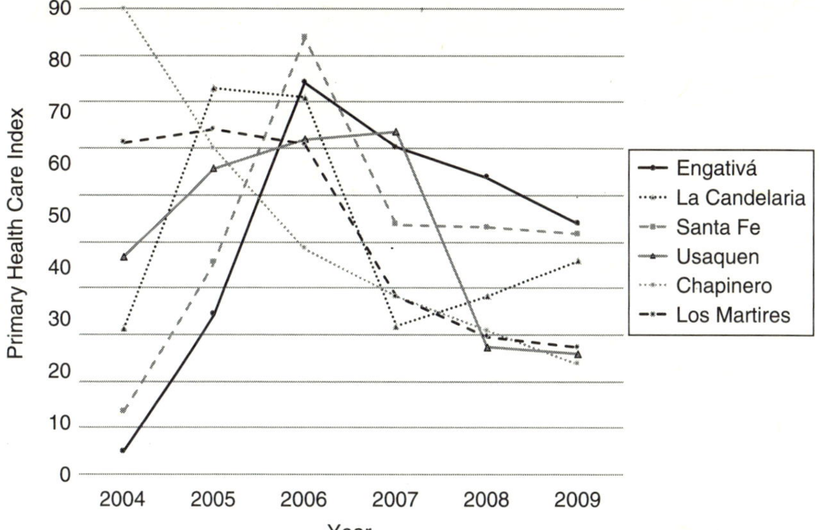

in the contributory scheme's enrolment percentage. Moreover, a general improvement in health outcomes was identified, with slight reductions in the under-5 mortality rate, infant mortality, and mortality due to acute diarrheal disease. The decline between the two periods was greater in the case of death due to pneumonia, at 75%, and the prevalence of acute malnutrition decreased 25% from the first period. Exclusive breastfeeding showed a slight increase in prevalence, and diphtheria, pertussis, and tetanus vaccination coverage increased 25% from the first period.

The analysis of the PHC program's contribution to health outcomes using multivariate regression models showed that there was a statistically significant reduction in risk probability between 2003 and 2007 in the group of localities with greater coverage intensity in indicators such as under-5 mortality (13.8%), infant mortality due to pneumonia (37.5%), acute malnutrition in children under-5 (5.5%), and diphtheria, pertussis, and tetanus vaccination coverage (4.9%). Although there was a decline in infant mortality and an increase in the prevalence of breastfeeding, they were not statistically significant. In the case of mortality due to acute diarrheal disease, an increase was found, but was not statistically significant (Table 5.1).

Table 5.1 Poisson models, 2003 and 2007, and relative difference model, 2007/2003

Indicators	2003			2007			Relative difference 2007/2003		
	RR*	[95% conf. interval]		RR	[95% conf. interval]		RR	[95% conf. interval]	
Under-5 mortality rate									
Group	0.915	0.773	1.084	0.879	0.765	1.011	0.862	0.780	0.953
QLI	1.004	0.948	1.062	1.024	0.957	1.096	0.968	0.946	0.990
Scheme membership	0.987	0.974	1.001	0.986	0.972	1.001	0.998	0.993	1.003
Sewerage coverage	1.003	0.970	1.036	1.010	0.937	1.089	1.000	0.972	1.029
Infant mortality									
Group	1.067	0.892	1.277	0.951	0.819	1.104	0.968	0.870	1.078
QLI	0.969	0.912	1.029	1.014	0.945	1.087	0.947	0.925	0.970
Scheme membership	0.997	0.983	1.012	0.990	0.974	1.005	1.003	0.998	1.009
Sewerage coverage	1.037	1.001	1.074	1.003	0.925	1.086	1.026	0.995	1.057
Infant mortality due to acute diarrheal disease									
Group	1.367	0.272	6.866	2.052	0.290	14.50	1.078	0.353	3.294
QLI	1.936	1.302	2.877	1.704	0.744	3.900	1.750	1.297	2.360
Scheme membership	0.860	0.788	0.939	0.885	0.743	1.056	0.871	0.813	0.933
Sewerage coverage	1.127	0.807	1.575	0.599	0.303	1.183	0.940	0.726	1.210
Infant mortality due to pneumonia									
Group	0.957	0.474	1.932	0.629	0.314	1.262	0.625	0.400	0.976
QLI	1.025	0.825	1.275	0.909	0.653	1.264	0.849	0.770	0.936
Scheme membership	0.972	0.924	1.023	1.011	0.940	1.088	1.011	0.990	1.033
Sewerage coverage	1.137	0.987	1.309	0.664	0.484	0.912	1.006	0.893	1.133
Acute malnutrition									
Group	0.866	0.795	0.944	0.723	0.662	0.790	0.945	0.894	1.000
QLI	0.865	0.843	0.888	0.824	0.799	0.849	0.907	0.890	0.925
Scheme membership	1.029	1.023	1.035	1.030	1.023	1.036	1.011	1.007	1.015
Sewerage coverage	0.910	0.893	0.928	1.155	1.113	1.199	1.033	1.017	1.048

Indicators	2003			2007			Relative difference 2007/2003		
	RR*	[95% conf. interval]		RR	[95% conf. interval]		RR	[95% conf. interval]	
Breastfeeding									
Group	0.954	0.903	1.007	0.961	0.921	1.003	0.968	0.935	1.004
QLI	0.994	0.977	1.011	0.977	0.960	0.994	0.987	0.974	1.002
Scheme membership	0.996	0.992	1.000	1.004	1.001	1.008	1.001	0.997	1.004
Sewerage coverage	0.982	0.971	0.994	1.019	0.994	1.044	0.992	0.981	1.002
Diphtheria, pertussis, and tetanus vaccination									
Group	0.879	0.859	0.900	1.051	1.030	1.072	1.049	1.034	1.063
QLI	0.872	0.865	0.879	0.867	0.860	0.874	1.009	1.003	1.015
Scheme membership	1.029	1.027	1.031	1.029	1.027	1.031	0.998	0.997	0.999
Sewerage coverage	0.948	0.944	0.953	0.991	0.980	1.000	1.001	0.997	1.005

RR: Risk ratio

Source: Table from Mosquera, P.A., Hernández, J., Vega, R., Martínez, J., Labonté, R., Sanders, D., & San Sebastián, M. (2012, Aug 16). Primary health care contribution to improve health outcomes in Bogota-Colombia: A longitudinal ecological analysis. *BMC Family Practice*, 13(1), 84.

Discussion and Conclusions

The cases studied show that despite the fact that the district health policy has sought to develop a CPHC approach, in practice a hybrid PHC model has been implemented: comprehensive in certain components such as community participation and intersectoral collaboration, selective in the sense of cost-effective and vertical interventions under the PIC and the POS, and traditional primary care provided at the first level of medical care.

Despite the fact that the PHC strategy designed in Bogotá sought to guarantee the right to health and refocus the provision of health services at the district level, these goals have been undermined due to the focus on the program of community health managers. The role of these managers is to induce demand for social and medical services and promote community participation in order to identify needs, albeit with serious limitations on making decisions and on the ability to act on them.

The segmented and hybrid model that was developed seems to be the result of the permanent tension between contextual factors, the content of social and health policies, and the process of PHC implementation at different levels, which all reflect the competing interests of the actors involved. The national health policy's neoliberal approach, based on social risk management, managed health care, the deterritorialization of services, the SGSSS's focus on profitability, and the EPSs' discretionary provision of services and the lack of importance given by it to PHC in the SGSSS have imposed structural limitations on the ability to develop a CPHC approach. Added to these health-policy limitations are the limitations of social policy, such as deregulation of the labour market, which causes instability in the personnel that manage the strategy's operations; the focus on national social risk management and welfare services, which conflicts with the focus on social rights at the district level; and shortcomings in the professional and technical training of personnel, which hinder the adoption of the values and principles of CPHC during its implementation, especially in terms of its family- and community-centred approach.

While the PHC strategy developed in Bogotá has been a priority for the last two district governments and has been developed in this adverse climate, certain shortcomings have also been detected in the DHS's own implementation process, such as the complexity and conceptual confusion in relation to the Quality of Life and Health Promotion Strategy (the other guiding strategy for the implementation of the district health policy); the fragmentation of care due to social determinants, such as health care in microterritories; the rigidity of health-service guidelines, which focus on vertical planning; the gaps in health-service coordination between the POS and the PIC; the lack of sufficient mechanisms to reduce turnover of personnel; the lack of continuity in the training of personnel; and shortcomings in building effective community participation and developing intersectoral collaboration.

The conclusions of this study show that the tensions between the context and the content of social and health policies at the national and district level have resulted in hybrid PHC at the locality level. Thus, the State Social Enterprises have attempted to refocus their care models, which have been in a permanent state of dilemma over offering comprehensive care and ensuring their survival in the marketplace.

Moreover, given that the insurance model of the Colombian healthcare system divides health into public goods (public health) and private goods (individual medical care), the public resources that fund public health services are managed by the State Social Enterprises, and the public resources that fund individual medical care for those enrolled in the two insurance system schemes (subsidized and contributory) are managed by insurance companies (EPSs). The EPSs are usually private and contract out individual health services to public or private healthcare providers under a plan of apparent market competition, which segments and fragments care and prevents the territorialization, coordination, and integration of individual and public care.

These factors explain why the PHC model that was ultimately implemented in Bogotá has ended up being comprised only of teams of health promoters (generally nursing assistants) coordinated and supervised by professional medical and nursing personnel, despite the model's formulation as CPHC centred on the family and community and involving the creation of interdisciplinary basic health-care teams comprising physicians, nurses, health promoters (paid CHWs), and other support personnel. The funding of the basic health-care teams' personnel could be guaranteed by the DHS only for the health promoters, who, in the context of the division of health into public goods (public health) and private goods (individual medical care), are classified as public-health personnel who can be funded by public resources managed directly by the DHS. In accordance with statutory standards, the EPSs are responsible for funding the basic health-care teams' medical and nursing personnel to carry out health services. However, the EPSs never agreed to incorporate private resources with DHS resources to fund these medical personnel and thereby guarantee the formation of truly interdisciplinary basic health-care teams. Therefore, in practice, the resulting PHC model that was implemented was one of health promoters (managers).

The results of this model indicate that the work of health promoters can be effective in improving the health of the target population, despite the health-care system's segmentation and fragmentation. This was suggested by the study's findings in child health indicators, even though these were for the general population and not just the target population. These findings concur with those of other studies that have found PHC to have an effect on the reduction of infant mortality in different contexts (Macinko, Marinho de Souza, Guanais, & da Silva Simões, 2007; Perry, Shanklin, & Schroeder, 2003; Bixby, 2004).

PHC models comprising only health promoters have proven to be effective in other contexts, as indicated by the *Lancet* study (Haines et al., 2007), by Gogia & Sachdev (2010), and in several countries in Latin America (although not necessarily in big cities), including Brazil (Svitone, Garfield, Vasconcelos, & Craveiro, 2000). Sometime after the creation of the Community Health Workers program, the Brazilian Ministry of Health, seeking to refocus basic PHC, integrated this program with the Family Health Program, forming multidisciplinary basic health teams comprising a physician, a nurse, and four health promoters who worked at a basic health-care centre and were assigned to approximately 600 to 1,000 families (Escorel, Giovanella, Mendonça, & Senna, 2007; de Sousa & Hamann, 2009).

A PHC strategy based on the work of CHWs that is adequately formulated and implemented in terms of efficacy in health care, promotion, prevention, community participation, and intersectoral collaboration can be a model to keep in mind in the case of general PHC implementation in Colombia's market-oriented health insurance system. Nevertheless, a fully comprehensive approach, with interdisciplinary basic health-care teams assigned to microterritories, would be possible only under a new health-care system that is able to overcome the commercialization of health and its accompanying problems of segmentation and fragmentation.

REFERENCES

Apraez, G. (2010). Evaluación de la atención primaria de la salud en Colombia como política de salud 1939 - 2008. Doctoral Thesis in Public Health. Universidad Nacional de Colombia. Retrieved from http://www.bdigital .unal.edu.co/2725/

Bixby, L.R. (2004, Feb). Evaluación del impacto de la reforma del sector de la salud en Costa Rica mediante un estudio cuasiexperimental. *Pan American Journal of Public Health, 15*(2), 94–103. http://dx.doi.org/10.1590/S1020 -49892004000200004 Medline:15030654

Centro de Estudios e Investigación en Salud Fundación Santa Fe de Bogotá. Universidad de la Sabana. (2008). Consultancy's research brief assessing the primary health care strategy adopted in Bogotá, D.C., under the framework of the General System of Social Security in Health and in compliance with the Development Plan 2004–2008. "Bogotá sin Indiferencia, un compromiso social contra la pobreza y la exclusión social". (Unpublished document).

Colombia. Congreso de la República. (1993). Ley 100 de 1993 "Por la cual se crea el Sistema General de Seguridad Social."

Cueto, M. (2006). Los orígenes de la Atención Primaria de Salud y la Atención Primaria Selectiva de Salud. In Marcos Cueto and Víctor Zamora Mesía (Eds.), *Historia, salud y globalización* (pp. 27–58). Lima: IEP, UPCH.

DANE–SDP. (2011). *Departamento Nacional de Estadísticas, Secretaría Distrital de Planeación*. Encuesta Multipropósito para Bogotá.

D'Elia, Y., Negri, A., & Castañeda, M. (2002). Documento de Trabajo. Estrategia de Promoción de la Calidad de Vida. La construcción de políticas públicas por la calidad de vida desde una perspectiva de derecho y equidad. GTZ Agencia de Cooperación Alemana y Ministerio de salud y Desarrollo social de la República Bolivariana de Venezuela.

de Sousa, M.F., & Hamann, E.M. (2009, Oct). Programa Saúde da Família no Brasil: uma agenda incompleta? *Ciencia & Saude Coletiva, 14*(Suppl 1), 1325–35. http://dx.doi.org/10.1590/S1413-81232009000800002 Medline:19750338

Escorel, S., Giovanella, L., Mendonça, M.H.M., & Senna, M.C.M. (2007). O Programa de Saúde da Família e a construção de um novo modelo para a atenção básica no Brasil. *Revista Panamericana de Salud Pública, 21*(2), 164–76. http://dx.doi.org/10.1590/S1020-49892007000200011

Gogia, S., & Sachdev, H. (2010). Visitas domiciliarias por parte de personal sanitario comunitario para prevenir la mortalidad neonatal en los países en desarrollo: revisión sistemática. *Bulletin of the World Health Organization, 88*(9), 658–66. http://dx.doi.org/10.2471/BLT.09.069369 Medline:20865070

Haines, A., Sanders, D., Lehmann, U., Rowe, A.K., Lawn, J.E., Jan, S., …, & Bhutta, Z. (2007, Jun 23). Achieving child survival goals: Potential contribution of community health workers. *Lancet, 369*(9579), 2121–31. http:// dx.doi.org/10.1016/S0140-6736(07)60325-0 Medline:17586307

Hernández, M. (2002, Jul–Aug). Reforma sanitaria, equidad y derecho a la salud en Colombia. *Cadernos de Saúde Pública, 18*(4), 991–1001. http:// dx.doi.org/10.1590/S0102-311X2002000400007 Medline:12118306

Hernández, M., Obregón, D., & Miranda, N. (2002). *La Organización Panamericana de la Salud y el Estado colombiano: Cien años de historia 1902–2002*. Bogotá, D.C., Editorial Carrera 7.

Labonté, R., Sanders, D., Baum, F., Schaay, N., Packer, C., Laplante, D., … Pooyak, S. (2008). Implementation, effectiveness and political context of comprehensive primary health care: Preliminary findings of a global literature review. *Australian Journal of Primary Health*, *14*(3), 58–67. http://dx.doi.org/10.1071/PY08037

Macinko, J., Almeida, C., & de Sá, P.K. (2007, May). A rapid assessment methodology for the evaluation of primary care organization and performance in Brazil. *Health Policy and Planning*, *22*(3), 167–77. http://dx.doi.org/10.1093/heapol/czm008 Medline:17400576

Macinko, J., Marinho de Souza, M.F., Guanais, F.C., & da Silva Simões, C.C. (2007, Nov). Going to scale with community-based primary care: An analysis of the family health program and infant mortality in Brazil, 1999–2004. *Social Science & Medicine*, *65*(10), 2070–80. http://dx.doi.org/10.1016/j.socscimed.2007.06.028 Medline:17689847

Ministerio de Salud. (1989). *Memoria al Congreso 1988–1989*. Bogotá, Colombia: Imprenta Nacional.

Ministerio de Salud. (1990). *Reorganización del Sistema Nacional de Salud. Una respuesta al cambio social. Memoria analítica de la Ley 10 de 1990* (2 vols.) Bogotá: ACOMSAP.

Ministerio de Salud. (1992). *Salud para Todos. Memorias 1991–1992*. Santa Fe de Bogotá.

Mosquera, P., Granados, G., & Vega, R. (2008). La estrategia de atención primaria en salud (APS) para Bogotá y su relación con la disminución de inequidades en los resultados en salud. *Rev Gerenc. Polit. Salud*, *7*(14), 88–109.

Mosquera, P.A., Hernández, J., Vega, R., Martínez, J., Labonté, R., Sanders, D., & San Sebastián, M. (2012, Aug 16). Primary health care contribution to improve health outcomes in Bogota-Colombia: A longitudinal ecological analysis. *BMC Family Practice*, *13*(1), 84. http://dx.doi.org/10.1186/1471-2296-13-84 Medline:22898368

Organización Panamericana de la Salud/Organización Mundial de la Salud. (1978). Declaración de ALMA-ATA. Conferencia Internacional sobre Atención Primaria de Salud, Alma-Ata, URSS, 6–12 de Septiembre de 1978 (Centro de Prensa).

Organización Panamericana de la Salud/Organización Mundial de la Salud (1989). Resolución XV: Desarrollo y fortalecimiento de los sistemas locales de salud en la transformación de los sistemas nacionales de salud, aprobada por la XXXIII Reunión del Consejo Directivo de la OPS. En: Desarrollo y fortalecimiento de los sistemas locales de salud. Washington.

Panamerican Health Organization [PAHO] (1986). Carta de Ottawa para la promoción de la salud. Retrieved from http://www1.paho.org/spanish /HPP/OttawaCharterSp.pdf.

Perry, H.B., Shanklin, D.S., & Schroeder, D.G. (2003, Dec). Impact of a community-based comprehensive primary healthcare programme on infant and child mortality in Bolivia. *Journal of Health, Population, and Nutrition*, *21*(4), 383–95. Medline:15038594

Restrepo, H. (1992). Las políticas de promoción de la salud en la Organización Panamericana de la Salud. In: Colombia-MS/OPS. Conferencia Internacional de Promoción de la Salud. Santa fé de Bogotá, November 1992.

Secretaría Distrital de Salud de Bogotá. (2004). Salud a su Hogar: Un modelo de Atención Primaria en Salud para garantizar el derecho a la salud en Bogotá (Unpublished document).

Secretaría Distrital de Salud de Bogotá. (2008). Plan de Salud del Distrito Capital 2008–2012. (Unpublished document).

Secretaría Distrital de Salud Dirección de Salud Pública (2010a). Lineamientos del ámbito familiar, Programa Salud a su Casa. (Unpublished working paper).

Secretaría Distrital de Salud Dirección de Salud Pública. (2010b). Coberturas programa Salud a su Casa.

Shi, L., Starfield, B., Kennedy, B., & Kawachi, I. (1999, Apr). Income inequality, primary care, and health indicators. *Journal of Family Practice*, *48*(4), 275–84. Medline:10229252

Svitone, E.C., Garfield, R., Vasconcelos, M.I., & Craveiro, V.A. (2000). Primary health care lessons from the northeast of Brazil: The Agentes de Saúde Program. *Revista Panamericana de Salud Pública*, *7*(5): 293–302. https:// dx.doi.org/10.1590/S1020-49892000000500002

Testa, M. (1983). Atención ¿Primaria o Primitiva? de Salud. Retrieved from http://www.saludcolectiva-unr.com.ar/docs/SC-176.pdf.

Vega, R.R., Acosta, N., Mosquera, P., & Restrepo, O. (2008). La política de salud en Bogotá, 2004–2008. Análisis de la experiencia de atención primaria integral de salud. *Medicine and Society*, *3*(2), 126–44.

Vega, R.R. (2009). Los orígenes y desarrollos de la APS en Colombia. In R.Vega Romero, N. Acosta, P. Mosquera,, & O. Restrepo (Eds.), *Atención primaria de salud: Estrategia para la transformación del sistema de salud y el logro de la equidad en salud* (pp. 53–82). Bogotá, D.C.: Unión Gráfica.

Vega, R.R., Acosta, N., & Mosquera, P. (2009). Modelo conceptual y filosófico de la APIS en Bogotá. In R. Vega Romero, N. Acosta, P. Mosquera, & O.

Restrepo (Eds.) *Atención primaria de salud: Estrategia para la transformación del sistema de salud y el logro de la equidad en salud* (pp. 82–102). Bogotá, D.C.: Unión Gráfica.

Vega, R.R., Acosta, N., Mosquera, P., & Restrepo, O. (2009). *Atención primaria de salud: Estrategia para la transformación del sistema de salud y el logro de la equidad en salud*. Bogotá, D.C.: Unión Gráfica.

Vega, R.R., Martínez, J., & Acosta, N. (2009). Evaluación rápida del desempeño de la red pública de servicios de salud de Suba en el logro de los atributos de la Atención Primaria de Salud – APS. *Revista Gerencia y Políticas de Salud, 8*(16), 165–90.

Vega, R.R., Hernández, J., & Mosquera, P. (2012). Una explicación desde el contexto y contenido de las políticas de salud al modelo híbrido y segmentado de atención primaria en salud en Bogotá. *Saúde em Debate, 36*(94), 392–401. http://dx.doi.org/10.1590/S0103-11042012000300011

World Bank (2016). Profile of Colombia. Retrieved from http://data.worldbank.org/country/colombia

SECTION TWO

Community Engagement

There is a large body of health-promotion literature on community empowerment and capacity building that distils to improving the knowledge, analytical skills, local leadership, internal and external resource mobilization, and organizing abilities of disadvantaged communities. The narrative literature review that began this project found that health-system reforms consistent with comprehensive primary health care (CPHC) (in contrast to "selective" primary health care that focuses on specific diseases or interventions) were more likely when there was strong community participation that continued to hold governments accountable. The evidence-informed argument this literature presents is that improvement in empowerment reduces vulnerabilities to disease threats by increasing both material and immaterial (psychosocial) resources for health.

Not all community engagement starts from scratch. Several of our country studies noted the existence of formal participation structures within the CPHC systems they were researching. Not all of these were effective, however, and only when they were functioning well were there evident pay-offs in health outcomes or health-centre use.

The *Revitalizing Health for All* (*RHFA*) team in **South Africa** examined how community health worker (CHW) programs under different institutional environments affected community participation and intersectoral actions for health. Not only was the study interested in how CHW efforts promoted these two components of CPHC, but also how community dynamics interacted with CHWs in doing so. The research team found that although there are formal local-government participation structures (such as ward committees), these structures often function poorly. As a result, two of the communities studied had no mechanism by which members could voice their health needs and concerns. Typically, as a result, community needs were not addressed. The lack of functioning participatory structures, in turn, weakened the perceived legitimacy of CHWs in their community work. In contrast, a third case study in the Eastern Cape site demonstrated more responsiveness to community needs largely as a result of a well-established and supported process that had not explicitly commenced around health issues but which had carefully engaged communities over a relatively long period. The relatively stable nature of the Eastern Cape community, in contrast to the more fluid population flows in the other two cases, led to more and stronger social-network bonds, improving the social cohesion and social capital of residents. These qualities were associated with effective community participation and some indicative efforts at intersectoral actions for health. Rolling out CPHC reforms in South Africa, then, requires not only adept CHWs and good participatory mechanisms; it must also account for constraining community factors that inhibit participation, and give particular emphasis to the importance of supporting the development of social networks in areas where they may be weak.

The research team in **Kenya** similarly found a strong relationship between increased community empowerment (capacities) and reduced health vulnerabilities. Specifically, community engagement ensured that the needs of disadvantaged groups were heard and incorporated at the planning level through specific structures, including a complaints board in local villages, a position for more senior (and paid) community health extension workers on the health/hospital management boards, and the requirement for public feedback on how the health system has responded to the concerns raised by community members. The team's evaluation of the country's relatively new Community Strategy Approach (CSA), which embodies most of the same principles of CPHC, had demonstrable impacts not only on health-care delivery but also on the social determinants of health. The team undertook two tasks at the same time: a comparison of how well the CSA was being implemented by three different groups (including the team's own Great Lakes University of Kisumu's Tropical Institute of Community Health and Development); and a comparison between sites selected for implementation and those that were "nonintervention." In all districts studied, the implementation (intervention) sites performed better on most health-system output measures than the nonintervention (control) sites. Significantly, sites with the more comprehensive form of, and longer exposure to, the CSA outperformed other sites on most, although not all, health measures. Key elements of CPHC that were part of the CSA implementation (notably the establishment of governance and management structures at the subcommunity level via community health committees populated by stakeholders from a variety of areas, with human resources allocated to support these committees) had the strongest correlations with two key outcomes: antenatal care (ANC) visits and use of insecticide-treated nets. A subsequent study undertaken the following year using similar methods, but with a much smaller sample, was able to administer pre- and post-intervention surveys and to compare results between CSA-implementing intervention sites and non-intervention controls. Compared with control sites, this study found statistically significant improvements in a number of health indicators (for health facility delivery, ANC, water treatment, and insecticide-treated net use) for the rural implementation sites. Findings for the peri-urban and nomadic implementation sites were more mixed, but still indicative of the positive role the CSA can play in the renewal of a comprehensive PHC system in Kenya.

This approach is similar to that used in the remote First Nations Island Lake community of Garden Hill in **Canada**, explored by the Canadian Aboriginal research team.[1] This study was designed to identify the health beliefs and values of the residents of the Island Lake First Nations communities in order to create a governance model for a CPHC system that best reflects their identified values. The Garden Hill focus groups began by generating an extensive list of determinants of their health, which included food, physical activity, hygiene, mental health, community participation, equity, and accessibility. Based on the themes developed, the community agreed on a definition that best represented their understanding of health:

> Health is living in a community where basic necessities are affordable and the community is set up and safe so that people can be active, eat healthy, and keep themselves and their community clean. Traditional ways are respected and supported, and the roles of parents and families are strengthened. The community is independent and has strong leadership that engages community members and advocates for better social and environmental conditions, and safe and accessible health care.

---

1 The team was unable to contribute a chapter to this book, but did provide a summary of their study that we draw upon here.

As in other Aboriginal communities in Canadian provinces, and similar to the experiences captured in Chapter 3's account of the Australian Ingkintja program, a key element of health for focus group participants was others' recognition of and respect for self-determination in First Nations communities.

Research out of **Bangladesh**, in turn, found that the absence of opportunities for members of the community to participate in decision-making processes on health issues within their community (even via the simple presence of a complaints or suggestion box) had a direct impact on their use of facilities and uptake of health-promotion messages. By contrast, an urban health centre, which ran a daily "health education get-together" on its premises with health assistants present for feedback, attracted strong community participation, and individuals expressed their satisfaction with the hospital administration involving the community and delivering health education. This study's comparison of "high-performing" and "low-performing" *upazilas* (subdistricts) also found striking socioeconomic gradients in access to quality care, with most persons in the "high-performing" (also higher-incomed, better educated, and urban) setting preferring private over public facilities. Both subdistricts, however, reported surprisingly low rates of facility births and ANC, indicating that for a number of structural reasons explored in this chapter, inequities in basic health-care access (or acceptability) persist. Thus, even while some progress on the community-participation dimension of CPHC was made in one of the *upazilas*, there were still severe deficits in basic PHC.

The study findings are critical of the country's top-down approach to health-care planning and the fragmentation across different government sectors of responsibility for PHC, comprehensive or otherwise. It also cautions that an emphasis on community insurance schemes (such as the one developed in the Safe Motherhood program in DRC) risks increasing population inequities in health-care access, since wealthier communities will be better able to subsidize services than poorer ones. It concludes more optimistically with a robust set of recommendations for more effective and empowering reforms, re-emphasizing the need for greater community voice and the information citizens need to exercise that voice critically and effectively.

6 The Role of South Africa's Government in Strengthening Community Participation

NONHLANHLA NXUMALO, JANE GOUDGE, AND LIZ THOMAS

Background

South Africa's history has had a significant impact on the general health of its population, its health policies, and its services. Eighteen years after apartheid-related discriminatory and restrictive laws and policies, inequality continues to permeate all aspects of South Africa's society and the country's development efforts. These inequalities also extend to health status, in which black African and rural households bear a disproportionate burden of ill health (Bradshaw et al., 2008; Gilson & McIntyre, 2007; Coovadia, Jewkes, Barron, Sanders, & McIntyre, 2009). Despite various policy changes, the country's government has struggled to realize improved health outcomes. The country is in the centre of four concurrent epidemics (Bradshaw et al., 2006). The burden of non-communicable diseases continues to grow while poverty-related health challenges such as infectious diseases and maternal deaths remain widespread (Norman et al., 2007). HIV and tuberculosis remain the concomitant epidemics that present a major public health challenge; South Africa accounted for 17% of the global burden of HIV infection in 2007, with an estimate of about 5.5 million people (South African Department of Health, 2007; United Nations Programme on HIV/ AIDS [UNAIDS] & World Health Organization [WHO], 2007).

Owing in part to the country's level of poverty, derelict environment, and the effect of HIV/AIDS (particularly in rural, peri-urban, and informal dwellings), maternal and infant mortality rates in South Africa (a middle-income country) are worse than those of several low-income countries (Chopra, Daviaud, Pattinson, Fonn, & Lawn, 2009; Karim, Churchyard, Karim, & Lawn, 2009). Instead of experiencing a decline in child mortality since the Millennium Development Goals baseline was established in 1990, the country has seen an increase, with 69 deaths under-5 years of age per 100,000 live births (WHO, 2008). Despite the establishment of progressive health-care policies by the post-apartheid government in 1994 such as free PHC, the anticipated benefits have not been realized. Part of this is due to the inadequate quality of health care and inequitable access to services (Coovadia & Bland, 2008; Puoane, Tsolekile, Sanders, & Parker, 2008). Another contributor is the upstream determinants of health that are beyond the role and capacity of the health sector, such as those related to social and economic factors (Mayosi et al., 2009; WHO Commission on Social Determinants of Health, 2008).

The social and political context of South Africa provides a picture of a country that has a range of challenges in its efforts to reduce historical inequities. Informal settlements, homelessness, unemployment, and the lack of access to basic services are but some of the stark features of poverty that post-apartheid South Africa has inherited. Most of these features manifest even more prominently in the major cities of South Africa, where 16% of the total population resides in informal settlements, representing an estimated 2.4 million households (South African Cities Network [SACN], 2006). One quarter of Johannesburg's informal households are within and on the outskirts of its urban areas (City of Johannesburg, 2008). The process of internal and cross-border migration into Johannesburg has therefore contributed to increasing urbanization, and municipalities have steadily become incapable of responding to the multiple needs of these communities (Vearey, 2010). Consequently, the South African approach to addressing informal settlements has been the market-driven model, in which residents are relocated to "greenfield" sites. According to Huchzermeyer (2004), this process of moving communities undermines the existing community structures, prospects, and ideals for self- and community-improvement and the vulnerable livelihoods that rely on these informally established community networks and land-use patterns.

Inclusive in the efforts to overhaul the health system, the post-apartheid government ensured that PHC, delivered through the district health system, was the central aspect of its health policy (Coovadia et al., 2009) in alignment with the principles of PHC promoted at Alma-Ata. It envisioned and established a system that was based on community health centres. This vision is reflected in its policy in which children under 5 years of age and pregnant mothers receive free treatment

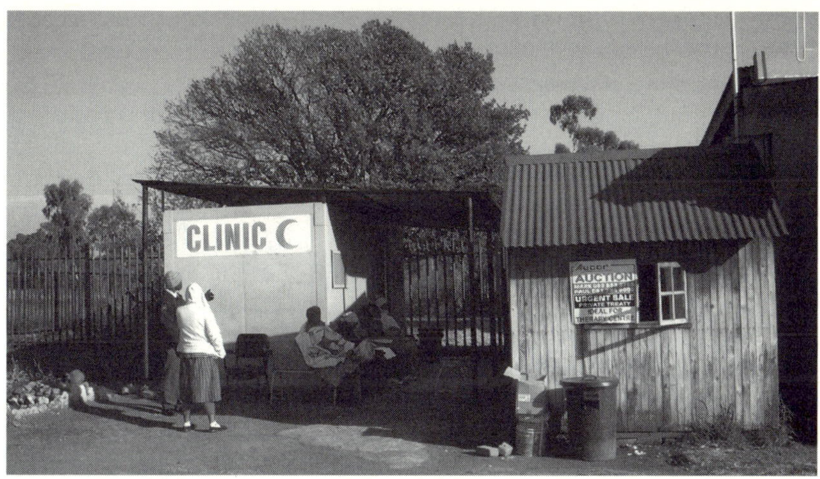

Eikenhof Clinic, South Africa

(Coovadia et al., 2009). As with other governments that have attempted to transform their health systems and implement PHC, the South African government has faced challenges, including a shortage of health professionals, the historical inequity in the distribution of resources, and weak managerial capacity and health-system leadership (Kautzky & Tollman, 2008). In response to these inefficiencies and the lingering remnants of apartheid, many service-oriented civil-society organizations have emerged to fill some of the implementation gaps.

Despite the challenges, efforts to strengthen and revitalize PHC are visibly continuing. Central to these efforts was the service agreement signed between the minister of health and the president of South Africa in October 2010 (Downing, 2010). Continued commitment to these efforts was further evidenced when the minister of health established a task team to provide advice on the re-engineering of PHC in South Africa (Barron, 2010). Part of this re-engineering will be rooted in community-based services; there will be a shift from the current PHC model in which the health system waits for users to access it. The new model would constitute a PHC team of health workers consisting of one professional nurse leading the team, one staff nurse, and four to six community health workers (CHWs) on the front line, actively going to communities and households (Ministerial Technical Task Team, 2010).

The mapping exercise of CHWs in South Africa by van Pletzen, Colvin, and Schneider (2009) provides an insight into the extent of reform that will be necessary to enable CHWs to provide effective PHC services. What remains evident is that the CHW terrain still constitutes a sector where CHW roles vary significantly and are not formalized or refined. The reality is a workforce that provides services that are as specific as HIV/TB-related activities to the more generalist, such as home-based care (Lehmann & Sanders, 2007). CHW roles become even more complex and blurred when one considers that the work they are expected to provide varies widely due to the needs of patients and households (van Pletzen et al., 2009). Although they also act as advocates for households and demand better services on behalf of their clients, this role is unrecognized and unofficial and, if pursued, has been reported at times to lead to conflict with formal sector providers (van Pletzen et al., 2009).

The realization that CHWs are crucial to the provision of PHC including a range of other caring services has led to the revision of South Africa's CHW policy, which is still under review. This review is being run parallel to the revitalization process of PHC. What is highlighted in the current CHW policy framework is that CHWs will take on a more integrated role. The policy denotes that CHWs will play a role in mobilizing communities to be more responsible for their health and social needs. This role pertinently speaks to the principles of CPHC. The recognized importance of community participation is based on the premise that for any community to achieve the health gains advanced in the Declaration of Alma-Ata (i.e., health for all), communities should have the right to plan and implement their own health-care programs (WHO, 1978). Community participation provides communities the platform to hold authorities of services accountable. In addition, an involved community has the potential to ensure that those sectors act on the social determinants of health (SDH). However, despite support and acknowledgment of the positive role of community participation in the implementation of CPHC, the extent to which a community's involvement can change policies towards more equitable health care still remains unknown and, in fact, is marred with challenges.

Although various CHW programs such as the Western Kenya Kisumu PHC project (Aga Khan Health Service, Kenya, n.d.) and India's Jamkhed Comprehensive Rural Health Project (Arole & Arole, 1975; Arole & Arole, 2000) provide lessons regarding the value of community participation, they fall short in exploring and explaining what determines the extent

Table 6.1 The social dimensions of community participation and health to which CHWs might contribute

Social cohesion	The extent of engagement and the sense of trust that individuals have within their communities. A more cohesive society, in which there is a strong sense of group identity, tends to be more sensitive to common well-being. A sense of community elicits the extent to which individuals feel that they have an influence on their immediate environment.
Social capital	The levels of social and civil trust in communities, including the existence of social networks. These factors influence coordination and cooperation for mutual gain, including resources useful for health.
Social networks	Linked set of social interactions and personal relationships, both of which have been linked to health outcomes. Social networks are the webs from which particular forms of social support (emotional, instrumental, informative, and appraisal) are drawn.

to which communities can mobilize to determine their own services and why. Community participation has been rendered a "complex and delicate process" (Zakus & Lysack, 1998). Terms such as "social cohesion," "social networks," and "social capital" have been used, often interchangeably, to explain the nature of communities and the existing factors that drive communities to participate (Table 6.1). This chapter uses three CHW programs in South Africa to examine the factors that enable and/or constrain effective community participation.

Research Questions and Methods

This research examined three case studies to compare the institutional environments and community contexts behind the implementation of CHW-provided services and explored how the services contributed to CPHC. In an effort to find answers, the study examined social cohesion and social capital within the communities where CHWs operated and how these impacted community participation. Along with this inquiry, the investigation looked at how the extent of community participation impacts the services provided by CHWs and the facilitation of intersectoral action (ISA), another key element of CPHC.

The focus on community participation was based on three premises. First, learning about the factors that contribute to successful facilitation of community participation can provide lessons regarding which elements and structures enable communities to be involved in decision making.

Second, learning about the impact of community participation would help to decipher whether it is a strategy to support in communities or a resource to use for engagement with government sectors. Finally, if community participation is indeed deemed a useful mechanism for accessing services and resources, the lessons learned could guide CHWs on how to utilize this platform, which would further determine whose role it should be to support and implement community participation.

The research was qualitative and used case-study methodology to analyse and compare the role, function, and context of three CHW programs in two provinces in South Africa. This allowed for an in-depth examination of the organizational and contextual factors associated with outcomes of community participation. Data collection took place during 2010.

Selection of case studies

The selection of cases was designed to better understand the reasons for success and failure. The size of the organization, type of services provided, nature of funding received, and the number of CHWs in the organization were considered. One successful organization with an established national reputation (Case Study 3) was selected for comparison with two less successful organizations (Case Studies 1 and 2). For the purpose of this chapter, we will name each case study according to their core work. Case Study 1 is the Home-based Care (HBC) Program; Case Study 2 is the Information Dissemination Program, and Case Study 3 is the Child Care Program. Further description of these case studies is provided below.

Data collection and analysis

A range of methods was used to collect data. These included key-informant interviews with government, NGO managers, and other key stakeholders. The activities of CHWs were assessed using participant observations during their household visits, focus-group discussions with CHWs, and the use of maps to capture CHW networks of work-related contacts. In total, 23 participants were interviewed, 74 participant observations were conducted in households across the three case studies, and three focus-group discussions were conducted, one with CHWs from each of the selected case studies.

Transcripts and field notes were analysed to assess the factors that were seen to facilitate successful community participation and ISA at a community level. The data were compared within and between cases. *ATLAS.ti* was used to assist with the identification of a priori and emerging themes in each of the case studies. Themes were examined comprehensively by returning to the original data to test the emerging analyses, and divergent evidence was examined in depth.

Results and Analysis

Description of the communities and the CHW programs

Community participation in the study was observed through the experiences of the CHWs. Although this chapter uses the community context to explore the dynamics regarding community participation, it is through this cadre that community participation is articulated.

The HBC (see Figure 6.1) and Information Dissemination programs (see Figure 6.2) were located in the Gauteng province within the metropolitan area of Johannesburg. Both programs provided services to communities that lived in informal settlements on the periphery of the metropolitan area. A large proportion of the residents of both communities were recent migrants from other South African provinces who were seeking work.

The communities serviced by CHWs in the HBC and Information Dissemination programs had common characteristics. Both were informal settlements that were located on the margins of Johannesburg, far from formal infrastructure and public transport. They also faced similar social, economic, and health circumstances. The high level of poverty was exacerbated by unemployment and high levels of chronic and infectious disease. Due to the lack of financial means, households were often unable to access health and social welfare services, which were mostly concentrated in the central parts of the city. Access problems were exacerbated for clients who were not physically mobile, whether due to illness or disability.

The Child Care Program (see Figure 6.3) was located in the province of Eastern Cape and operated in a small town we shall anonymize as X. The dense rural settlements served by the town had been established during the apartheid government's separate development policy. Many of the families in this area had been resident there for some time.

Figure 6.1 Home-based Care Program

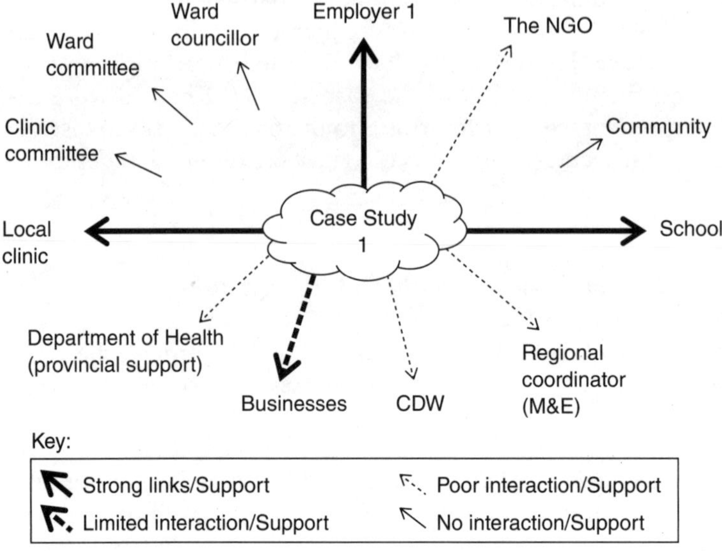

Figure 6.2 Information Dissemination Program

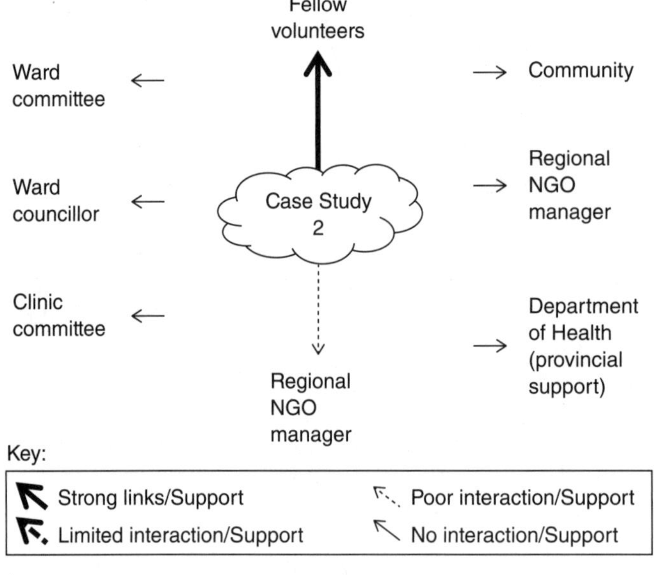

Figure 6.3 Child Care Program

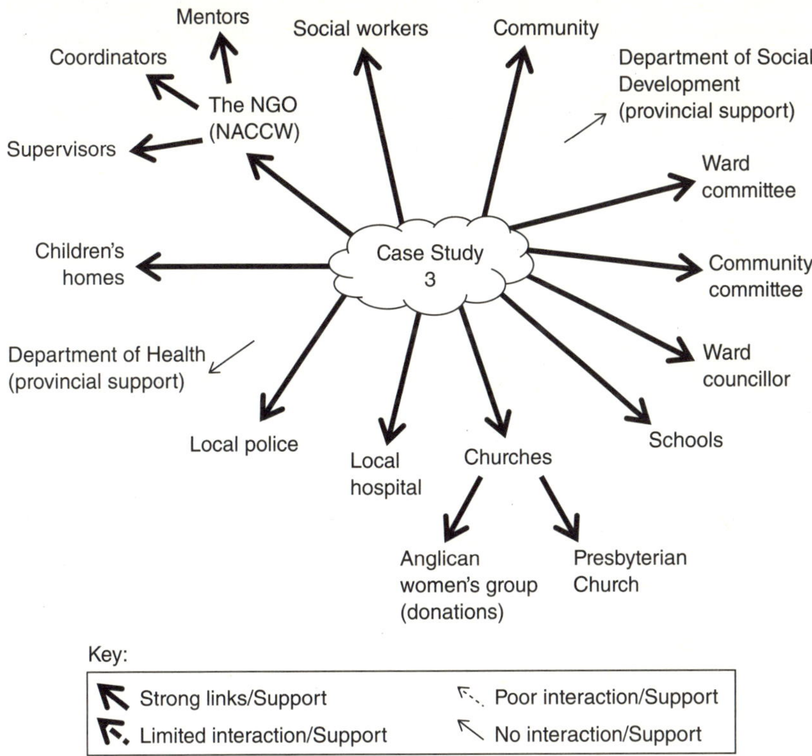

A substantial proportion of those in the community depended on remittances from family members working in other provinces such as Gauteng. As in the Gauteng case studies, poverty was also pervasive. Deprivation, associated with high unemployment, limited the households' access to key services. This was mostly because major government departments and services were accessible only in the closest major town, requiring a two-hour journey. The lack of financial means rendered the households dependent on the services and interventions of the CHWs to help them access services.

The households in all three case studies required identity documents and birth certificates to obtain food parcels and cash grants (meant to help reduce food insecurity) and to travel to services such as clinics and other social services. This requirement for official documents proved to be a barrier to accessing the necessary services. Many individuals in the case-study communities struggled to obtain these documents. As shown further on in this chapter, CHWs in the Child Care Program played a crucial role in facilitating access to official documentation and services by using collective community resources through community participation.

Social cohesion enables community participation

It was evident that the extent and nature of social networks established within the communities contributed to a level of social cohesion. This cohesion provided a favourable environment for effective community participation, as illustrated in the community serviced by the CHWs from the Child Care Program. This community shared a long history and had managed to forge strong bonds and trust over time. The social networks that were created over generations allowed the community to generate and share collective resources. The existence of avenues for community involvement offered the CHWs in this case study an enabling environment to provide services that address the SDH in the community.

An example of how the CHWs used the social capital in the community involved a case in which a homeless elderly woman was too frail and poor to take care of her orphaned grandchildren. The CHWs, through a community committee, were able to identify a neighbour who agreed to take over the guardianship of the children:

> During the time when the grandmother was struggling to take care of the children, I eventually found the neighbour … I asked the neighbour if she could take over the care of the family and the children … If the children do not have other family around, you ask the neighbours, as community members, to look after the family and the children. *(Focus-group discussion – Child Care Program CHW)*

This example illustrates one of the factors that contribute to effective community participation. In fact, this experience also shows that existing resources in the community were not necessarily material or monetary. Although vulnerable, this community was still able to share resources such as offering care and skills, which are often necessary when caring for young children.

The Gauteng communities did not have the same communal resources. The instability of a community that was made up of an amalgamation of different and mobile households and individuals resulted in little trust between community members where households had conflicting needs. The lack of shared experiences and history rendered social networks weaker, and thus social capital was poor. The lack of trust also made it difficult for communities to share any existing collective resources. The stark differences in the range of social networks established in the case studies illustrate how a community with a denser profile of social networks provides a richer environment for community-based organizations, thereby increasing the potential for ISA to address multifaceted needs. While the CHWs from the Child Care Program benefited from the strong links and networks in the community, the Gauteng programs had to deal with communities that had weaker structures. This factor is one reason why the CHWs failed to engage with, and provide comprehensive services to, their respective communities in the Gauteng programs.

Formal community participation structures:
A resource for the community

Formal community participation structures established by local governments provide communities with a platform to interact not only with the greater community but also with the authorities that provide services. Although these community committees (either clinic committees or ward committees) were available across the three case studies, the extent of their effectiveness varied. An active ward committee in the community of the Child Care Program enabled it to make decisions collectively regarding community needs. In addition, an involved ward councillor (a local political appointee who coordinates the input of different sectors in ward-committee meetings) acted as an enabling link to the different service providers and the community:

> We use the ward committee to communicate with the community. For instance when the NGO coordinators wanted to open a Safe Park for children in these locations (townships), they worked hand-in-hand with the ward committees and with the councillor. *(Focus-group discussion – Child Care Program)*

Although a resource for the community, the ward committee was also a resource for the CHWs in the Child Care Program in two ways. First, it provided the CHWs with a link to the community through which they could communicate emerging problems in the community and harness a collective effort to address those issues. (An example is the case of the aforementioned elderly woman, who was in need of shelter. Through their relationship with the ward councillor, the CHWs requested that the local government authorities identify land where they could build a home for the woman. Through the assistance of their NGO, they managed to obtain building material and to identify people with building skills in the community, and they built the elderly woman a new home.) Second, the interaction with existing social networks, such as community leaders (e.g., ward councillors), afforded the CHWs legitimacy and recognition as community agents who had the potential to assist households and individuals in need.

The Gauteng communities had a different experience. The absence of both shared needs and a mobilized community made efforts to stimulate community participation difficult. An attempt by one of the clinic nurses to establish a clinic committee, which would have enabled community members to voice their needs with regards to health care, failed. One community representative explained,

> I've been trying to mobilize a clinic committee. I've got about five members; but they have not been coming because sometimes some of them get employment and they have to work ... And you know, being a poor community, people want to do something for something in return. I remember when the notice was put up about wanting people to form a clinic committee, people used to come in and ask if there was some sort of stipend, and when I said no, they never came back. *(Key-informant interview, clinic nurse – Information Dissemination Program)*

In addition, with regard to assisting households to access services, the limited ability of the CHWs to provide tangible interventions did very little for their legitimacy in the community; hence the lack of confidence in their services. Consequently, the CHWs in the Gauteng case studies lacked the influence to mobilize the community and generate responses from the sectors in their respective areas.

> We do try our best but, once we have referred them, we really can't guarantee that they will receive any help or find anyone who is relevant for their problem. *(Focus-group discussion – Information Dissemination Program)*

Political affiliation has an impact on commitment of ward councillors

Failure to benefit from the community structures and to use them to access the different sectors made it difficult for the CHWs in Gauteng to affect ISA. This situation was exacerbated by politically appointed ward councillors who focused more on political activities, which resulted in a lack of active community participation:

> If at least there was a functional ward committee where we could vent and report these issues and have people that are supposed to deal with these issues, then that would at least help, but sometimes we don't hear from Mr. X [ward councillor] for months. I am yet to hear of any ward committee meeting taking place. *(Key-informant interview, clinic representative – HBC Program)*

In addition, many of the residents felt that political alignments of the ward councillors compromised their level of commitment to their communities, with their commitment being swayed towards those community members who were loyal to them:

> The councillor also calls meetings with his own people and they make their own decisions without calling the rest of us ... He is a member of Political Party A so he tends to engage with those that are also members. What is he then? Is he here to rally Political Party A members or is he a councillor to deal with issues of the community? *(Focus-group discussion, CHWs – Information Dissemination Program)*

In other instances, community members felt that ward councillors served those that they were more likely to relate to. A community member explained, "Politically, our ward councillor this side is a Political Party B councillor, so it's difficult to get him on board. He can't relate to the issues in this community" (key-informant interview, NGO manager – HBC Program).

The community in the Eastern Cape experienced similar dynamics. There was the view that the political choices affected not only the quality of services rendered to communities but also the level of accountability, primarily because people appointed to positions of authority were not well suited for the nature of the work. One of the NGO representatives expressed this sentiment: "There is no political accountability because the vote of the people is still a vote for a party, and that party ends up choosing or deploys someone ... but it is not really the community that votes for this councillor" (key-informant interview, NGO representative – Child Care Program).

This potential partnership affected the level of service provision as well as who received services: "The community constantly complains that the things don't get done unless you know so and so, or you are related to the ward councillor. That is the deep reality which we have in [X]" (key-informant interview, NGO representative – Child Care Program).

Interestingly, the CHWs in this particular community [X] had not been deterred from using the existing community structures. The strength of their social networks and social capital enabled them to circumvent this potential circumstance. "The team has formed really good relationships with the police, the school principals, with some of the key people in the hospital, the clinics. These relationships facilitate many referrals" (key-informant interview, NGO Representative – Child Care Program).

As illustrated by the community serviced by the Child Care Program, it is evident that the community and the CHWs were able to harness ISA efforts due to strengthened social networks and established social capital. As these factors were limited in the Gauteng communities, there was little evidence of community participation as a tool for empowerment to reduce their vulnerability and to address the SDH.

Discussion

The enabling effects of social cohesion and social capital

The community that was serviced by the CHWs in the Child Care Program had long-established social networks and relationships. The strong social cohesion strengthened the extent of community involvement and the establishment of social capital, which the community could share when community members were in need. These factors provided the CHWs from this case study a favourable environment to link to and mobilize the community.

The Eastern Cape case study illustrates that social capital can be generated by the existence of diverse and active social networks, and that communities can use these networks to support households. This finding is in line with findings in other research that suggest that communities with strong social networks are more likely to address poverty and other factors that result in vulnerability (Moser, 1996). More important, the Child Care case study echoes the lessons from various South African microcredit projects: that where there is a scarcity of other forms of capital, social capital can provide a cushion to vulnerable communities to mitigate social and economic barriers (Gilbert & Walker 2002; Pronyk et al., 2008).

In contrast, the nature of the communities in the Gauteng case studies determined the extent of social networks and social capital – which, in turn, determined the extent to which the CHWs could mobilize the community to address community problems. The less social cohesion there was, the less the communities found space to create or use community-participation structures. Some authors are of the view that the extent of poverty, unemployment, and segregation, as well as constant episodes of moving and displacement, erodes any possibility of developing social networks (Beyers et al., 2008). Conflict, poor leadership, and lack of control of resources exacerbate the poor potential for collective involvement (Havemann & Pridmore, 2005). This was certainly the case in the Gauteng communities. Although the community in the Eastern Cape experienced similar poverty and unemployment, the presence of sustained generations contributed to the growth of complex social networks, strengthening social cohesion. In contrast, the communities in the Gauteng case studies were made up of residents who came in at different times, from different parts of the country and other countries, which resulted in weak social networks and conflicting priorities. The Gauteng communities illustrate what King, Samii, & Snilstveit (2010) explained as the disadvantage of marginalized communities – that social networks are difficult to generate in communities that have to endure the manifestations of poverty, which lead to degeneration of the social fabric, lack of power, and, in Woolcock & Manderson's (2009) view, low levels of trust and tolerance.

The legitimate status of CHWs in fostering links
with sectors and the community

The efforts by the Child Care Program to establish strong relationships with various government departments contributed to the responsiveness of these departments to community needs. The extensiveness of these relationships enabled CHWs to foster ISA and to harness the different sectors to operate in a comprehensive fashion. It was evident that the CHWs in this case study had established a legitimate status in the community, hence generating a level of respect. Their position in the community as effective agents enabled them to link households to services. Moreover, it fostered a community that heeded their calls. These findings highlight that CHWs who have a good standing in the community have the potential to generate a community response that can further their effectiveness in assisting households. Poor relationships and links in the communities in Gauteng, however, provided little opportunity for the CHWs to harness intersectoral responses.

Sociopolitical context affects the provision of comprehensive services

The experiences of the community, including the CHWs across the case studies, indicate the constraining effect of political dynamics that manifest at the community level. In the advent of the revitalization of CPHC in South Africa, this factor needs attention, particularly with regard to the district health systems. The community in the Eastern Cape, partly due to the influence of the CHWs, was able to withstand and circumvent the potentially negative impact of local politics and decision making, primarily due to the strengthened relationships and networks it had.

Conclusion

Across the three case studies, the experiences of the communities and the CHWs show that community participation is an important strategy for accessing comprehensive services and for holding service providers accountable. It also shows that although a mobilized community has the potential to harness collective resources, poor communities, which are often fragmented, have conflicting needs and limited resources. These challenges limit the ability of such communities to mobilize their populations and harness collective resources. The study therefore raises an important inquiry: To what extent is it the role of government to assist communities to strengthen social networks and, consequently, social capital? The plans to revitalize CPHC in South Africa acknowledge the role of CHWs. If the government is to implement this intervention, it is important to recognize the constraining factors of community participation in poor communities and the extent to which they can inhibit the ability of CHWs to facilitate ISA and address the SDH.

REFERENCES

Aga Khan Health Service, Kenya, Community Health Department. (n.d.).
  Policy brief no.3. Best practices in community-based health initiatives: Sustaining community-based health initiatives. Mombasa: Aga Khan Health Service.

Arole, M., & Arole, R. (1975). A comprehensive rural health project in Jamkhed (India). In K.W. Newell (Ed.), *Health by the people* (pp. 70–90). Geneva: World Health Organization.

Arole, M., & Arole, R. (2000). Jamkhed, India: The evolution of a world training center. In D. Taylor-Ide & C.E. Taylor (Eds.), *Just and lasting change: When communities own their futures* (pp. 150–60). Baltimore: John Hopkins University Press.

Barron, P. (2010). *Re-engineering PHC in South Africa*. South Africa: Innovative Pharmaceutical Industry Association. Unpublished document.

Beyers, M., Brown, J., Cho, S., Desautels, A., Gaska, K., Horseley, K., & Anderson, S.M. (2008). *Life and death from unnatural causes: Health and social inequity in Alameda County*. California: Alameda County Public Health Department.

Bradshaw, D., Chopra, M., Kerber, K., Lawn, J.E., Bamford, L., Moodley, J., …,Velaphi, S. (2008). Every death counts: Use of mortality audit data for decision making to save the lives of mothers, babies, and children in South Africa. *Lancet, 371*, 1294–304.

Bradshaw, D., Nannan, N., Laubscher, R., Groenewald, P., Joubert, J., Ngilana, B., & Schneider, M. (2006). *South African national burden of disease study 2000. Estimates of provincial mortality: Summary report*. Parow: Medical Research Council.

Chopra, M., Daviaud, E., Pattinson, R., Fonn, S., & Lawn, J.E. (2009, Sep 5). Saving the lives of South Africa's mothers, babies, and children: Can the health system deliver? *Lancet, 374*(9692), 835–46. http://dx.doi.org/10.1016/S0140-6736(09)61123-5 Medline:19709729

City of Johannesburg. (2008). *Draft Integrated Development Plan review*. Johannesburg.

Coovadia, H., & Bland, R. (2008, Sep 13). From Alma-Ata to Agincourt: Primary health care in AIDS. *Lancet, 372*(9642), 866–8. http://dx.doi.org/10.1016/S0140-6736(08)61373-2 Medline:18790293

Coovadia, H., Jewkes, R., Barron, P., Sanders, D., & McIntyre, D. (2009, Sep 5). The health and health system of South Africa: Historical roots of current public health challenges. *Lancet, 374*(9692), 817–34. http://dx.doi.org/10.1016/S0140-6736(09)60951-X Medline:19709728

Downing, R. (2010). *Delivery agreement signed to improve service delivery*. Business Day. Rosebank.

Gilbert, L., & Walker, L. (2002, Apr). Treading the path of least resistance: HIV/AIDS and social inequalities a South African case study. *Social Science & Medicine, 54*(7), 1093–110. http://dx.doi.org/10.1016/S0277-9536(01)00083-1 Medline:11999505

Gilson, L., & McIntyre, D. (2007). Post-apartheid challenges: Household access and use of health care in South Africa. *International Journal of Health Services*, 37(4), 673–91. http://dx.doi.org/10.2190/HS.37.4.f Medline:18072315

Havemann, K., & Pridmore, P. (2005). *Social cohesion: The missing link to better health and nutrition in a globalized world*. Paper presented at New Frontiers of Social Policy: Development in a Globalizing World, Arusha, Tanzania. Retrieved from http://siteresources.worldbank.org/INTRANETSOCIAL DEVELOPMENT/Resources/Havemannpaper.rev.pdf

Huchzermeyer, M. (2004). *Unlawful occupation: Informal settlements and urban policy in South Africa and Brazil*. Trenton, NJ: Africa World Press.

Karim, S.S. A., Churchyard, G.J., Karim, Q.A., & Lawn, S.D. (2009, Sep 12). HIV infection and tuberculosis in South Africa: An urgent need to escalate the public health response. *Lancet*, 374(9693), 921–33. http://dx.doi. org/10.1016/S0140-6736(09)60916-8 Medline:19709731

Kautzky, K., & Tollman, S. (2008). A perspective on primary health care in South Africa. In P. Barron & J. Roma-Reardon (Eds.), *South African Health Review 2008* (pp. 17–30). Durban: Health Systems Trust.

King, E., Samii, C., & Snilstveit, B. (2010). Interventions to promote social cohesion in sub-Saharan Africa. *Journal of Development Effectiveness*, 2(3), 336–70. http://dx.doi.org/10.1080/17449057.2010.504552

Lehmann, U., & Sanders, D. (2007). *Community health workers: What do we know about them? The state of the evidence on programmes, activities, costs and impact on health outcomes of using community health workers*. Geneva: World Health Organization, Evidence and Information for Policy, Department of Human Resources for Health.

Mayosi, B.M., Flisher, A.J., Lalloo, U.G., Sitas, F., Tollman, S.M., & Bradshaw, D. (2009, Sep 12). The burden of non-communicable diseases in South Africa. *Lancet*, 374(9693), 934–47. http://dx.doi.org/10.1016/S0140 -6736(09)61087-4 Medline:19709736

Ministerial Technical Task Team. (2010). *Re-engineering PHC in South Africa: Summary of principal recommendations*. South Africa: Ministerial Technical Task Team.

Moser, C. (1996). Confronting crisis: A comparative study of household responses to poverty and vulnerability in four poor urban communities. Environmentally sustainable development studies and monographs series, 7. Washington, DC: World Bank. http://dx.doi.org/10.1596/0-8213-3562-6

Norman, R., Bradshaw, D., Schneider, M., Joubert, J., Groenewald, P., Lewin, S., …, Pieterse, D., & South African Comparative Risk Assessment Collaborating Group. (2007, Aug). A comparative risk assessment for South Africa in 2000: Towards promoting health and preventing disease. *South African Medical Journal*, 97(8 Pt 2), 637–41. Medline:17952221

Pronyk, P.M., Harpham, T., Busza, J., Phetla, G., Morison, L.A., Hargreaves, J.R., …, & Porter, J.D. (2008, Nov). Can social capital be intentionally generated? A randomized trial from rural South Africa. *Social Science & Medicine, 67*(10), 1559–70. http://dx.doi.org/10.1016/j.socscimed.2008.07.022 Medline:18771833

Puoane, T., Tsolekile, L., Sanders, D., & Parker, W. (2008). Chronic non-communicable diseases. In P. Barron & J. Roma-Reardon (Eds.), *South African health review* (pp. 73–87). Durban: Health Systems Trust.

South African Cities Network. (2006). *State of the cities report*. Johannesburg: Author.

South African Department of Health. (2007). *National HIV and syphilis prevalence survey in South Africa 2006*. Pretoria: Department of Health.

United Nations Programme on HIV/AIDS & World Health Organization. (2007). *2007 AIDS epidemic update*. Geneva: Joint United Nations Programme on HIV/AIDS. Retrieved from http://data.unaids.org/pub/EpiSlides/2007/2007_EpiUpdate_en.pdf.

van Pletzen, E., Colvin, C.J., & Schneider, H. (2009). *Community care workers in South Africa: Local practices, case studies from nine provinces*. Cape Town: School of Public Health & Family Medicine, University of Cape Town.

Vearey, J. (2010). *The persistent urban challenges of migration and informal settlements in the context of HIV: Towards the development of a framework to guide the appropriate and equity promoting urban health and developmental of local government within Johannesburg, South Africa*. (Doctoral dissertation). School of Public Health, University of the Witwatersrand: Johannesburg.

Woolcock, G., & Manderson, L. (2009). Introduction: Social capital theory in critical perspective. In G. Woolcock & L. Manderson (Eds.), *Social capital and social justice: Critical Australian perspectives* (pp. 3–17). Darwin: Charles Darwin University Press.

World Health Organization. (1978). *Primary health care report of the International Conference on Primary Health Care, Alma Ata, U.S.S.R.* Geneva: Author.

World Health Organization. (2008). *Global tuberculosis control: Surveillance, planning, financing*. Geneva: Author. Retrieved from http://data.unaids.org/pub/Report/2008/who2008globaltbreport_en.pdf

World Health Organization Commission on Social Determinants of Health. (2008). *Closing the gap in a generation: Health equity through action on the social determinants of health: Final report of the Commission on Social Determinants of Health*. Geneva: Author.

Zakus, J.D.L., & Lysack, C.L. (1998, Mar). Revisiting community participation. *Health Policy and Planning, 13*(1), 1–12. http://dx.doi.org/10.1093/heapol/13.1.1 Medline:10178181

7 An Assessment of the Contribution of the Community Strategy Approach to Comprehensive Primary Health Care in Kenya

JACK BUONG, CLEMENTINE GWOSWAR, AND DAN KASEJE

Background

In Kenya, the PHC model was first established in 1974 as a Ministry of Health (MoH) pilot project in the district of Kakamega. The Kakamega experience was one of the models discussed during the International Conference on Primary Health Care at Alma-Ata. Although the pilot project demonstrated admirable results, the results were not sustained, since the findings of the project were not translated into national health policy (Were, 1984).

Over the years that followed, many Kenyan health indicators remained poor. Nyanza Province, the site of this study, and North Eastern Province are significant contributors to the country's poor performance. For example, the infant mortality rate of Nyanza is 119 per 1,000, against the national rate of 72 per 1,000 (Otieno & Opiyo, 2004). Malaria is the most prevalent disease. The HIV infection rate sits at 15% (National AIDS & STI Control Programme, 2005), and prevention of mother-to-child transmission, as well as voluntary counselling and testing uptake, are low. The contraceptive prevalence rate sits at 46%, and only 44% of women deliver babies with skilled birth attendants present (UNICEF, 2012).

In spite of decades of effort to improve health in Kenya through selective PHC activities and health-sector reforms (Ministry of Health, 2005), health indicators worsened. Poor performance of the District Health System (DHS) is partly caused by selective PHC initiatives, which, despite achieving high levels of coverage, have had poor outcomes in terms of mortality. Werner & Sanders (1996) attributed these poor outcomes, in part, to selective PHC ignoring the wider social determinants of health (SDH). Even interventions in child and maternal health care are selective in most cases, undermining health systems' capacities to work intersectorally. This situation is exacerbated by the fact that insufficient information is available for an evidence-based management of the health system. Another notable inadequacy is limited community participation in formal health systems, thus denying the system an opportunity for timely feedback from those who access care or preventive services.

History of PHC in Kenya

In the 1970s, there was a perception that "modernization" on its own was not producing dignified living for the majority of people. A focus on PHC emerged from the realization that the dominant medical model was failing to meet the major health needs of populations; the system could treat disease for some but it could not build health for all. A comprehensive approach to PHC attempts to move beyond the boundaries of the narrow biomedical framework and place the social, economic, and environmental contexts of people's lives within the picture of disease and health. It emphasizes the notion that technical "solutions," such as pharmaceuticals and clinical interventions, will not be adequate in improving health without the creation of healthy environments.

PHC started in Kenya in the 1960s, but the first community-based PHC project supported by its MoH was implemented in Kakamega District, Western Province, between 1974 and1982. The project offered fresh ideas, mechanisms, strategies, and approaches that could lead to essential health care for all (Were, 1984). Although the MoH approved the PHC approach in 1982 (Were, 1984) and established a unit (known as the community health unit [CU]) at headquarters to institutionalize it, no policy guidelines were elaborated to guide its implementation on a large scale. With health indicators in the country either stagnant or declining, the government realized it needed to revisit and clarify the contributions of past health-system efforts that had led to health improvements in order to plan for more effective health services in the future (Chen, Hill, Murray, & Garenne, 1993). Strengthening the health systems has been identified as a key intervention for reducing child mortality as well as promoting health growth and development (Bryce et al., 2003). In Kenya health services are provided through a network of more than 4,700 health facilities countrywide, with a public sector system accounting for about 51% of these facilities (National Coordinating Agency for Population and Development, Ministry of Health, Central

Bureau of Statistics, & ORC Macro, 2005). The National Health Sector Strategic Plan II (Ministry of Health, 2005), implemented between 2005 and 2010, sought to "reverse the trends" in health indicators. It provided a framework to ensure a functional health system through good governance, management, and an effective information system. The MoH looked for partners who had developed community approaches to health-care issues and could provide technical support on how to strengthen the DHSs and the network of more than 4,700 health facilities countrywide, with a public sector system accounting for about 51% of these facilities (National Coordinating Agency for Population and Development, Ministry of Health, Central Bureau of Statistics, & ORC Macro, 2005). The Tropical Institute of Community Health and Development (TICH) at the Great Lakes University of Kisumu (GLUK) was identified as one such partner and was asked to evaluate the community strategy approach (CSA), a revitalization of Kenya's earlier experiences in CPHC that was initiated by TICH in 2003 in six of the then 12 districts of Nyanza Province.

GLUK worked with the DHSs to develop, test, and scale up the CSA in six districts in Nyanza Province. These included Nyando, Siaya, Suba, Kisumu, Rachuonyo, and Bondo districts. Key elements of the CSA included the following:

- Development of committees at the village, community, and health-facility levels as governance and link structures, bringing service providers and consumers into the decision-making process together.
- Identification, training, and deployment of community health extension workers (CHEWs). A CHEW is a community health worker with certification in nursing or public health, and employed by the MoH. Each community unit is staffed by community health workers (CHWs) and one CHEW. A community unit (CU) is the lowest level of health care in the Kenyan health system, providing PHC to a local population of 5,000 people. CHEWs act as facilitators of dialogue at the community level and provide support to CHWs.
- Identification, training, and deployment of CHWs to support households in health-improvement initiatives, to maintain the village register as part of a community-based information system, and to facilitate dialogue at the household and divisional level through community structures.
- Establishment of village registers of all households to provide community-based information on all health-status aspects targeted for

improvement. The household registers are updated by the CHWs every six months to monitor change in health-seeking behaviour. This community-based information is analysed and displayed on chalk boards at sites agreed upon by the community, such as the health facility.
- Analysis and display of relevant health facility data on chalk boards by the nominated health worker at the link facility.
- Use of suggestion boxes at health facilities for client satisfaction comments. These are analysed monthly by a facilitating agency.
- Hosting of "dialogue sessions" based on data from the community and health facilities, depicting the current situation regarding elements targeted for improvement. These sessions are held monthly at the household, community, and health-facility level and every four months at the subdistrict/subcounty level.

The evaluation of the TICH-piloted CSA found that the approach was effective in strengthening the link between the community and the health facilities. The evaluation results were fed into the implementation plan for the National Health Sector Strategic Plan II, which focuses on the Kenya Essential Package for Health (KEPH). The KEPH includes service targets for maternal and child health, communicable conditions, control of noncommunicable diseases, reductions in behavioural risk factors, and stronger intersectoral collaboration with respect to water, pollution, housing, nutrition, and a number of other health-determining conditions (Ministry of Medical Services & Ministry of Public Health and Sanitation, 2013).

The MoH has been rolling out the CSA throughout the country with other development partners. However, little is known about how well the roll-out has been facilitated by the MoH and other development partners or what the results have been. It is also not clear whether and how effectively the CSA can be applied in contexts different from that in Nyanza Province where it was piloted.

Research Questions and Methods

Awareness is growing among politicians, policymakers, health-care providers, and researchers that the evidence base to support the theory and practice of strengthening health systems is not strong, especially in low- and middle-income countries. Moreover, the scientific foundations for this type of research are in need of significant development and improvement. The CSA as an effort to strengthen the health system is rapidly emerging as one of the most dynamic and complex areas of health research.

The purpose of the current study was to evaluate the uptake of the key elements of the CSA as well as to assess its sustainability in terms of implementation and contribution to CPHC outcomes. To do so, four basic questions were posed:

1. What components of the TICH-developed CSA model have been implemented and sustained by the MoH and other partners in the districts where TICH is not involved?
2 What has been the experience (i.e., successes, challenges, and best practices) of its implementation by the MoH and other partners (apart from TICH)?
3 To what extent does evidence-based participatory planning, a key element in the CSA model, improve accountability and responsiveness in health-service delivery at the district level?
4 What improved maternal and child health outcomes (improvement being one of the important goals of the Kenya Essential Package for Health) have been achieved and sustained in the districts implementing the CSA?

Study design

The research used a mixed-methods comparative case-study design to compare areas in which the TICH and MoH are involved together with areas in which the MoH is implementing the CSA with other partners or on its own. Qualitative methods of data collection included key-informant interviews (N = 7), focus-group discussions (N = 14), health-facility assessments (N = 21), and observational field notes. The quantitative method consisted of a cross-sectional household sample survey (N = 3,694) in seven districts, which was designed to assess health measures associated with the KEPH program in order to answer research question 4. These methods were intended to provide evidence as to the effectiveness of CPHC in improving the population coverage by the KEPH when implemented jointly by MoH-TICH as compared to the MoH with other partners or on its own; in effect, to determine if one implementation model was more effective than others.

Data was collected at different times throughout 2009 in the seven selected districts because they had been either TICH pilot districts or had other partners involved in implementing the community strategy. Nyanza Province provided the three TICH-supported districts (Suba, Bondo, and Rachuonyo) and is notable for also having the highest poverty-index ranking of any province in Kenya (United Nations Development Programme, 2005). The comparison implementation districts were randomly selected: three from Central Province (Thika, Nyandarua North, and Nyandarua South) and one from North Eastern Province (Garissa). North Eastern Province is a semiarid region and is sparsely populated with nomadic communities. Central Province ranks higher in socioeconomic status than the other provinces and has a greater population density. A multistage sampling technique was used to select samples from the three different provinces. Cluster sampling of villages was used to randomly select households to participate in the household survey.

The intervention sites in each province and district were those where CSA implementation activities were supported, which had established CUs, and had trained and continuously supervised CHEWs and CHWs. A total of 78 CUs and 33 health facilities were visited for the study. Matched nonintervention sites (those without specific CSA implementation activities) were also identified in each of the seven districts and included in the survey portion of the research to allow for some comparison with those sites actively implementing the CSA irrespective of the supporting agency.

Quantitative data were entered and analysed statistically using *SPSS*; qualitative data were analysed to identify factors influencing the implementation outcomes. The study was approved by the GLUK and Kenya Medical Research Institute research and ethics boards.

The study arose from a participatory research initiative in which communities using health facilities were key partners in the study's design and implementation. Communities participated as partners and suggested methods of data collection, such as a suggestion box, to monitor client satisfaction, instead of using exit interviews. Communities and service providers participated in identifying performance-measurement indicators for inclusion. In addition, they participated in data collection, collation, and use in dialogue meetings, which in turn led to planning for and actions on the key issues discussed during the dialogue. Community members were therefore able to manage the information, feeding it back to the health system for strategies to improve key health indicators. Focus-group discussions were also held as part of the study process, giving community members an opportunity to participate in decisions affecting their health. These methods brought together the community, service providers, and MoH management to discuss evidence of their performance and to inform continuous improvement of the selected key health indicators, such as immunization, client satisfaction, and antenatal care (ANC) attendance.

Results and Analysis

Implementation of the CSA was based on five elements: the proportion of CUs established (based on the target of one CU/5,000 population); the establishment of governance and management structures (i.e., community health committees [CoHCs], health-facility management committees [HFMCs], and district stakeholders forum); the proportion of trained and active CHEWs and CHWs against prescribed targets; the existence of a community-based health information system (CBHIS); and the number and level of dialogue sessions held. Since the establishment of a CU is basic to all other elements, implementation coverage was estimated across the country's provinces and used as a key marker for CSA roll-out (Figure 7.1).

The study findings reported in this chapter cover Nyanza Province, which had the highest community-strategy implementation rate at 31.8%; Central Province, ranked third in coverage at 19.4%; and North Eastern Province, with 10.8% coverage (Ministry of Health, 2010). At the time of our study, none of the provinces had achieved a CU implementation rate of 50% or higher.

As noted in the research design, there were three categories of CSA implementation that spanned the seven different districts. GLUK, through TICH, supported Bondo, Suba, and Rachuonyo districts. The Ministry of Public Health and Sanitation supported Garissa and Thika districts; while other nonprofits supported the Nyandarua South and Nyandarua North districts. The functionality of these three differing implementation structures was rated by the number and frequency of CoHC meetings, the presence of minutes, and the attendance and community representation at the meetings. By using these criteria, the functional performance rates of CoHCs were highest for the TICH-supported districts, followed by the MoH- and non-profit–supported districts (see Figure 7.2, organized by implementing agency from left to right). A similar pattern was found in the presence of functioning CUs. In all districts, the HFMCs and the district stakeholders were assessed as "functional."

Generally, more than 70% of the governance and management members at various levels of the CSA understood their roles and responsibilities and how the various levels are related. Some concern, however,

Figure 7.1 Community health unit implementation by province (2010 data)

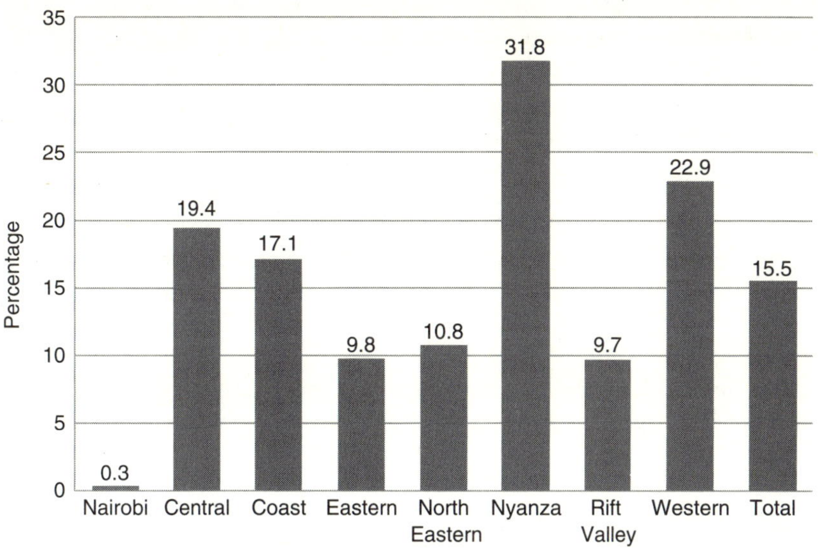

Figure 7.2 Percentage of functionality ratings for community health committees (CoHCs) and community health units (CUs) by district

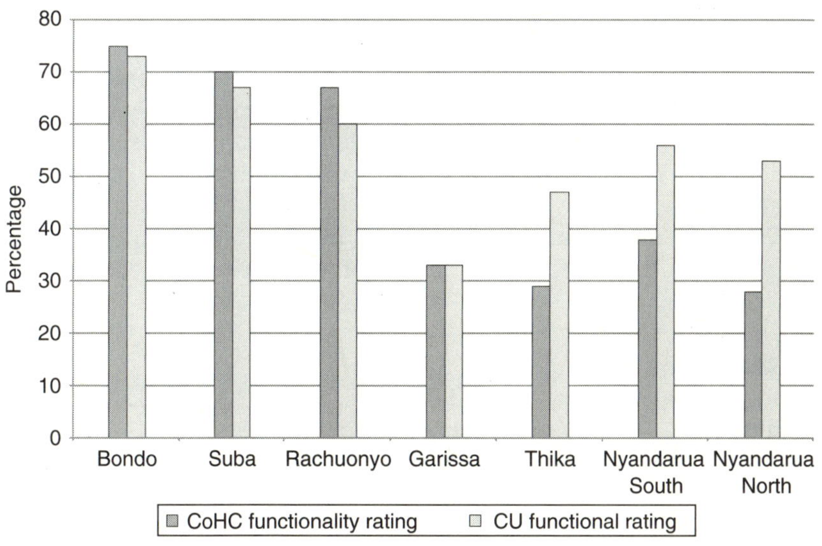

was noted about the role of CoHC members. As one of these members said, "They [CU staff] were trained. They have the concept. They have the content. But they are not driving this … I think the community health committees should be driving this [CSA implementation]."

CSA IMPLEMENTATION

As with most elements of health-systems delivery, the capacity and capabilities of human resources are key to CSA implementation. CHWs in particular are key to the success of the CSA. Our assessment, based partly on the number and content of training sessions, found that more than 80% of the CHWs could account for what they do during their household visits. One CHW gave the following examples:

> [We do] defaulter tracing both for tuberculosis patients and immunization. Once [we] go round and check from the cards [we] will be able to know and take up the matter with the patient. Also, for water treatment, [we] pick [up] the tabs from the CHEWs and go out and distribute them. [We] are also able to talk comfortably about the message of latrines – that these people can make simple latrines to prevent outbreak of diarrheal or any other disease. [We] also talk to the community about nutrition, the need to keep their homes clean, and slashing and destroying used containers that can harbour mosquitos.

The CBHIS is another basic component of the CSA. Its elements were ranked and scored (weighted) as 1 = Available; 2 = Available and linked to the facility's health management information system; and 3 = Available, linked, and used for dialogue. Bondo district ranked highest in CBHIS at 86%, which indicates data was continuously collected, made available, linked to health facility information, and used for dialogue with community members either during household visits or dialogue days (see below). Suba scored second best in CBHIS performance at 72% (once more indicating that TICH districts were outperforming the others), while performance for the other districts ranged between 50% and 60%.

DIALOGUE DAYS

Dialogue sessions were assessed differently at the household and community level. The household dialogue level was assessed by identifying the portion of households visited by CHWs during which a dialogue took place about a health concern associated with the KEPH program.

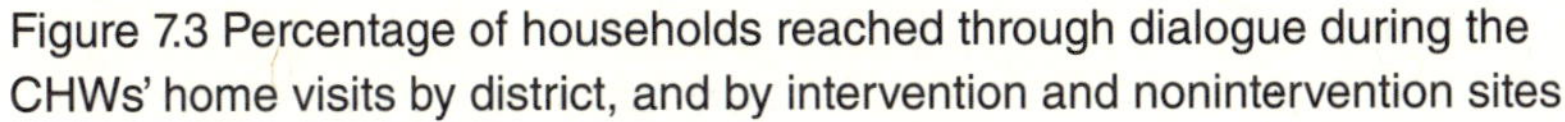

Figure 7.3 Percentage of households reached through dialogue during the CHWs' home visits by district, and by intervention and nonintervention sites

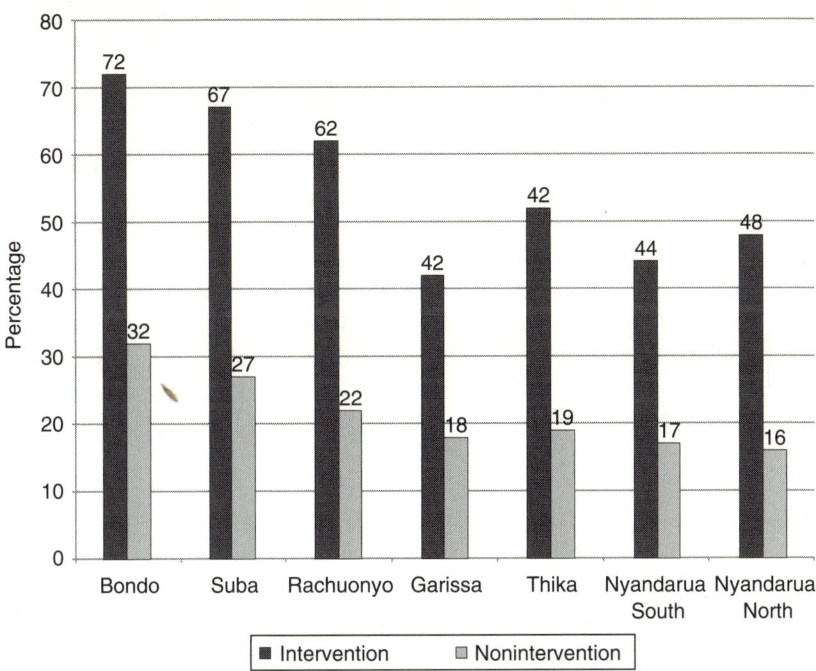

This assessment covered both intervention sites in the seven districts, as well as nonintervention sites (Figure 7.3). Predictably, the level of household visits by CHWs that included dialogue was much higher for intervention sites; with the TICH-supported CSA districts showing a greater portion of visits with dialogue than the MoH- and nonprofit-supported districts.

At the CU level, dialogues were evaluated based on the duration and frequency of the dialogue days. Dialogue days were held regarding CSA elements targeted for improvement and for which community members and/or health-facilities staff had identified a concern. The CSA advises that these dialogue sessions ideally should be held monthly at household, community, and health-facility levels, and every four months at the subdistrict level. Only the TICH-supported districts convened dialogue days: Bondo held 56 such days over a two-year period; Suba had 30 over 18 months; and Rachuonyo had 12 over a one-year period. Dialogue at the CU level, however, was observed in all the health facilities visited during the study.

Qualitative analysis of observational and interview findings suggests that the dialogue sessions with community members did lead to improvements in the CSA implementation plans. As one individual involved with a HFMC noted,

> There has just been a monthly dialogue day at the community level. People come and say what they know about the facility; how the services can be improved. We also display the charts showing how we are performing – you see the children are not coming for immunizations, women are not delivering in the facility, etc. Then they will tell us why; whether it is the staff attitude at the facility or the quality of treatment. Then we see what to do and discuss other issues like latrine coverage, water treatment – how best they can be done.

KEPH outcomes

One of the premises of the CSA is that it should improve KEPH outcomes. Table 7.1 provides a descriptive summary of key indicators based on the KEPH and chosen as important measures by community members and CU staff involved in the study. As Table 7.1 shows, there were some differences by districts. Consistent with the premise, the three TICH-supported districts, which scored best on CSA implementation, performed slightly better than other districts on three measures (ANC attendance, use of insecticide-treated nets [ITNs], and household safe water). TICH-supported districts, however, performed poorly on the health-facility measure, a finding that could be explained, in part, by the TICH-supported districts being the poorest.[1] These findings nonetheless suggest that KEPH measures differ little by implementing agency.

Across all seven districts, several strong correlations were found between KEPH measures and several elements of the CSA (Table 7.2). Strengthened governance, particularly the presence of CoHCs and stakeholder fora, was correlated with greater ANC attendance of 4 times or more ($r = 0.750$) and ITN use ($r = 0.906$). Similarly, CHW use correlates

---

1 Since the TICH districts had also been previously surveyed, establishing a baseline, it is important to note that health-facility delivery in the 2009 survey had risen by 2% to 5% across the three districts.

Table 7.1 KEPH measures (%) by CSA-implementing districts

Measure	Bondo	Suba	Rachuonyo	Garissa	Thika	Nyandarua South	Nyandarua North
ANC attendance (4+ times)	67	66	64	54	63	58	57
Health-facility delivery	34	32	34	28	46	50	49
Immunization coverage	83	84	63	77	91	87	83
Proportion of households with safe water	75	79	65	52	72	65	67
Use of ITNs for mothers and < 5 years	67	66	64	54	65	58	58
Vitamin-A uptake < 5 years	77	80	78	65	80	79	80

Table 7.2 Correlation of community-strategy elements with KEPH measures

	Structures[1]	CHWs	CHEWs	CBHIS
Correlation with health outcomes	$(r)^2$	(r)	(r)	(r)
Immunization coverage	0.375	0.032	0.205	*0.607*
ANC attendance (4+ times)	*0.750*	*0.510*	0.091	0.000
Use of ITNs for mothers and < 5 years	*0.906*	*0.615*	0.496	0.000
Health-facility delivery	0.354	0.320	0.258	0.000
Proportion of households with safe water	0.471	*0.600*	0.258	0.382
Vitamin-A uptake < 5 years children	*0.540*	*0.734*	0.592	0.000

1 Refers to the establishment of governance and management structures: community health committees, health-facility management committees and district stakeholders forum.
2 Strong Pearson's correlations (> .5) are *italicized*.

strongly to ITN use (r = 0.615), households with safe water (r = 0.600), and vitamin A uptake (r = 0.734). CBHIS is strongly correlated only with one measure: immunization coverage (r = 0.607). Although correlation is not causality, the logic of the relationships indicates that certain of the CSA elements are positively influencing desirable health-system outputs. While the Pearson's test found only a weak correlation between CHWs and immunizations, qualitative accounts indicated otherwise and underscored the findings on ITNs and safe water, as one health-facility staff noted:

> Yes… the immunization coverage went up with the community strategy by involving CHWs. Children are now coming and, as of last week, measles coverage was at 81%, and latrine coverage and water treatment have also increased. The use of ITNs has gone up because of behaviour changes … Nutrition has improved because of kitchen gardening, and there is increased demand for service delivery at the facility.

Finally, data on a number of measures compared intervention with nonintervention sites. Although it is likely that there was some spillover from the intervention to the nonintervention sites on some of the outcomes (notably knowledge of family planning, CHW visits, and travel distance to health facilities), the differences between the two were striking (Figure 7.4).

General implementation experiences

Based on observational data gathering during the study, evidence-based participatory planning improvements were noted in more than half of the health facilities. MoH policy documents were made available at the health-facility level, and raised health workers' awareness of the policy issues and current trends regarding health indicators. Links between the health-facility management information system and the CBHIS appear to have been strengthened, improving the completeness of health data. The use of this data to trigger dialogue in the CUs has also inculcated a culture of dialogue for continuous health-system improvement. As one individual working in a health facility noted about the supply chain,

> There is improvement … when you are criticized to change your attitude, or there is a lack of drugs. Then you try to improve on that. When the nets are not there you call … so that whatever makes them [community members] not visit the facility is made available.

Health facilities have become more sensitive to the needs of the community, in part by providing space on HFMCs for (paid) CHEWs, who are able to more rapidly convey any concerns identified by CHWs and community members. HFMCs also meet more frequently now for planning, implementation, monitoring, and feedback. These changes have been accompanied by a progressive improvement in staff attitude and commitment based on achievement; a culture or a system rewarding performance is now in place. In virtually all the health facilities, order

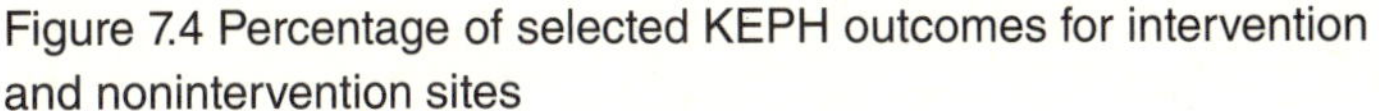

Figure 7.4 Percentage of selected KEPH outcomes for intervention and nonintervention sites

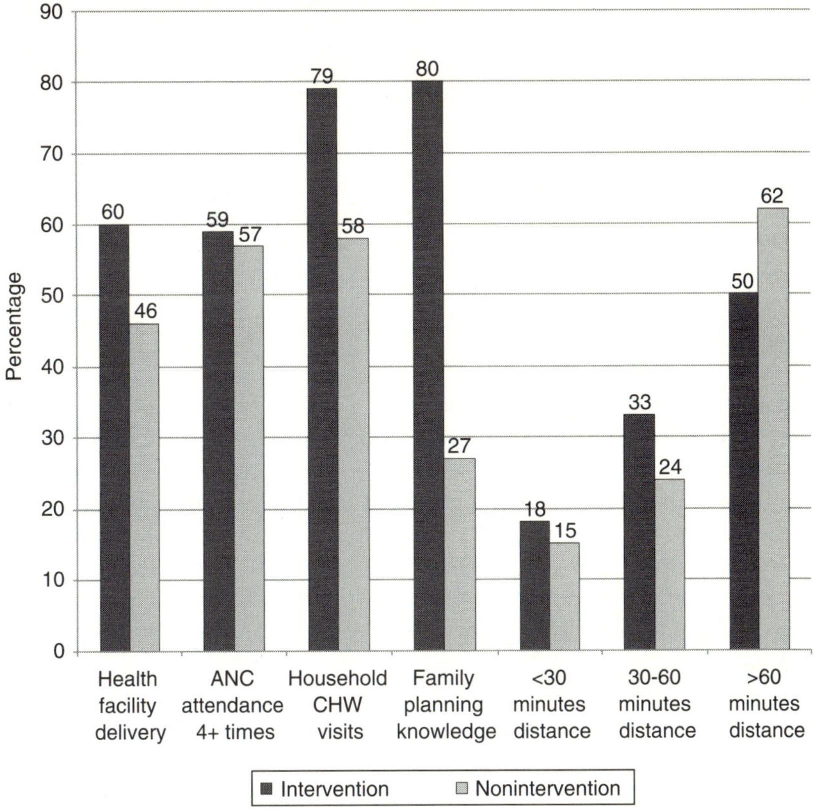

and punctuality were observed. There was significant improvement in accountability and responsiveness of district health-service delivery; community members in the CUs expressed the feeling that health workers in the health facilities are now accountable.

With the improvements have come some challenges. As one key informant noted, "It has become tricky. Now that everything is being rolled down to the health-facilities level, it's the facilities which are to make annual work plans to capture all that they want to do, and all the ministry does is approve."

Another participant, in a detailed account of what happens in the process of establishing CUs, complained that, "Finally, MoH through partners is expected to support our dialogue and outreach activities financially; however, the financing has not been very positive."

Another study participant reported how the lack of motivation by CHWs was partly an effect of the community's misunderstanding of their work:

> The community members think we are employed and paid a salary, but us we know we are volunteers, yet during the household visits, the household members tell us that we are "eating" [paid] from the data we collect from them.

Discussion

Relative to the idealized components of CPHC that informed this study, several findings from our study are worth noting. First, health-facility assessments and a review of dialogue-day content found that many of the CUs in our study reflected on SDH in their planning exercises. As well, and in keeping with the CPHC intent of reducing health disparities among population groups, the CSA employed in our study sample targeted disadvantaged communities and engaged them in planning at the CU level to identify their priority needs. Our study also found that outreach programs and home visits, which are associated in the literature with improved health outcomes,[2] were evident in the CSAs in all seven districts, and notably so in the TICH-supported districts (which reported the highest CSA-implementation levels). Although the CSA made all these improvements possible, it was noted that developing relationships within communities took time and they often started with addressing priority issues identified by the community. These issues were not necessarily the same ones identified by local service providers. Our study also found some evidence of intersectoral work that addressed the SDH. As one of facility health worker commented,

> When we make our AOP [Annual Operating Plan], we meet with partners who are also making their annual work plan regarding what they want to do in the district, so we include them in our work plans.

---

2 See Chapter 2, this book.

Finally, one of the key findings from our study is that, with a few exceptions, the districts with the highest CSA implementation levels (which happened to be those supported by TICH) and longest exposure to the CSA (with the TICH districts being among those involved in the TICH's earlier pilot CSA work) also performed better on most measures than the other districts. Since the CSA is very much predicated on the principles of CPHC, this finding bodes well for the continuing roll-out of the CSA in Kenya as a tool for CPHC revitalization.

Conclusion and Recommendations

Although the descriptive nature of most of our findings from this study prevents us from drawing any generalized conclusions, it nonetheless supports the larger literature on how CPHC can contribute to reducing health inequities and improving health-system performance. The process of undertaking this study is also informing the scale-up of the CSA in Kenya. Here are a few observations:

- Research design for CPHC should consider the context of the research area and provide room for justifiable flexibility. Through the implementation processes in this study, communities significantly contributed to new research questions in order to achieve the CPHC elements and health outcomes they desired. The community continued to be involved in the research design and in planning for the community survey, as well as in participating in stakeholder fora to influence policy and interventions.
- Involving research users in every stage of the research process created a higher demand for the use of findings. The principal stakeholders, including the MoH and CUs, continued to be involved in several aspects of the proposed scaling-up phase of the study, such as taking responsibility for ensuring the necessary service coverage in their own villages and units, continuously assessing improvements in health outcomes in their areas of responsibility, and following up on proposed actions.
- Greater involvement of team leaders resulted in better collaboration by various health personnel and stakeholders. Team leaders' influence was expanded, and they communicated more widely, bringing on board all health personnel.
- Dialogue day and case study data revealed that prompt and appropriate responses to health issues within the community were realized where CUs were formed.

The research team formulated recommendations based on the findings from this study. Foremost, the CSA should play a key role in the renewal of CPHC in Kenya, as it represents an integrated approach to a multidimensional and multisectoral health program aimed at ensuring communities have increased access to health services. The results further emphasize the importance of continuous supervision and close ties between district-level health-management teams, health workers at the health-facility level, and CHEWs, CoHCs, and CHWs at the community level to achieve sustainable CSA activities.

ACKNOWLEDGMENTS

We would like to acknowledge the strong collaboration of the MoH and GLUK, which made the whole research process a participatory one. Prof. Dan Kaseje, the research mentor and the GLUK team leader, used his capable technical and managerial skills to oversee the entire study with enthusiasm, energy, and rigour. Finally, we express our gratitude to the respondents from the households and the community health workers, who gave their time freely and cooperated with us in making this study possible. The results of this study will be used to improve the DHS and eventually improve the health outcomes of residents through the community strategy approach.

REFERENCES

Bryce, J., el Arifeen, S., Pariyo, G., Lanata, C., Gwatkin, D., Habicht, J.P., & Multi-Country Evaluation of IMCI Study Group. (2003, Jul 12). Reducing child mortality: Can public health deliver? *The Lancet, 362*(9378), 159–64. http://dx.doi.org/10.1016/S0140-6736(03)13870-6 Medline:12867119

Chen, L.C., Hill, A.G., Murray, C.J., & Garenne, M. (1993). A critical analysis of the design, results and implications of the mortality and use of health services surveys. *International Journal of Epidemiology, 22*(Suppl 1), S73–S80. http://dx.doi.org/10.1093/ije/22.Supplement_1.S73 Medline:8307678

Ministry of Health. (2005). *Reversing the trends: The Second National Health Sector Strategic Plan of Kenya.* Nairobi: Author.

Ministry of Health. (2010). *The Third National Health Sector Strategic Plan of Kenya.* Nairobi: Author.

Ministry of Medical Services & Ministry of Public Health and Sanitation. (2013). *Transforming health: Accelerating attainment of health goals. Kenya Health*

Sector Strategic and Investment Plan (KHSSP) July 2013–June 2017. Retrieved from http://www.who.int/pmnch/media/events/2013/kenya_hssp.pdf

National AIDS & STI Control Programme. (2005). *AIDS in Kenya: Trends, interventions and impact* (7th ed.). Nairobi, Kenya: National AIDS and STI Control Programme, Ministry of Health.

National Coordinating Agency for Population and Development, Ministry of Health, Central Bureau of Statistics, & ORC Macro. (2005). *Kenya service provision assessment survey 2004.* Nairobi, Kenya: Author.

Otieno, F., & Opiyo, S. (2004). Introduction. In Central Bureau of Statistics [Kenya], Ministry of Health [Kenya], and ORC Macro. *Kenya demographic and health survey 2003* (pp. 1–12.). Calverton, Maryland: Author.

UNICEF (2012). *Kenya: Statistics.* Retrieved from http://www.unicef.org/infobycountry/kenya_statistics.html

United Nations Development Programme. (2005). *Linking industrialization with human development.* Retrieved from http://hdr.undp.org/sites/default/files/kenya_2005_en.pdf

Were, M. (1984). *Primary health care in Kenya.* Baltimore: John Hopkins University Press.

Werner, D., and Sanders, D. (1996). *The politics of primary health care and child survival.* Palo Alto: Health Wrights.

8 Developing a Comprehensive Primary Health Care Model for Bangladesh

TAUFIQUE JOARDER, ANWAR ISLAM, AND AFTAB UDDIN

Background

Since its independence in 1971, Bangladesh has made significant progress in many areas of social development, including health. Gross national income per capita (by Atlas method) increased from around US$220 in 1980 to US$1,080 by 2014. Life expectancy at birth increased from 55 years in 1980 to 71 years by 2014. Similar progress has been seen in child health. For instance, the infant mortality rate and under-5 mortality rate per 1,000 live births, which were 134 and 199 in 1980, decreased to 32 and 40, respectively, in 2014. Modelled estimates for the maternal mortality ratio also declined from more than 550 per 100,000 live births in 1990 to 170 in 2013. The total fertility rate also dropped to 2.2 in 2013, from 6.4 in 1980 (World Bank, 2015).

Bangladesh was one of the signatories of the Declaration of Alma-Ata in 1978. Guided by its principles, Bangladesh adopted primary health care (PHC) as the key approach to reach the declaration's target of "Health for All" by 2000, a goal later iterated by the World Health Organization with the same deadline. To reach this goal, *upazila* health complexes (UpHCs), which are small health complexes with 50 beds (few UpHCs have a lower number of beds), were instituted and now function in 424 *upazilas* (subdistricts) of Bangladesh (Government of Bangladesh, 2014). UpHCs act as the hub of PHC delivery and the first point of referral. All treatments in these facilities are supposed to be free of charge. Above the UpHCs, there are district-level secondary-care hospitals, regional teaching hospitals, and national specialized institutions for tertiary-level specialized care with modest user fees (Osman, 2004). On average, each UpHC covers a population catchment area of 320,444. Below the level of UpHCs, at *union* level, there are smaller health centres. Below the *unions*, the government has established 13,240 community clinics, each covering a population of 6,000 (Government of Bangladesh, 2014).

While many of the improvements in basic health indicators such as total fertility rate, maternal mortality ratio, and infant mortality rate have been attributed to Bangladesh's PHC system, the critical issue of equity across socioeconomic strata still remains. The health system faces challenges in terms of shortages and maldistribution of staff, skills-mix imbalances, negative work environments, and weak knowledge bases, all obstacles identified by the Joint Learning Initiative (2004). Despite gains in health indicators, PHC coverage is below 50%, and a wide array of problems exists, including lack of medicine, absence of doctors and other providers, under-the-table payments, lack of cleanliness, lack of privacy and confidentiality, neglect and maltreatment of patients, lack of health-system responsiveness towards the nonmedical expectations of patients, and discriminatory treatment of patients.

All of these problems create hurdles to the development of an efficient and effective health system in Bangladesh. Persistent inequalities exist between the rich and the poor. While most of the achievements are celebrated at an aggregate national level, there is clear underperformance in achieving health for all, with the most vulnerable groups (i.e., poor, women, children, and disabled) at the losing end (Osman, 2004).

Studies in Bangladesh highlighted that health centres in the public sector are not used by all segments of the community. Service-provider inefficiencies were the reported cause of this situation. As a result, there has been increased utilization of health facilities in the private formal and informal sectors. According to Cockcroft, Andersson, Milne, Hossain, and Karim (2007), the whole group of "unqualified practitioners" in the private sector provides 60% of treatment services in rural Bangladesh. This statistic underscores the fact that the conventional PHC delivery system in the public sector is inadequate in catering to the needs of the community, as almost 85% of the Bangladeshi population visit private-sector providers, with informal providers being the first resort (Bangladesh Health Watch, 2008). Although the public sector employs about 38% of the registered doctors (Government of Bangladesh, 2014), the high rate of absenteeism makes them ghost doctors (existing in registers, but not in person), adding to the plight of the health-care system.

The above context and the prevailing constraints demand reform of the delivery of health services to all in Bangladesh, making health services universally acceptable, available, and accessible. To meet this challenge, this project was conceptualized to develop a reformed PHC model appropriate to the context in Bangladesh and one that is more comprehensive in nature.

Research Questions and Methods

The principal objective of this project was to design a *comprehensive* primary health care (CPHC) model appropriate for Bangladesh. This required

- reviewing the historical evolution of the PHC system in Bangladesh;
- analysing the existing PHC system and its comprehensiveness by measuring the performance of existing PHC delivery centres and identifying weaknesses in the country's existing PHC delivery system;
- measuring the equity status in PHCs in terms of SDH; and
- making recommendations for designing and developing an acceptable CPHC model for Bangladesh.

Data for the mixed-method (quantitative and qualitative) study was collected in three distinct phases. The first phase of the study comprised a literature review and key-informant interviews to understand the historical evolution of PHC in Bangladesh. Key informants were selected purposively and included one government high official in charge of PHC delivery in Bangladesh, three veteran public-health professionals who had been involved in early PHC policy formulation and implementation in Bangladesh, and one public administration specialist from the University of Dhaka who did extensive ground work on health policy of Bangladesh.

The second phase was entirely quantitative, involving the administration of a cross-sectional survey in 20 UpHCs. Ten UpHCs were selected within the vicinity of the capital city of Dhaka, and the other 10 from the distant, hard-to-reach district of Barisal. To evaluate their performance, the "goals" and "functions" of a health system as outlined in the World Health Report on improving health systems performance (World Health Organization, 2000) were considered. We determined the average rating of three goals and four functions of the health system for each UpHC. To evaluate them, we used both the weighted and

Table 8.1 *Upazilas* selected for study near Barisal
and Dhaka regions

District	*Upazila* health complex			
Barisal	Agailjhara Babuganj Bakerganj	Banaripara Gaurnadi	Hizla Mehendiganj	Muladi Wazirpur
Barguna	Bamna			
Dhaka	Dhamrai Dohar	Keraniganj	Nawabganj	Savar
Gazipur	Kaliakair			
Manikganj	Harirampur			
Narsingdi	Belabo			
Narayanganj	Bandar	Sonargaon		

simple average method. Expert opinions were sought to determine what weight should be given to the goals and functions. Most of the experts suggested that "goals" should be given more weight than "functions," arguing that whatever these functions may be, they would be worthless should the desired outcomes not be achieved. Hence, 60% weight was given to the "goals" and 40% to the "functions." Using these weights, we obtained a score for each UpHC. These were expressed in an index (where 100 is the base category). Data were generated by interviewing the *upazila* health and family planning officer (UH&FPO, the head of the UpHC), the medical officers (the registered medical doctors), the administrative staff, and the patients. Based on the index, the 20 UpHCs were ranked, and the "highest performing" and the "lowest performing" UpHCs were selected for in-depth study.

The third phase was the in-depth study carried out in the low-performing and high-performing UpHCs and their catchment areas (Table 8.1). This study contained three parts: a qualitative study at the UpHC; a household survey in a randomly selected village within the UpHC's catchment area; and a participatory rapid appraisal (PRA) in the same village. The qualitative study involved observation of the UpHC and its functions for 15 days as well as in-depth interviews with the local government leader, the UH&FPO, medical officers, medical assistants (paramedics), field staff, and purposively selected inpatients and outpatients. A village was randomly selected from the list of villages falling within the catchment area of the UpHC. From that village, using systematic random sampling, 5% of the total population was interviewed to investigate "equity in health service utilization." In the selected village, a PRA session was arranged in which 30 people from different socioeconomic strata participated.

UpHCs were selected based on some assumptions. It was assumed that the *upazilas* near Dhaka would perform better due to their proximity to the capital, drawing on the increased availability of health personnel, more frequent external monitoring, and better communication as opposed to the UpHCs in and around Barisal.

A range of tools and techniques (e.g., checklists, semistructured questionnaires, PRA guidelines) were pretested and employed to collect data. Qualitative data were collected using checklists and PRA tools, and quantitative data were collected using a semistructured questionnaire. The lead researcher made quality-control visits during data collection. PRA was conducted by the lead researcher with assistance from the qualitative-data collector and the field-research assistant. The interviews were all audio recorded and transcribed. Qualitative data were coded according to inductive and a priori themes using *ATLAS. ti* 5.5 software. Quantitative data were analysed using *SPSS* 13.0. Respondents agreed to take part in the research by giving their verbal informed consent.

Results and Analysis

The analysis of evolution of PHC in Bangladesh reveals certain characteristics. From the early 1980s to the early 1990s, emphasis was primarily on infrastructure development. Most health-care delivery institutions were established during that period. However, from the early 1990s, there was a paradigm shift in policy, focusing on system issues rather than infrastructure, as vertical program initiatives began, such as demand-side interventions, emergency obstetric care, and the Bangladesh integrated nutrition project. The first evaluation of the national health for all strategy was conducted in 1986. It identified some bottlenecks in implementing PHC in Bangladesh. According to the report, inadequacy in the managerial process, lack of adequate resources, bias towards curative medicine, and lack of coordination and community involvement posed hindrances to putting PHC into action. Based on the report's recommendations, the government of Bangladesh initiated an "Intensified PHC Program" in two *upazilas* in different districts. The program was gradually extended across the country. In the late 1990s, successful initiatives were undertaken, such as an urban primary health-care project, an example of good cooperation between government and NGOs. In 2009, a decision was made to establish a community clinic for every 6,000 people in rural Bangladesh to cater to the PHC needs at the grassroots level. Finally, Bangladesh succeeded in adopting its first national health policy, which was approved in Jatiyo Sangsad (Bangladesh Parliament) on 31 May 2011.

Our screening survey revealed Dhamrai UpHC in Dhaka District as the "highest performing" (index value 68.30) and Mehendiganj UpHC in Barisal District as the "lowest performing" (index value 43.82). (See Table 8.2.)

Accordingly, in-depth studies were carried out in the Dhamrai and Mehendiganj *upazilas* using a household survey in two PRA villages. The villages selected randomly from these two *upazilas* were Kashipur (in Dhamrai) and Charlata (in Mehendiganj).

Dhamrai is one of the five *upazilas* (subdistricts) of Dhaka District, situated 20 kilometres west of the capital city of Dhaka. The UpHC is situated in Islampur, adjacent to the Dhaka-Aricha highway, one of the busiest highways in the country, and is located at the border of Dhamrai, at the bank of the Dhamrai River. It was established in 1965 as a 31-bed hospital, upgraded to 50 beds in 2008. Dhamrai is easily accessible by both road and river.

Mehendiganj is one of the nine *upazilas* of Barisal District, located in the south of Bangladesh, crisscrossed by many rivers, making it difficult to access. The city of Barisal itself is approachable by road (and river), but Mehendiganj can be reached only by river. It takes two hours on average to get to Mehendiganj from Barisal City by motor launches. It takes much longer by other vehicles, such as traditional boats. Mehendiganj UpHC was also a 31-bed facility, but was recently upgraded to a 50-bed facility; construction work was still taking place at the time of data collection, hindering treatment temporarily.

Kashipur falls under the catchment area of the "highest performing" Dhamrai *upazila*, whereas Charlata is within the "lowest performing" Mehendiganj *upazila*. The educational qualification and average monthly household income of the villagers correspond with the performance of the *upazilas* they fall under. Table 8.3 details the sociodemographics of the two villages.

Table 8.2 Index of performance of 20 UpHCs

Name	Health status	Responsiveness	Fairness in finance	Stewardship	Financing	Service provision	Resource generation	Performance index
Sonargaon	5.00	7.03	3.50	2.49	2.50	7.41	8.00	51.45
Savar	7.50	6.28	6.00	3.36	2.50	8.07	9.00	62.49
Kaliakair	8.50	6.99	1.50	3.40	3.75	7.26	5.00	53.38
Harirampur	5.50	6.07	9.50	3.54	2.50	6.24	6.50	60.93
Dhamrai	8.50	6.83	5.50	7.63	3.00	8.50	7.50	68.30
Nawabganj	8.50	5.74	1.50	3.64	3.00	6.71	7.50	52.33
Keraniganj	3.75	5.86	5.00	3.10	5.00	7.93	6.75	52.00
Dohar	8.00	6.25	4.00	2.91	3.50	7.10	7.50	57.51
Belabo	6.00	4.88	4.00	2.60	5.50	6.89	7.00	51.74
Bandar	2.50	6.17	6.50	3.56	3.50	7.77	7.00	52.16
Wazirpur	7.50	6.36	3.50	1.23	4.50	7.19	6.50	54.15
Muladi	8.00	5.61	5.00	1.44	4.00	8.50	9.00	60.16
Babuganj	6.50	4.00	7.50	1.66	4.00	6.46	6.00	54.12
Agailjhara	8.50	4.57	3.50	1.06	4.00	6.44	6.00	50.63
Gaurnadi	9.00	5.10	0.50	1.24	4.50	7.88	8.50	51.32
Banaripara	8.00	4.78	7.50	1.38	6.50	7.76	6.00	62.19
Bakerganj	7.00	4.51	3.50	1.07	4.50	5.79	6.00	47.39
Hizla	8.00	4.51	4.50	1.03	5.00	6.56	6.50	53.12
Mehendiganj	5.00	4.36	2.50	1.84	3.50	8.25	6.50	43.82
Bamna	7.00	4.29	2.50	1.07	5.00	6.71	7.00	47.36

Table 8.3 Sociodemographic characteristics of the respondents

Variable: number (%)	Kashipur (Dhamrai)	Charlata (Mehendiganj)	Total
Number of respondents	100 (44.44)	125 (55.56)	225 (100)
Age in years: mean (SD*)	41.13 (11.38)	42.27 (10.63)	41.76 (10.96)
Gender			
Male	44 (44)	81 (64.8)	125 (55.6)
Female	56 (56)	44 (35.2)	100 (44.4)
Age of marriage: mean (SD)	17.3 (4.09)	18.63 (3.18)	18.04 (3.67)
Number of family members: mean (SD)	5.27 (2.51)	5.67 (1.88)	5.49 (2.18)
Educational qualification			
Illiterate	48 (48)	95 (76)	143 (63.6)
Primary (classes 1–5)	43 (43)	29 (23.2)	72 (32)
Secondary (classes 6–10)	6 (6)	1 (0.8)	7 (3.1)
Higher secondary (classes 11–12)	3 (3)	0 (0)	3 (1.3)
Average household income per month in Taka: mean (SD)	14015 (22157.11)	4576.8 (3994.37)	8771.56 (15744.91)
Occupation (multiple response allowed)			
Farming on own land	46 (46)	39 (31.2)	85 (37.8)
Agricultural labourer	7 (7)	11 (8.8)	18 (8)
Day labourer	16 (16)	31 (24.8)	47 (20.9)
Poultry farmer	4 (4)	0 (0)	4 (1.8)
Dairy farmer	3 (3)	0 (0)	3 (1.3)
Service holder	21 (21)	19 (15.2)	40 (17.8)
Small trade** or business holder	23 (23)	75 (60)	98 (43.6)
Lives abroad	32 (32)	10 (8)	42 (18.7)
Other	1 (1)	3 (2.4)	4 (1.8)

*SD = standard deviation
**Small trade includes village tea stalls, small grocery shops, itinerant vendors, etc.
While similar in many respects, Charlata respondents differ from those in Kashipur
in being poorer, less educated, and less engaged in agriculture, while a much higher
number report being involved in trade or business.

Table 8.4 details data from a sample of 225 respondents. It demonstrates that individuals in Kashipur self-reported their health status as better compared to respondents in Charlata. Individuals in Charlata, despite the low quality of care, tended to visit the UpHC more often, possibly because they did not have any alternative. The qualitative part of this study indicated that the on-site health-education session was satisfactory in Dhamrai, but community-based household visits by government health educators were more frequent in Charlata. The use of safe water and sanitation and hygiene practices have improved over

Table 8.4 Health status and access to health care

Variable	Kashipur (Dhamrai)	Charlata (Mehendiganj)
Self-reported health status (number, %)		
Bad	1 (1)	23 (18.4)
Moderate	71 (71)	101 (80.8)
Good	28 (28)	1 (0.8)
Who usually treats the patient (number, %)		
Traditional healer	1 (1)	4 (3.2)
Village doctor	40 (40)	79 (63.2)
Private hospital/clinic	99 (99)	1 (0.8)
Union subcentre	0 (0)	10 (8)
UpHC	0 (0)	108 (86.4)
Ever visited the UpHC		
Yes	61 (61)	125 (100)
No	39 (39)	0
Anyone ever visited to deliver health education		
Yes	4 (4)	125 (100)
No	96 (96)	0 (0)
Uses safe water (tube-well or boiled water)		
Yes	100 (100)	125 (100)
No	0 (0)	0 (0)
Has sanitary latrine at home		
Yes	99 (99)	112 (89.6)
No	1 (1)	13 (10.4)
Washes hands with soap before eating or cooking and after latrine use		
Yes	98 (98)	116 (92.8)
Sometimes	1 (1)	1 (0.8)
No	1 (1)	8 (6.4)
Where the last child was born		
Home/ paternal home	85 (92.4)	123 (100)
Private hospital/ clinic	7 (7.6)	0 (0)
Received antenatal care		
Yes	17 (18.5)	15 (12.2)
No	75 (81.5)	108 (87.8)
Vaccination status of the child		
Vaccinated	74 (80.4)	121 (98.4)
Not vaccinated	18 (19.6)	2 (1.6)
Availability of medicines at UpHC		
Always available	1 (1)	0 (0)
Sometimes available	7 (7)	0 (0)
Rarely available	92 (92)	125 (100)

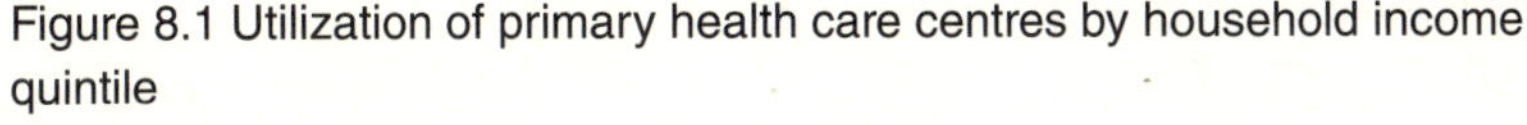

Figure 8.1 Utilization of primary health care centres by household income quintile

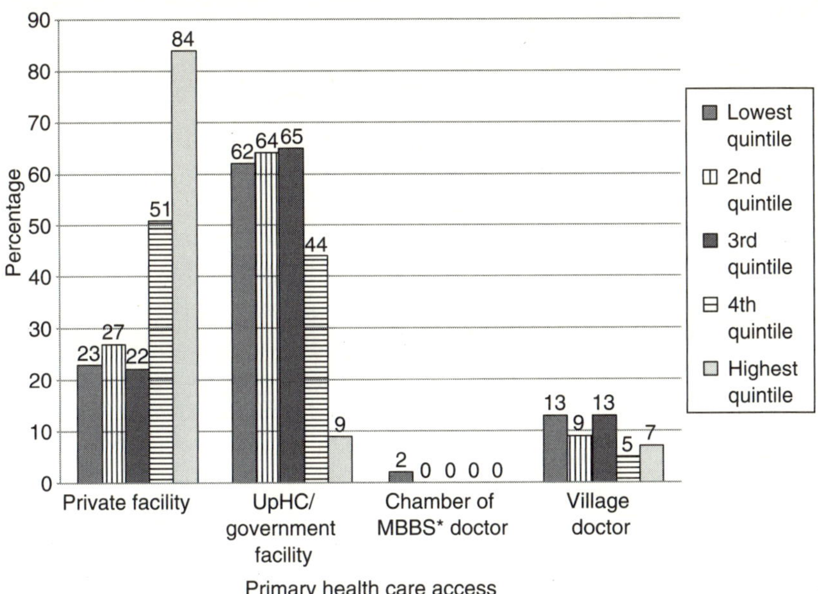

*Bachelor of Medicine, Bachelor of Surgery (basic medical graduation degree)

past years, which is supported by the study findings as well. But the low rate of ANC is still staggering, with more than 80% of women going without such care, and 90% to 100% delivering at home. The Expanded Program on Immunization has traditionally been one of the most successful health programs, having been delivered via a close partnership between government and NGOs. The lack of availability of drugs created a sorry figure in both health complexes, and the qualitative part of this study revealed ignorance among physicians about any such thing as an "essential drug list."

EQUITY ACROSS SOCIAL DETERMINANTS OF HEALTH

UpHCs were mostly used by individuals from the three lowest income quintiles, whereas individuals from the two highest income groups mostly visited private facilities when seeking care. Another feature in the utilization of UpHCs was the difference in the gender of the

Table 8.5 Gender difference in utilization of UpHCs

	Went to UpHC	Did not go to UpHC
Male	58.6%	41.0%
Female	41.4%	59.0%
Total	100.0%	100.0%

Table 8.6 Use of mass media disaggregated by village

	Kashipur	Charlata
Television	100 (100%)	5 (4.0%)
Radio	0 (0%)	119 (95.2%)
Newspaper	0 (0%)	1 (0.8%)

(Pearson Chi-square P-value < 0.05)

patients: 58.6% of those who had visited the health complexes were male (Table 8.5). Despite deliberate efforts by service providers to maintain privacy for female patients, the social norm of discouraging females from being referred to male physicians might be the reason for low utilization by females.

Every individual had access to some source of information through mass media. Forty-three percent of households had at least one mobile phone among family members. The type of mass media providing the most health information varied between the two villages (Table 8.6). Kashipur, being close to Dhaka, had better network access to television, while radio was the main source of information in Charlata.

Sixty-three percent of respondents of Kashipur said that there had been no decision-making fora on health, while 35% expressed ignorance of any such fora. In Charlata, all the respondents confidently said that there had never been any such forum. Our qualitative interviews discovered that the Expanded Program on Immunization camps, a potential source of community decision making, were usually arranged in the courtyards of local elites. Some families felt discouraged from going to the households of these individuals due to local politics or social issues.

These problems were expected to be solved with the introduction of community clinics, which could be used for Expanded Program on Immunization initiatives and for community-based health fora. The government relaunched community clinics in 2009 for every area with a population of at least 6,000. Community clinics are designed to be run by community groups, each consisting of 11 members. Only two

Table 8.7 Suggested mechanisms for client feedback

Suggestion	Percentage
Government staff can visit households to receive complaints	0.5
Install a complaint box	6.7
Local government members can be involved	0.4
Appoint someone to receive complaint	92.4

of those members can be from the government health department; the other nine are selected from the community. The government has issued specific guidelines on membership of community groups. In brief, these groups must consist of local government members, local elites, retired teachers or government staff, and land owners, among others. One of the two government members must be a health assistant, and the other a family welfare assistant. These 11 members self-appoint a president, vice-president, secretary general, and treasurer. Community clinics thus are regarded as a potential source of community participation in decision making on health services.

The client-feedback mechanism was found to be unsatisfactory in all UpHCs (Table 8.7). The formal mechanism for providing feedback was to deposit a written complaint to the UH&FPO in a complaint box or directly with the doctor. However, no written complaints were ever deposited, for a number of reasons. First, the population's literacy level is too low to lodge a written complaint. Second, lodging a complaint letter is not common in Bangladeshi culture; indeed, people are hesitant in general about writing anything that leaves their name on record. Third, doctors occupy a very high position in Bangladesh's social hierarchy, so people feel they cannot write anything against them. In addition, even though the UH&FPO indicated that lodging written complaints was the feedback mechanism, most individuals were not even aware this mechanism existed. Instead, in the event of serious issues, individuals typically would address local leaders. Hence, in the case of incidents such as serious mishandling of a patient or the death of a patient due to physician negligence, individuals would resort to going to their local leaders. It was expected that the local leader would go forward and talk to the UpHC authority.

Regarding their ability to hold the decision makers accountable, one patient from Mehendiganj acerbically remarked, "Here we get some medication, however trivial it might be; that's all we can expect. How can we hold these important persons responsible?" There was no formal way to challenge the accountability of UpHC personnel. As a result, a set of informal ways had evolved, ranging from shouting and quarreling to even physically abusing the health-care providers. We heard many stories from the patients about negligence and misbehaviour of the health-care providers, which the patients were powerless to address. According to the patients, "Accountability is there, but it can be sought only by the influential people; not by the common patients."

As there was no social health insurance or community-based health insurance coverage in either of the *upazilas*, health-care payment was on an out-of-pocket only basis. In most of the UpHCs, user fees are not imposed, and health care is supposed to be absolutely free of cost as long as the required service is available. Mehendiganj was an exception, as it was under a pilot project to evaluate imposing user fees at the UpHC level. Though the pilot project was already formally concluded at the time of our data collection, the Mehendiganj UpHC authority continued collecting user fees because a government directive had not been issued to withdraw them. Each patient had to pay 3 Taka (approximately 4 cents) for entry into the health centre. In addition, they had to pay for laboratory facilities, indoor facilities, and other hospital facilities according to rates set by the government. They received only free medication, on condition of availability.

In both UpHCs, we found patients who had been encumbered with impoverishing health expenditures. One patient described the story of his nephew:

> Both his kidneys have stopped functioning. Every day my sister has to bring him to Dhaka city. They have attached a pipe to his mouth, which needs to be cleaned every day. Fortunately, she has another son who lives abroad and supports the treatment; not everyone has that luck. Still they had to sell their calf and much of their properties to get their son treated.

Common complaints in Mehendiganj and, to a lesser extent, in Dhamrai included shortages of medicine and patients having to find and purchase medicines on their own.

In addition to the user fees, patients in Mehendiganj vehemently complained of doctors taking on private-practice consultations in the UpHCs and during office hours. One patient commented,

> We have to buy all the medication. On top of that we have to bear the doctor's fees, otherwise the doctor doesn't tend to the patient sincerely.

Sometimes they even unnecessarily send the patient to Barisal [nearest district town] just to harass us. That certainly costs us a lot more than the doctor's fees. We most despise such practice during office hours. If we do not give them the private practice fee of 20 Taka [approximately 30 cents] and buy a user fee ticket of 3 Taka, then we have to wait hours after hours while the doctors remain busy with their private-practice patients.

We found claims of private practice during office hours to be true. When we asked the doctors about their private practice in the health centre and during office hours, they responded amiably, outlining their part of the story. Private practice by public-service doctors is not prohibited after office hours and outside the hospital premises. In fact, it is rather widely practiced all over the country as a means for ill-paid doctors to augment their livelihood. Mehendiganj is a desolate island, disconnected from surrounding small islands, and it cannot be approached easily by patients whenever they desire or need care. Therefore, doctors made themselves available to help those who managed to come to the island during regular office hours and were willing to be treated privately. If these doctors, like those in other parts of the country, practiced in the evening hours, they would not have patients, because of the geography of the region. Therefore, a posting in Mehendiganj itself was difficult for doctors; how could they afford further disadvantage in being deprived of their legitimate income through private practice? The exceptional geography and conditions of the area compelled the doctors to take on their private practice during office hours and, as they could not leave the office during that time, they saw their private patients on the health-centre premises. They claimed that they attended both the private patients and general patients simultaneously, with equal importance. They opposed the accusation of discrimination against general patients.

DEVOLUTION OF HEALTH SERVICES

Each UpHC has a health management committee that includes the member of parliament, *upazila* chairman (a local government leader), UH&FPO, *upazila* nirbahi officer (the administrative head of the *upazila*), and other government high officials at the *upazila* level. There is no direct link between the community and the health management committee, except for the involvement of the member of parliament and the *upazila* chairman. These public representatives are not formally linked to the community in terms of health issues unless an individual approaches them on his/her own. In addition, these members are not formally empowered by the state regarding their administrative domain of involvements, roles, and responsibilities.

Most of the key informants and health personnel opined strongly in favour of delegating more authority to the UpHC administration. As one key informant explained,

> Suppose the ceiling fan of the patient waiting area has gone out of order. They repeatedly come to me and complain. If I send a requisition to the authority for it to be fixed I have to go through protracted administrative hassles. It may take even such a long time that summer may subside. By the time the fan is repaired there is no necessity for a fan anymore, because it is winter. The patients are not going to understand my limitations; they will simply blame me.

Another key informant shared his experience of visiting health centres in Malaysia and Thailand where, he claimed, "health centres enjoy much more autonomy both in terms of finance and recruitment. They can raise their own money, spend it according to need, and can employ the type of personnel particularly required for that health centre."

Although the health personnel demanded autonomy, they did not agree with the idea of complete devolution, by which local leaders would have administrative superiority over health-sector personnel. During the regime of General Hussain Muhammad Ershad such reform was attempted and faced strong opposition from the doctors. "Doctors will never agree to be held accountable by less educated local leaders," mentioned one of our key informants, who spent his whole career in PHC delivery before retiring. He added, "Although there are examples of such local-level committees supervising the health facilities in developed countries, it will not work in the Bangladeshi context where local leaders are rather more corrupted on top of being uneducated."

There were some preventive programs in the UpHCs designed through a top-down approach from the Directorate General of Health Services (DGHS). Every UpHC is instructed to maintain a disease profile, which is supplied by the DGHS. However, the list of diseases in the disease profile often did not contain the name of a certain disease that might be prevalent in that particular area. No epidemiological survey had been conducted to formally identify locally endemic diseases or environment-specific injuries in order to devise appropriate prevention and control strategies. An example of this is kala-azar (visceral leishmaniasis), which was endemic in Dhamrai. Treatment of kala-azar was available in the UpHC, but there was no facility for diagnosing it by the simple Aldehyde Test. Mehendiganj, surrounded by water and having many ponds, had an alarming number of drowning cases; intubation facilities and oxygen supplies, which are critical for treating drowning cases, were absent. Snake bites arising from chars (a newly emerged strip of sandy land rising out of the river bed above the water level) were also common, and yet there was also a chronic shortage of polyvalent antivenoms, which are essential for snake-bite treatment.

Promotion of food supply and proper nutrition was found to be grossly neglected in PHC delivery everywhere, although some vertical and temporary nutrition projects were implemented without any follow-up and scaling-up mechanism. In Dhamrai UpHC, we found a tin shed that had previously been used as a "nutrition unit" under a vertical nutrition project. During our observation, this shed was being used as a recreation room for the nurses. Remarks by the UH&FPO on the facility reflected a lack of ownership over such vertical projects: "It was their [donor/government] project. As the project is over, the necessity of the building is over as well." There was no facility for growth monitoring of newborns, supplementary feeding, breastfeeding counselling, or any other nutrition-related activities in the centre, let alone initiatives for household food security, which was one of the commitments of PHC. The only nutrition-related activity remaining at the *upazila* level was staff carrying out growth monitoring of pregnant mothers.

Despite a shortage of medicines, necessary surgical instruments, and required health workforce, Mehendiganj UpHC was found to possess an "ambulance." The UH&FPO of Mehendiganj, however, pointed out,

> Yes, there is one ambulance … But where is the road here in this desolate island to run this ambulance? Each UpHC was allotted one ambulance, so we also got one. No one even thought where the ambulance will run and how patients will be carried from here to somewhere else; there is no road connection from Mehendiganj to any place.

Mehendiganj is, rather, in need of a water ambulance. Critical patients have no way to get to the UpHC other than waiting for the steamer to arrive. Relatively solvent patients hire speedboats from Barisal to carry them. There are 13 *unions* under Mehendiganj *upazila*, among which only three are connected by roads, but these are unpaved. Moreover, the roads are too narrow for the ambulance. Therefore, patients usually travel to the health centre by "rickshaw-van," while the ambulance, along with its driver, lies idle, without any visible utility.

SUGGESTIONS AND RECOMMENDATIONS BY RESPONDENTS

The existing PHC model in Bangladesh is based on scenarios from the past when communicable diseases were more prevalent. In accordance with the epidemiological transition pervading Bangladesh, emphasis is now necessary on noncommunicable diseases, elder health, psychiatric disorders, and different types of disabilities. Improving urban primary health care, establishing a nutrition unit in each UpHC, and ensuring availability of essential drugs were also suggested as vital. As well, study participants implied that the list of available drugs should be regularly updated and displayed. Provision for alternative resources was also suggested (e.g., a chlorine solution could be locally produced for infection prevention).

Our UpHC patient-respondents made innovative suggestions about how they could attain their health entitlements. Information is imperative in empowering the community; mass media can play a pivotal role in informing people of their health entitlements. In addition, communication materials regarding entitlements and aimed at changing patient behaviour towards those entitlements can be developed and disseminated. Information regarding available facilities at the health centres can also be included with the health communication materials. Currently these materials focus only on health practices, such as handwashing and sanitary latrine use. There is already a wide network of government health workers who are primarily responsible for disseminating health-education messages. These health workers can play a fundamental role by informing people of available services and their health-care entitlements.

To improve community empowerment, it was recommended that local government play a more active role. Respondents suggested that the local government could organize regular community meetings to discuss health issues. These meetings could also pave the way for members of the community to express their complaints and experiences regarding their encounters with health facilities.

Resources are allocated via a top-down approach, without a recognition of the needs of the particular area. Studies should be undertaken to determine the epidemiological patterns in an area to decide on what kind of drugs should be dispensed there and in which season. UpHCs or local authorities should be consulted before allocating certain resources, such as evidenced in the case of an ambulance delivered to a community without paved roads or petrol pumps. The health centre must have certain levels of autonomy over the resources it generates. Awaiting a central decision for petty expenditures compromises the quality of services and, at the same time, puts people at risk of being deprived of emergency medical services. Issues related to health should be brought under a unique coordinating body. For example, water and sanitation is closely related to health, and the activities of that department directly influence health outcomes. Therefore, there should be clear guidelines regarding coordination among different departments with mandates affecting health.

A separate cadre for nonclinicians responsible for public health administration, management, and research should be developed, to enable clinicians to conduct their clinical responsibilities. It was observed that field staff from both the health and family-planning departments were going to the same households with similar health messages. To avoid this duplication of service, waste of resources, tension between two cadres, and confusion among the community, the service providers suggested effective removal of the health-family planning dichotomy to create a single category of health worker.

Discussion and Conclusion

The household survey, qualitative interviews, and the PRA were conducted to examine the state of education concerning prevailing health problems and the methods of preventing and controlling them. Topics surveyed related to the promotion of food supplies and proper nutrition, the supply of safe water and basic sanitation, maternal and child health care (including family planning), immunization against major infectious diseases, the prevention and control of locally endemic diseases, the treatment of common diseases and injuries, and the provision of essential drugs. In terms of water, sanitation, and immunization the findings were satisfactory, although the village under the "highest performing" *upazila* fared slightly better in most of the indicators.

The nutrition component is not functioning in most of the UpHCs, including in the two UpHCs where we conducted our study. The supply of safe water and basic sanitation is not the responsibility of the health sector, but rather of the Department of Public Health Engineering. Maternal and child health care is delivered under the DGHS, whereas family planning is under the aegis of the Directorate General of Family

Planning. Although both the directorates are under the Ministry of Health and Family Welfare, the placement of these components under different directorates creates resource mismanagement, professional schisms, confusion, frustration and, consequently, inefficiencies.

The fragmentation of PHC has also affected access to medicines. There is no recognized list of essential drugs, and the availability of drugs is unsatisfactory. A comprehensive approach would also take into consideration the recent trends of demographic and epidemiologic transitions: noncommunicable diseases, elder health, urban health, and the health concerns of disabled persons should be included in the package.

The survey also shed some light on the condition of the referral system, which, again, is related to a number of issues involving service delivery, accessibility, and equity in service utilization. The study found that there is no functional integrity in the referral system. Service delivery and utilization is inequitably distributed among the population along gender and income quintiles. Richer people can access health centres more quickly than the poor. Long waiting times, less contact time, lack of service-provider responsiveness, scarcity of medicine and equipment, unavailability of appropriate health professionals, and lack of trust provoke the people to bypass the lower referral level and seek care at distant health facilities, notwithstanding higher personal cost. Furthermore, it is difficult to refer patients to a higher health facility, as there is no appropriate referral facility in place.

Finally, an important component of our CPHC model is community empowerment and participation. Access to information, participation in decision-making fora, and the ability to challenge the transparency and accountability of decision makers were identified as important factors by our respondents. Adoption of these recommendations demands further operational research. For instance, studies should be commissioned to understand the variable dynamics of different components of CPHC and to identify the resources that may be required to upgrade the existing system to a comprehensive model.

ACKNOWLEDGMENTS

This research was conducted at James P Grant School of Public Health, BRAC University, Bangladesh. The authors want to acknowledge the contributions their colleagues at BRAC University, including Nahitun Naher, Shafiun Nahin

Shimul, AKM Shahidullah, Jahid Ali, and Hena Akhter. We also acknowledge the contribution of our respondents and other relevant persons from Dhamrai and Mehendiganj *upazilas*, Bangladesh.

REFERENCES

Bangladesh Health Watch. (2008). *The state of the health in Bangladesh 2007: Health workforce in Bangladesh: Who constitutes the healthcare system?* Dhaka: James P Grant School of Public Health.

Cockcroft, A., Andersson, N., Milne, D., Hossain, M.Z., & Karim, E. (2007, February 26). What did the public think of health services reform in Bangladesh? Three national community-based surveys 1999–2003. *Health Research Policy and Systems*, 5(1), 1–7. http://dx.doi.org/10.1186/1478-4505 -5-1 Medline:17324263

Government of Bangladesh. (2014). *Health bulletin 2014.* Dhaka. Retrieved from http://www.dghs.gov.bd/images/docs/Publicaations/HB_2014 _2nd_Edition_060115.pdf

Joint Learning Initiative. (2004). *Human resources for health: Overcoming the crisis.* Boston: Harvard University Press.

Osman, F.A. (2004). *A study of the health policy process: Policy making in Bangladesh* (1st ed.). Dhaka, Bangladesh: A H Development Publishing House.

World Bank. (2015). *World development indicators.* Retrieved from http://data .worldbank.org/data-catalog/world-development-indicators

World Health Organization. (2000). *The world health report 2000: Health systems: Improving performance.* Geneva: Author.

SECTION THREE

Community Health Workers

In the countries where our funded projects undertook research, a diversity of community health workers (termed in different contexts as health extension workers, lay workers, or outreach workers) could be found contributing to CPHC. Several *RHFA* projects focused on community health workers: one each in Iran and India, two in Ethiopia, and one centred on the Māori of Aotearoa/New Zealand. This focus is unsurprising given the importance of community health workers (CHWs) as first contacts and (in some instances) primary-care providers in PHC services and the role CHWs play in linking people to formal health systems, in facilitating action on local social and environmental determinants, and in being conduits for community participation.

The **Iranian** study on *behvarz* (the Farsi name for CHWs, meaning "good skills") examined the barriers and enablers of rural CHWs in delivering CPHC over the last three decades. *Behvarz* are almost equally divided between men and women, with men primarily dealing with environmental health issues, and women with maternal and child health issues – a gendered division of labour common throughout similar programs in areas where more traditional patriarchal norms still prevail. Unlike many programs, however, *behvarz* are paid employees of the Iranian health system who act as important agents of change in their societies. They do so by mobilizing community resources, attending social events, consulting with religious leaders, acting as advocates on different issues for their communities, and building intersectoral and collaborative team action. Based on text analyses, interviews, and secondary data, there was substantial evidence of CPHC in the *behvarz* program, including significant improvements in rural health outcomes that were strongly related to the program. Over time, the mandates of *behvarz* expanded to incorporate new roles in school, occupational, mental, and elder health, indicative of its aim to be comprehensive. The findings of the Iranian team reinforced the importance of employing *behvarz* from within geographic or cultural communities, while also cautioning about such workers becoming burdened with an ever-growing list of functions, from primary care to social determinants of health.

India's accredited social health activists (ASHA) program is a cornerstone of a renewed effort (the National Health Mission) to revitalize a weak public health system. Relying on volunteer village-level female health workers, it has shown positive outcomes in different states of the country. Our study team was based in a district in North Bihar, one of the least developed regions in the country, and found that the role and training attributed to CHWs are keys to ensuring their status, and thus their credibility and effectiveness, within the communities they serve. Our team revealed weaknesses in this training, and in the recruitment and operational roles of many of the ASHAs. Support of ASHAs by village councils was often lacking, while the financial incentives offered to ASHAs (such as payment tied to immunization or ensuring prenatal visits) limited the ability of ASHAs to engage in community-defined SDH. If provided quality training and appropriate pay, CHWs such as ASHAs can act as health promoters precisely where promotion should be targeted: within local communities, schools, and even homes. Providing them a voice in health-care planning is also important, as they are the interlocutors of the community they serve. Significantly, our study led to improvements in the program, and our team discovered that the ASHAs themselves were organizing into a union to advance their own role and status within the health system.

Our **Ethiopian** team based in Jimma worked with health extension workers (HEWs) to see how coverage and comprehensiveness of PHC services delivered in rural settings could be improved. As with the *behvarz* program in Iran, the HEW program in Ethiopia is widely regarded as one of the more ambitious initiatives to expand PHC coverage in recent years. Similar to the Iranian program, HEWs in Ethiopia are trained paid staff of the country's public health system. Our Jimma team found that, despite many uphill battles, the HEWs were continuously working towards ISA for improved CPHC services. For instance, the HEWs worked with the educational sector, primarily with schools, delivering health activities and messages on a weekly basis (e.g., delivering immunizations and discussing nutrition and ways to improve access to a safer water supply). They also worked with agricultural development

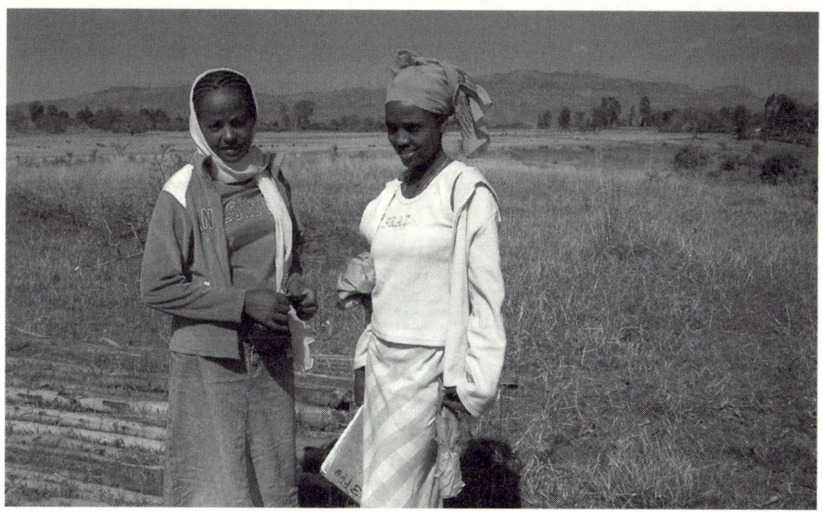

Health extension workers on their way to home visits, Southwest Ethiopia

agents to campaign on methods to prevent malaria and ensure food security and thus prevent malnutrition. The HEWs were able to work with almost all cultural, religious, and administrative structures but had little impact on ISA other than those just mentioned. This seemed largely due to the sheer difficulty in mobilizing intersectoral collaboration at higher levels, which was beyond the capacity of the HEWs. One interesting finding was that HEWs quickly became identified as the "go to" people for any new initiative that required local intersectoral collaboration (regardless of which sector it emanated from). While this development embodied the goal of CPHC in having PHC serve as a conduit for ISA, it also increased the risk of the workloads of and demands upon HEWs becoming unmanageable – reflecting the similar caution expressed about the expanding mandate of *behvarz* in Iran.

The Tigray-based team in **Ethiopia** investigated the contribution of HEWs in improving the utilization of maternal health services in three districts in Northern Ethiopia. These services included family planning, antenatal care, birth assistance, postnatal care, and HIV testing. The team employed mixed methods, including a qualitative component that explored community participation and ISA advanced through the work of HEWs, and a cross-sectional survey to examine how effectively the program enabled access to services. Although not presented in this book, the team's qualitative study did find instances of increased community participation via the HEWs and, as with the Jimma study, documented local examples of intersectoral collaborations. The team's principle findings arose from the survey, which is the focus of their chapter. When compared to findings from earlier surveys, the Tigray study found substantial increases in access to family planning, ANC, and HIV testing following the introduction of the HEW program. There was little change in utilization of health facilities for delivery, however, with the exception of the "model families" who participate with the HEWs as voluntary health workers within local villages.

One of our Indigenous teams in **Aotearoa/New Zealand** was unable to contribute a chapter but did prepare a short report summarizing its key findings:

The Role of the Community Health Worker
in a Māori Person's Health Journey[1]

We conducted a case study of a Māori CPHC provider in Aotearoa/New Zealand – Kokiri Marae Health and Social Services (KMHSS). KMHSS is a long-established urban health provider based at a marae (a Māori meeting place) located in an industrial area of New Zealand's capital city, Wellington. KMHSS has a strong reputation for effectively engaging with Māori whānau (extended families), principally through the work of Māori community health workers (CHWs). Four key findings arose out of our study on the role of the Māori CHW.

First, Māori CHWs provide culturally distinctive care that is centred on the person and the whanau rather than on the health system. Second, CHWs play a vital role in improving access not only to health care but also to social services in general and to the social determinants of health. Third, CHWs add significant value as team members of Māori CPHC, improving both service delivery and links with other agencies. Finally, there are significant challenges facing both CHWs and KMHSS, which employs them, with regard to the underresourcing of the CHW role.

---

1 The researchers on this project who prepared this summary were Tania Forrest, Pat Neuwelt, Rowena Gotty, and Sue Crengle.

Our study found that Māori, as is likely the case for others who experience poverty and high health needs, are unable to manoeuvre in the complex systems of "care." CHWs serve as an important "bridge" between agencies, services, communities, and people with health needs. Indigenous CHWs engage in therapeutic relationships with people with whom they share community links, cultural knowledge, and similar life circumstances. They are in the strongest position of anyone in the CPHC team to hold that therapeutic relationship, if they are carefully chosen for the role.

Māori and other nonprofit CPHC providers in New Zealand committed to reducing health inequities employ CHWs to ensure their services are accessible, appropriate, and comprehensive for populations with the worst health outcomes and lowest rates of health-service utilization relative to their need. As one CHW interviewed in this study noted, before the CHW service was instituted, Māori people were sent here and there for medical tests "… but really it's about housing, income, stress, and all that." In the words of one client interviewed, "I was chasing the medication path [to deal with] my asthma, but I knew it was mainly the problems with the damp and coldness of the house. The [CHW] helped us get into another place and helped with the housing people and all that." Another study participant also emphasized how CHWs ensured a comprehensive approach to health: "Since I met [the CHW], it's like all these other services came with her."

Overall, Māori CHWs were found to be critical "access enablers." They play a valuable role in enabling multidisciplinary interventions to occur in a manner that is acceptable to the Māori and are integral to the implementation of "by-Māori-to-Māori" health-care delivery. They have become heavily relied upon for CPHC delivery to the Māori people. And yet, like many of their CHW counterparts in other countries, they are largely undervalued, underpaid, and underresourced, with insecure jobs. In New Zealand, this may relate to the fact that this profession remains unregulated.

9 The Contribution of Community Health Workers to the Implementation of Comprehensive Primary Health Care in Rural Settings, Iran

SARA JAVANPARAST, FRAN BAUM,
AND GHOLAMREZA HEIDARI

Background

Iran is a country of mountains, plateaus, and deserts that borders on Iraq, Turkey, Pakistan, Afghanistan, Armenia, Azerbaijan, and Turkmenistan. In 2011, the Iranian population was 74,961,720, with 29% of the population living in rural areas (Statistical Center of Iran, 2012).

The Declaration of Alma-Ata adopted at the International Conference on Primary Health Care (World Health Organization [WHO], 1978) coincided with the Iranian revolution, which spawned enormous political and social changes within the country and became the basis for a major health-system reform. The primary aim of this reform was to improve access to health care for disadvantaged groups and to reduce urban-rural disparities in health outcomes. A new health system was developed for a more equitable allocation of health resources based on the principles of PHC, although Iran's experience with PHC pre-dated the Declaration of Alma-Ata. In 1972, the Iranian Ministry of Health, in collaboration with the WHO, undertook a project in Iran's province of Azerbaijan on health-service expansion that was principally based on a PHC approach.

Reforms to the health system saw a number of strategies adopted to address shortages in the health workforce and improve access to basic health-care services, particularly in underprivileged areas, including the integration of medical education and health-care services (Khojasteh, Momtazmanesh, Entezari, & Einollahi, 2009), establishment of a rural and urban PHC network, and development of the community health worker (CHW) program.

At Alma-Ata, CHWs were identified as one of the cornerstones of comprehensive primary health care (CPHC). More recently, the concept of "task shifting" developed by the WHO, has emphasized the expansion of tasks undertaken by CHWs to address the current shortage of human resources for health (WHO, 2008).

CHWs in rural Iran

Iranian CHWs, called *behvarz* in Farsi, are locally sourced and paid health workers with specialized training in rural health needs. The village health house is the most peripheral health-delivery facility in rural areas and the place from which the *behvarz* works. Each health house is designed to cover a target population of about 1,500. According to the most recent statistics, in 2007 there were an estimated 17,000 health houses in Iran with almost 31,000 male and female *behvarz* covering most of Iran's 65,000 villages (Ministry of Health and Medical Education [MOHME], 2008).

In recruiting *behvarz*, criteria such as age, gender, education, and area of residence are taken into consideration. The selection and recruitment process strongly reflects the WHO definition of CHWs as "members of the communities where they work... [and] selected by their communities" (WHO, 1989). There is strong evidence of the engagement of local people, religious leaders, and rural families in the selection of *behvarz*. By 2004, a more formal process involving *behvarz* recruitment committees was established in each district to identify villages that were short of *behvarz* and to advertise vacancies.

Behvarz deliver a wide variety of health programs. They also play a crucial role in implementing major components of CPHC, including community engagement, health promotion, and intersectoral collaboration. Close relationships and trust between *behvarz* and their surrounding communities facilitate their role as advocates for their community and build collaborative teams for action. Figure 9.1 shows the potential interrelationships between *behvarz* and the health system, as well as between *behvarz* and their own communities.

Since the establishment of the PHC system and the integration of many health programs within the system, the country has made impressive improvements on many health indicators. In particular, the gap between rural and urban areas in terms of various morbidity and mortality indicators has narrowed considerably. A study conducted by

Figure 9.1 The interaction between *behvarz* and the health system and rural community

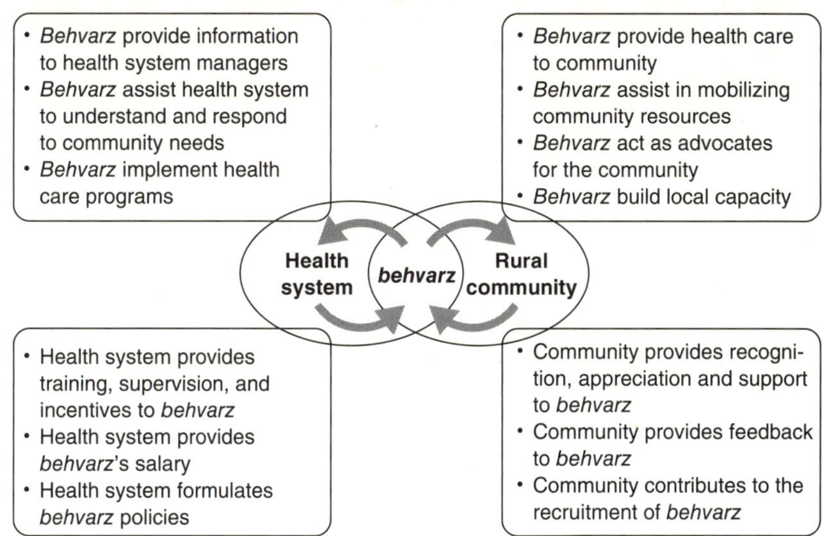

the Statistical Center of Iran between 1973 and 1976 revealed a striking difference in infant mortality rates between rural areas (130 per 1,000 births) and urban areas (13.9 per 1,000 births), attributable mainly to disparities in income, living standards, and access to basic health and social services (MOHME, 2005). This gap closed dramatically after the establishment of PHC in Iran, with its special emphasis on the rural poor. In 1985, rural infant mortality was almost twice that in urban areas (71 versus 33 deaths per 1,000 live births). This gap had narrowed by 1996, with 30.2 infant deaths per 1,000 live births in rural areas versus 27.7 in urban areas (Mehryar, 2004; MOHME, 2005). Rural infant mortality declined further to 23.7 deaths per 1,000 live births in 2003 (Mehryar, 2004). It has been suggested that the significant improvement in rural health outcomes is strongly related to the performance of community-friendly health workers (Mehryar, Aghajanian, Ahmad-Nia, Mirzae, & Naghavi, 2005), although it was unlikely to have been achieved through PHC alone as the period also saw economic growth, a rise in literacy rates, and improvements in rural infrastructure.

Research Questions and Methods

Despite the long experience with the CHW program in Iran and their recognition by health authorities, studies that assess program effectiveness are principally outcome oriented, with few studies assessing the program from the viewpoint of Iranian CHWs themselves. An exploratory study was undertaken to fill this gap by investigating CHWs' perceptions of their contribution to CPHC in Iran as well as of the barriers and enablers to their ability to implement PHC.

Different sources of evidence, including primary and secondary sources, were pursued. The study included a literature search and a review of policy documents, unpublished reports, and *behvarz* training materials that were available through Ministry of Health archives in Iran. Documentation analysis was complemented by a qualitative study to document the perceptions of *behvarz* of their role within rural communities and their contribution to improved health in that community over time.

Study participants were selected from 18 provinces in Iran. Ninety-one interviews were conducted by three research assistants residing in Iran between October 2009 and February 2010. Interviews were conducted at health houses in rural areas or in district health centres, depending on the preferences of the *behvarz*. Participants were asked questions concerning their recruitment, training, tasks and responsibilities, as well as support and supervision. Their perceptions of barriers to effective program delivery and suggestions for improvement were also sought. Interviews were recorded with the consent of participants, and interview files were transcribed by the three interviewers. All audio tapes were checked against the transcribed text by the principal researcher. Using qualitative content analysis, interview data were coded and main themes were created, based on the key concepts in the study questions. Since the transcripts were in the Farsi language, qualitative-analysis software could not be used and all data were categorized and coded manually. The key themes and illustrative quotes were translated into English by the principal researcher.

Ethics approval from the Iranian Ministry of Health and Flinders University ethics committees were obtained to gain access to *behvarz* policy documents and profiles to assist in conducting the interviews.

Results and Analysis

Both our policy review and interviews with *behvarz* undertaken in this study identified key elements of the *behvarz* program, including tasks

Table 9.1 Characteristics of *behvarz* interviewed

Gender		Age (years)				Work experience (years)			Marital status		Educational level			Place of residence	
		≤ 29	30–39	40–49	≥ 50	≤ 10	11–20	21–30	married	single	primary	secondary	tertiary	urban	rural
F	54	4	31	18	1	8	29	17	48	6	16	35	3	21	33
M	37	3	20	10	4	16	15	6	35	2	7	28	2	10	27

and responsibilities, recruitment, training, support, and supervision. The study placed a special emphasis on how the *behvarz* perceive factors that enable or constrain their ability to contribute to the implementation of CPHC and population health outcomes in rural areas. Table 9.1 shows the characteristics of the 91 participants interviewed in 18 provinces.

The large majority of the *behvarz* interviewed were married, which correlates with their age and years of work experience. While the minimum level of education required for admission into the *behvarz* training program is completion of secondary school, this changed only in 2004. From 1996 to 2004, recruits were required to have a minimum level of primary school education only. The study cohort included older *behvarz*, who entered the CHW program with a primary education. More than two-thirds completed secondary school. It is interesting to note that one-third of the respondents reported their place of residence as "urban." While the *behvarz* program is strictly for the rural areas, some trainees live in urban areas. They may continue to live in their urban residence during their training period but are committed to residing in the village they serve for at least four years after completing their training. Typically, they are placed in villages in which they lived prior to their move to urban centres. The sampled individuals reporting urban residence would have completed this four-year commitment. These individuals travel to and from the health house on a daily basis. They generally have more years of work experience and are older. Typically, they move out of their communities to the nearest urban area because they have older children and wish to access better educational facilities for their children. During the interviews, some participants raised challenges brought on by their urban residence, such as difficulties balancing work requirements and family needs.

Behvarz *training (process and trend)*

From the inception of Iran's *behvarz* program, training has been a key component and has undergone regular review based on changes in health patterns, the qualifications of *behvarz*, and new demands related to their roles. The preservice training program is divided into three blocks over a two-year period and consists of theoretical and practical classes, as well as clinical placements in health houses and rural health centres. *Behvarz* are centrally trained at a district *behvarz* training centre, which is part of the district health system. *Behvarz* trainers have tertiary degrees in family health, disease management, environmental health, midwifery, and nursing. Students receive free training and financial support (free accommodation, meals, transport) throughout their training.

In-service training of *behvarz* has also been recognized in Iran and is formally planned and structured at regular intervals in the form of workshops, monthly meetings, and refresher courses, all aimed at integrating new policies and changes into the *bevharz*'s work.

This study investigated the quality of training courses (pre- and in-service) from the viewpoint of the *behvarz* and how they believe the training courses have impacted their daily performance. The majority of participants believed that the preservice training was comprehensive and included relevant topics that had a huge impact on their capacity to provide health-care services and that built their confidence and skills in communicating with rural people.

The friendly environment of the training centres, the nature of trainer-trainee relationships, and the presence of highly qualified trainers were particularly noted by most participants as features that made training an exciting period in their life and career, and that had a positive impact on learning and motivation: "Behvarz training centre was the most appropriate place for our training, we were as a whole family working together. It was not just about teaching and learning a few topics, it was more about learning life skills, so motivating ... " (male, 22 yrs.).

From the viewpoint of some participants, training courses broadened their understanding of *behvarz* roles and functions. "When I started the course, I thought we are supposed to work like a nurse but after that [training courses] I realized that health education, disease prevention, and promotion is our main job" (male, 34 yrs.).

Clinical placement in the health houses under the direct supervision of the trainers was cited as crucial in gaining work experience, building a relationship with the local community, and collaborating with other local organizations. "During our placement we got to know people and our future work environment. Direct supervision by trainers helped us build up our confidence and to be trusted by the people" (female, 29 yrs.).

While every effort is made to place students in their own villages, some – depending on the number of *behvarz* trainees in the training program at the time and the availability of health houses – have to be placed in a village that is not their own, although still nearby.

The study participants also identified a number of problems related to the preservice training. Centrally produced materials, booklets, and step-by-step guidelines were perceived as didactic by some participants, constraining the adult participatory learning and problem-solving capabilities of the students. This perspective was particularly prominent among younger participants with higher educational qualifications. "There are too many step-by-step guidelines and instructions that we have to follow, we are not given a chance to search, to think, and to analyze things" (male, 28 yrs.).

Behvarz roles and responsibilities

Initially the *behvarz* program focused primarily on infectious diseases and maternal and child health, but changing disease profiles have expanded the range of *behvarz* responsibilities. Figure 9.2 shows the increasing trend in the range and scope of *behvarz* roles that is well-reflected in their training content and topics.

Study respondents ranked their tasks and responsibilities according to importance, workload and time spent on each. Health education, maternal and child health, and environmental health were reported as the most time-consuming responsibilities. For example, "Mothers and children are the most important target groups, so we spend more time on their health care" (female, 44 yrs.), and "Health education is included in all other programs, so the time we spend on it is very high" (female, 38 yrs.).

The role of behvarz gender in providing care

This study revealed that although there is no specific gender-related policy, in practice, task allocation appears to be strongly influenced by cultural and religious beliefs; it often is thought that only female health workers should provide women's care: "Women prefer to be served by me [female *behvarz*] … When a woman comes for family planning services or prenatal care and I'm not in she leaves the health house and won't talk to our male *behvarz*. I think they feel more comfortable with me" (female, 43 yrs.).

Figure 9.2 *Behvarz* training and roles over time

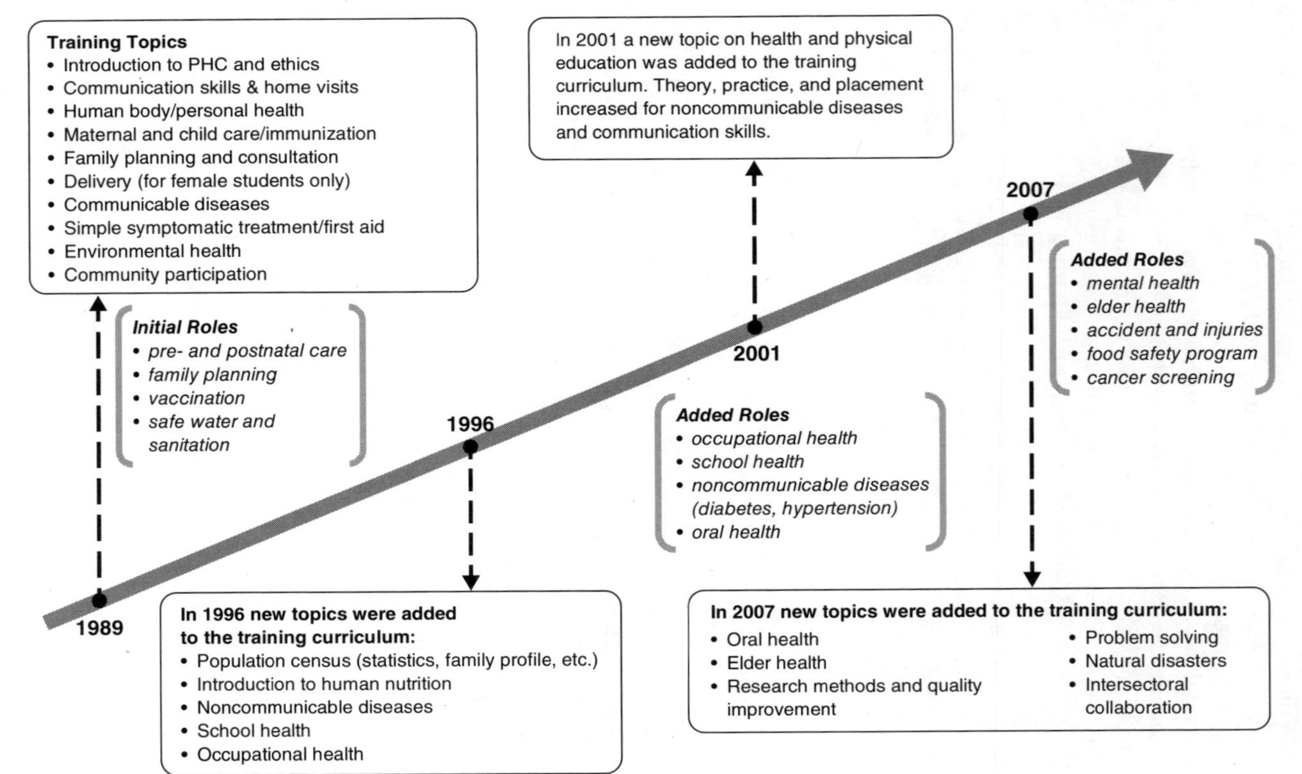

Female *behvarz* are generally responsible for tasks that are performed within the health house such as maternal and child health and recording data, while the male *behvarz* deal with activities outside the health house. "Our male *behvarz* does all the environmental and occupational health so I don't spend too much time on that. It is easier for them to take on the duties outside the health house" (female, 42 yrs.).

These activities include following up on cases of communicable disease, performing environmental checks (e.g., assessing the chloride level of drinking water in rural households, ensuring hygienic toilets, negotiating with other sectors for the collection of domestic waste), and engaging in occupational-health activities such as implementing food-safety programs.

Apart from the roles that are clearly identified in the *behvarz* program, other tasks are performed that are not recognized by the health authorities but which many *behvarz* strongly believe are crucial in building relationships with their rural community and improving program effectiveness. These tasks include attending social events in the rural area and consulting with religious leaders and other trusted people:

> We take advantage of every single opportunity to convey health messages to people so we must attend different social events like religious events or ceremonies. I believe it is part of our job … Or sometimes I've got an old lady coming to check her blood pressure, she wants to sit and chat with me for hours, I have to listen to her … I can't stop her because I have other duties to do. I have to respect her so she respects me back. *(male, 38 yrs.)*

Almost all respondents placed a special emphasis on "health education" as their principal role and as what they saw as the most important factor influencing rural health, followed by environmental health interventions that addressed basic determinants of health related to sanitation, potable water, road safety, and other physical risks. "All these changes that you see in the rural environment are the result of health education provided by us. People's beliefs and behaviour changed a lot and it makes everything easier for us" (male, 46 yrs.).

Behvarz perceptions about their contribution to rural health

The range and scope of activities undertaken by *behvarz* offer a good indication of their important contribution to rural health in Iran. There was general consensus among study respondents that the *behvarz* program has made a significant contribution to gains in rural health over the last few decades. A majority of respondents, particularly those who have been serving the community for many years, provided comparative data on major health indicators and how these indicators have improved as a result of their work in rural areas:

> I remember many years ago we had to go to people's houses and talk to them for at least one hour to convince them doing vaccinations for their children but now they chase us up. They've become much more sensitive to health issues and it all occurred due to our hard work and consistent education. *(male, 40 yrs.)*
>
> When I started my job about 20 years ago maternal mortality was very high but now we have no maternal death. Our prenatal care and health education for pregnant women have been very useful. There is a similar trend for the infant and under-five mortality rates. *(female, 46 yrs.)*

Study respondents demonstrated a broad understanding of social and environmental determinants of health and believed that the environmental-health program (including sanitation, safe water, food safety, and waste collection), done in collaboration with other sectors, has had a significant impact in reducing infectious disease over time: "I believe that what we have done in the area of environmental health is the most effective intervention… Now domestic waste is collected on a daily basis. You can't see animal waste in rural areas anymore and, as a result, the rate of diarrheal and other infectious diseases declined dramatically" (male, 44 yrs.).

Factors facilitating behvarz performance

Respondents identified some of the factors that facilitate successful implementation of the *behvarz* program in rural areas. These include building lasting and sustainable relationships with their communities based on trust and recognition, a sense of belonging, their strong motivation to serve rural people, and a high level of health knowledge and skills. "Being from this area helps me a lot. I know my people very well. People trust me which is very important" (male, 40 yrs.). "If a specialist prescribes a medicine for somebody here, s/he won't take the medicine unless s/he consults with me first even though I don't know what it is for … this is an example of how people trust me" (female, 44 yrs.). "Our training courses are very comprehensive so having knowledge and skills gives us enough confidence to work easily" (male, 31 yrs.).

Barriers affecting behvarz performance

Respondents cited workload, lack of a support system, and poor supervisory mechanisms as the most common barriers to effective implementation of the *behvarz* program in Iran. The majority perceived the heavy and increasing workload as a threat to the quality of health services. Integration of new programs within the Iranian PHC system, and the inclusion of extra forms and paperwork – leading to duplication – were frequently cited: "To be honest, we spend most of our time filling in forms and recording statistics; we have to record a child's injection on too many different forms which wastes our time" (male, 46 yrs.); and, "The variety of tasks makes us confused and tired ... On top of all these tasks other sectors expect us to help them in their projects because we are the only person who knows everybody in the village very well. Like last year we spent too much time collecting data for [a health-related organisation], with no payment ..." (male, 36 yrs.).

Insufficient support systems – including infrastructural support such as health house facilities, physical space, and maintenance; inadequate recognition by higher authorities; and poor incentives – were common challenges cited by a large number of *behvarz*. Most of the respondents felt that they were not fully supported by the health system: "We don't have enough space and educational materials in our health house for the educational classes. Sometimes, I have to pay out of my own pocket for the maintenance of the health house" (female, 43 yrs.).

Despite formal supervisory mechanisms being in place, as revealed in policy documents, poor-quality supervision was one of the barriers reported by *behvarz*. In most cases, supervisory teams do not provide sufficient technical and emotional support and are not educative. Instead, a large number of our respondents stated that supervisors mainly focus on their weaknesses rather than strengths. "Supervisors should provide advice and support but they only reflect on our weak points. They haven't solved my problems at all" (female, 28 yrs.). "We have supervisors from different units. Everybody expects us to do the best in their area of interest. Nobody considers our high workload and our expectations" (male, 28 yrs.). Table 9.2 shows other potential barriers reported by study participants.

Table 9.2 Perceived barriers to *behvarz* performance

Barrier	Quote
Lack of educational opportunities	… I started my job with a high school degree but now I have to get unpaid leave to be able to continue my education at the university level. Due to the financial problem this is not possible for me (male, 27 yrs.).
Lack of health house facilities and poor maintenance	It is about one year since the health house's window is broken. The fridge doesn't work properly and hasn't been fixed yet. Our sphygmomanometer is broken. I have followed up on these too many times with no success (female, 38 yrs.).
Job stress and mental-health issues	Expectations of *behvarz* and job stress are too high. Nobody cares about our mental health (female, 28 yrs.).
Lack of mechanisms for job promotion	There is no opportunity for job promotion. After 30 years we are treated the same as a newly employed *behvarz* (male, 34 yrs.).
Shortage in *behvarz*	We have been told that the standard number is 2 *behvarz* per 1,500 population but there is a 3,000 population in our village and we are only 2 *behvarz*. It doubles our workload (female, 32 yrs.).

Discussion

This review of *behvarz* policies supplemented by in-depth interviews with a broad range of *behvarz* highlighted some issues regarding Iran's CHW program and the extent to which it relates to the principles and desired outcomes of CPHC.

In many areas *behvarz* policies and practices are consistent with the principles of a CPHC approach as outlined in the Declaration of Alma-Ata. Table 9.3 demonstrates how well the *behvarz* program in Iran embodies the principles of CPHC. It is noteworthy that "weak presence" was not indicated for any of the principles.

CHWs are part of a systematic PHC strategy in Iran. The distribution, selection, and recruitment of *behvarz* from the communities they serve facilitate not only equity in access to health-care services based on rural needs but also, in practice, foster community participation. Almost all rural populations have easy access to basic health care via a trained and community-friendly health worker. Experiences from other countries have also shown that CHWs recruited from local communities have had greater impact on utilization of health-care services, creating better health awareness and improved health outcomes (Abbatt, 2005; Lewin

Table 9.3 Principles of comprehensive primary health care in the community reflected by the *behvarz* program in Iran

Principles of comprehensive PHC approach as stated in the Declaration of Alma-Ata	Evidence from *behvarz* policy review and interviews of how well the principles and elements of PHC are reflected in Iran		
	Strong presence	Some presence	Weak presence
Universal access and coverage on the basis of need (equity)	✓		
Comprehensive care with emphasis on disease prevention and health promotion	✓		
Community and individual involvement and self-reliance		✓	
Addressing social and environmental determinants of health		✓	
Intersectoral action for health		✓	
Appropriate technology and cost-effectiveness in relation to available resources	✓		
Equitable increase in population health outcomes	✓		

et al., 2005; Rosato et al., 2008). *Behvarz* interviewed in this study also believed that the recruitment strategy and being part of the community facilitated people's easy access to health-care services.

The provision of comprehensive initial and in-service training helps to ensure that *behvarz* are responsive to their communities' needs. Training content and task descriptions of *behvarz*, from the inception of the program in 1979, demonstrated the high priority given to disease prevention and health promotion as well as the management of common illnesses. Examination of *behvarz* training policies revealed that these were regularly reviewed and adjusted based on changing patterns of illness and population needs. *Behvarz* interviews also revealed training courses and the interaction with the trainers in *behvarz* training centres as strengths of the *behvarz* program in Iran. The benefits of the comprehensive training program are well reflected in *behvarz* skills and knowledge of primary health care. In many other countries, the initial induction and continuing training for CHWs has also been seen as a predictor of success (de Campos, Ferreira, de Souza, & de Aguiar, 2004; Abbatt, 2005; Lehmann & Sanders, 2007).

This study demonstrated a trend towards a more social approach to health. This shift is visible in the content of training curricula as well as in job descriptions. The inclusion of topics on social determinants of health (SDH) in *behvarz* training and job statements demonstrates the move towards a more comprehensive approach to PHC (Labonté et al., 2008). However, there was a general consensus among *behvarz* that the long list of basic health care tasks, in practice, may leave little time for *behvarz* to serve as agents for community development and change. The workload of *behvarz* and its increasing trend seem to be an issue of concern that needs to be considered by policymakers.

This study supported the earlier conclusions by Mehryar (2004) that Iranian health-system reform based on a PHC approach, and especially the emphasis on rural health provided by CHWs, accounts for the dramatic improvements in infant and maternal mortality rates and, particularly, for the convergence between rural and urban health indicators. This study allows us to make only tentative comments regarding the causal validity of the relationship between Iran's PHC program and these aggregated health improvements; although we can state that the recruitment and training of Iranian *behvarz*, in terms of content, skill sets, and the work they perform, is consistent with the types of health gains noted by Mehryar et al. (2005).

This study, however, highlighted some obstacles to the optimal functioning of the CHW program in Iran and in the process of translating policy into practice. The most serious problems concern support services, supervision, and workload. The amount of time *behvarz* spend in meeting cultural expectations, which are crucial in building trust and community engagement, does not appear to be sufficiently appreciated by the health system. An abundance of duplicative paperwork suggests the need for a comprehensive review of the reporting processes for all health programs running in health houses. Our finding is supported by a study undertaken in Iran's Kurdistan Province that investigated individual, work-related, and environmental factors impacting job satisfaction among CHWs (Arab, Pourreza, Akbari, Ramesh, & Aghlmand, 2007). It concluded that the high number of programs integrated within the PHC network and the lack of financial and nonfinancial incentives are factors that lead to job dissatisfaction among CHWs.

Little evidence was found in the policy documents about the quality and outcome of existing supervisory mechanisms. The quality and consistency of *behvarz* supervision and the extent to which the existing *behvarz* supervisory mechanism has assisted in resolving barriers, provided actual support, and sustained *behvarz* interest and motivation are issues that were not documented in the policy review. The interviews with *behvarz* highlighted pitfalls in the supervisory mechanisms. A large number of *behvarz* believed that supervisors were not supportive and felt they were only looking for negative aspects of their performance and not encouraging their positive work. The crucial role of effective supervision and support in the success of CHW programs, and in maintaining the motivation of the CHWs, is widely acknowledged in the literature (Ofosu-Amaah, 1983; Gray & Ciroma, 1988). These findings suggest that *behvarz* supervisory mechanisms (who should be supervisors and with what specific tasks) require health-authority attention to resolve these signals of dissatisfaction.

While the experience of the Iranian *behvarz* program may not be readily transferable to other settings that experience different patterns of health problems, varying economic and political factors, cultural determinants, population distribution, and resources available, the successes of the program do provide important lessons that certainly have some applicability to other settings, despite differing contexts.

Conclusion

To sum up, the Iranian CHW program provides a compelling example of how CHWs can be a crucial part of a CPHC strategy – in that *behvarz* provide basic health care but also work with community members and other sectors to address the SDH. The breadth of the tasks performed demonstrate that they contribute to rendering PHC in Iran more comprehensive than is often the case in national programs where services have tended to be more selective (WHO, 1989). The ongoing review and revision of training courses to ensure they match *behvarz* roles and responsibilities over time facilitated closing the gap between policy and practice. The *behvarz* were clear that the work they have done over the last three decades has made a significant contribution to improving the health of Iran's rural population. Lessons learned from this study of the Iranian CHW program may be applicable to programs in other countries that are aiming to ameliorate their health-worker shortage by increasing midlevel cadres while improving the retention of rural health personnel.

ACKNOWLEDGMENTS

We wish to express thanks to the research team in Iran — Sakineh Rezaei, Zohreh Rajabi, Mohammad Bazyari, and Javad Farahi Shahgoli — for their assistance in the implementation of the study and constructive comments on the instrument design and the collection of data. We would also like to acknowledge the participation of the Iranian CHWs who gave so generously their time to share their wonderful experiences and views with the research team.

REFERENCES

Abbatt, F. (2005). *Scaling up health and education workers: Community health workers*. London: DFID Health Systems Resource Centre.

Arab, M., Pourreza, A., Akbari, F., Ramesh, N., & Aghlmand, S. (2007). Job satisfaction on primary health care providers in the rural settings. *Iranian Journal of Public Health, 36*(3), 64–70.

de Campos, F.E., Ferreira, J.R., de Souza, M.F., & de Aguiar, R.A.T. (2004, March). Innovations in human resources development: The role of community health workers.

Gray, H., & Ciroma, J. (1988). Reducing attrition among village health workers in rural Nigeria. *Socio-Economic Planning Sciences, 22*(1), 39–43. http://dx .doi.org/10.1016/0038-0121(88)90033-X

Khojasteh, A., Momtazmanesh, N., Entezari, A., & Einollahi, B. (2009). Integration of medical education and healthcare service. *Iranian Journal of Public Health, 38*(Suppl 1), 29–31.

Labonté, R., Pooyak, S., Baum, F., Schaay, N., Packer, C., Laplante, D., …, & Sanders, D. (2008). Implementation, effectiveness and political context of comprehensive primary health care: Preliminary findings of a global literature review. *Australian Journal of Primary Health, 14*(3), 58–67. http:// dx.doi.org/10.1071/PY08037

Lehmann, U., & Sanders, D. (2007). *Community health workers: What do we know about them? The state of the evidence on programmes, activities, costs and impact on health outcomes of using community health workers*. Geneva: World Health Organization.

Lewin, S.A., Dick, J., Pond, P., Zwarenstein, M., Aja, G., van Wyk, B., …, & Patrick, M. (2005, Jan 25). Lay health workers in primary and community health care. *Cochrane Library*, (1): CD004015. Medline:15674924

Mehryar, A. 2004. *Primary health care and the rural poor in the Islamic Republic of Iran*. Washington, DC: World Bank. Retrieved from http://documents.worldbank.org/curated/en/605341468772180275 /Primary-health-care-and-the-rural-poor-in-the-Islamic-Republic-of-Iran

Mehryar, A.H., Aghajanian, A., Ahmad-Nia, S., Mirzae, M., & Naghavi, M. (2005). *Primary health care system, narrowing of rural-urban gap in health indicators, and rural poverty reduction: The experience of Iran*. Paper presented at XXV General Population Conference of the International Union for the Scientific Study of Population, Tours, France.

Ministry of Health and Medical Education. (2005). *Rural health in Iran*. Tehran: Author.

Ministry of Health and Medical Education. (2008). *The total number of behvarzes, behvarz training centres and district health centres in Iran, 1386*. Tehran: Author.

Ofosu-Amaah, V. (1983). National experience in the use of community health workers: A review of current issues and problems. *WHO Offset Publication, 71*, 1–49. Medline:6880399

Rosato, M., Laverack, G., Grabman, L.H., Tripathy, P., Nair, N., Mwansambo, C., …, & Costello, A. (2008, Sep 13). Community participation: Lessons for maternal, newborn, and child health. *Lancet, 372*(9642), 962–71. http:// dx.doi.org/10.1016/S0140-6736(08)61406-3 Medline:18790319

Statistical Centre of Iran. (2012). *Population and housing census 2011*. Tehran: Author.

World Health Organization. (1978). *Primary health care: Report of the International Conference on Primary Health Care, Alma-Ata, USSR*. International Conference on Primary Health Care, Alma-Ata, USSR. Geneva: Author.

World Health Organization. (1989). *Strengthening the performance of community health workers in primary health care. WHO Technical Report Series*. Geneva: Author.

World Health Organization. (2008). *Task shifting: Rational redistribution of tasks among health workforce teams: Global recommendations and guidelines*. Geneva: Author.

10 The Contribution of Accredited Social Health Activists in the Implementation of Comprehensive Primary Health Care in East Champaran District, India

ANIL CHERIAN, VANDANA KANTH, AND JAMEELA GEORGE

Background

The National Rural Health Mission, since renamed the National Health Mission (NHM), was launched in India to revitalize a crumbling public health-care system. It was implemented over a period of seven years, from 2005 to 2012. A cornerstone of the reforms was the introduction of a cadre of women from villages and hamlets. These women were called accredited social health activists (ASHAs).

The ASHA represents the latest in a long series of efforts by the government to incorporate a village-level health worker within the public health-care system in order to mobilize the community and increase community participation.

The set of reforms instituted under NHM must be viewed in the context of global efforts to revitalize the health-for-all strategy and to promote CPHC. The concept of CPHC involves equity in the access to health care, reducing vulnerability of communities to ill health through community empowerment, and an attempt to address the social determinants of health (SDH).

This study was carried out in Bihar, a state in the eastern part of India. It studied the ASHA program of the NHM in the district of East Champaran. This is one of the 38 districts of Bihar and is located in the north of the state, just below and bordering on Nepal.

In geographic terms, Bihar is the twelfth largest state in India. However it ranks as India's sixth most densely populated state with 1,102 persons per square kilometre, well above the national average of 325 persons per square kilometre (Dyson, Cassen, & Visaria, 2004). The population is growing at a rapid rate, with the decadal growth rate being 29%. This rapid growth also accounts for the fact that 58% of Biharis are below the age of 25 years. Bihar is one of the most underdeveloped states of India: until recent times, it was the byword for underdevelopment. Bihar hosts a caste-ridden and complex social stratification, weak infrastructure, poor governance, and widespread poverty (Timberg, 1982; Kumar, 2014.). Nearly 85% of the population is rural and largely dependent on agriculture and cattle rearing. The scheduled caste (the lowest-caste group) constitutes nearly one-fifth of all households (International Institute for Population Sciences [IIPS], 2007). The female-to-male sex ratio is 916:1,000, which suggests that there are gross gender inequities within the population. The Gender Empowerment Measure scored Bihar at 0.379 and ranked it 31 out of 35 Indian states and territories. Gender inequities are also reflected in the gender gaps in education and employment (Ministry of Women and Child Development, 2009).

The health status of the Bihari population at the launch of the NHM in 2005 was found to be poor, with high levels of mortality and a huge disease burden. The maternal mortality rate (MMR) was estimated to be 371 per 100,000 live births; the infant mortality rate (IMR), 61 per 1,000 live births (IIPS, 2007). The National Family Health Survey 3, which was the third in a series of national health surveys conducted in the country, revealed that 58% of the children under the age of 5 were underweight, of which 8% were severely underweight; both figures are above the national average (IIPS, 2007). The prevalence of vector-borne diseases – such as malaria, kala-azar (visceral leishmaniasis), filariasis, and other communicable diseases, including tuberculosis – is high.

Bihar has had its share of sociopolitical uprisings and reforms, largely associated with land or social-caste issues. Despite Mahatma Gandhi's civil disobedience movement, which ultimately led to the independence of India, Bihar remained neglected after Indian independence in 1947. Under the rule of the Indian National Congress party, the general government showed apathy towards Bihar; some government policies, such as "freight equalization," resulted in industry moving away from Bihar. The economic decline of Bihar and its disparity with the rest of India really became marked between 1980 and 2000, coinciding with the restructuring of the Indian economy and economic liberalization in the 80s. The incidence of poverty in Bihar has always been much higher than the national average, and, in 1983, 62% of the Bihari population was categorized as poor, against the national estimate of 44% (Mukherji & Mukherji, 2012). While the poverty in the Bihar region was primarily attributed to the lack of expansion of industry or the nonagricultural sector, others argued that the roots really remain in the absence of agrarian reform, the iniquitous and exploitative social structure, and the lack of political leadership (Sharma, 1995). But in 2005, Janata Dal, a socialist party under the leadership of Nitish Kumar, saw the government of Bihar become more progressive, encouraging and facilitating reforms within the state.

Village health workers

In India, the concept of the village health worker or part-time community health worker (CHW) has existed for more than 60 years. This cadre of health worker was introduced and found to be effective in NGO-run community-based health projects, although there is no evidence of village health workers being used before 1950. In 1967, a special commission constituted by the government of Bihar recommended that for effective relief work, the government should recruit, train, and organize village-level volunteers. In 1975, the Group on Medical Education and Support Manpower (Shrivastava Committee) recommended that a band of part-time, para- or semi-professional health workers be recruited from within the community itself to link local villages to the existing infrastructure of dispensaries and hospitals through a well-recognized referral system (National Institute of Health and Family Welfare, 2015).

These recommendations formed the basis of the ambitious but controversial "Community Health Worker Scheme" introduced in many parts of India, including Bihar, under the Integrated Rural Health Program in 1977 (Leslie, 1989). Two years later, it was converted into the "Community Health Volunteer (CHV) Scheme," since it was argued that the government did not, and should not, employ the personnel (i.e., "workers" as distinct from "volunteers") under the scheme. A few years later, in 1981, the scheme was renamed the "Village Health Guide Scheme" with the stated objective of placing "people's health in people's hands." It is important to note that these reforms came following the Declaration of Alma-Ata adopted in 1978. The scheme was financially supported entirely by the central government of India. The National Institute of Health and Family Welfare evaluated the CHV Scheme of 1979. One of its observations in the evaluation report was that "no systematic attempt had been made to bring about greater involvement of the community in the selection of the CHVs and ensuring their participation in the supervision of [the CHV's] work" (Kumar, Ramaiah, Maru, & Bhatt, 1979).

The Village Health Guide Scheme was discontinued in 2002 following the report of a three-panel committee, in view of its failure to meet its objectives. This came as a major setback to the PHC program, and subsequently some 10,000 village health guides were rendered jobless in Bihar. The central government withdrew financial support for the scheme but recommended that the states continue to finance it, if they wished, from their own revenues.

The government of Chhattisgarh state decided to continue the CHV program, introducing a new scheme called the *Mitanin* program in May 2002. It was operationalized across the state in a phased manner. In Chhattisgarhi, the term *Mitanin* refers to a female friend. Under this program, women were selected by the village through the *panchayat* (a local self-government body) and trained. Eventually, more than 60,000 *Mitanins* were trained (State Health Resource Centre, 2003).

Although not officially acknowledged, a quick comparison of the ASHA program under NHM and the *Mitanin* program in Chhattisgarh suggests that the latter was in many ways the prototype on which the ASHA program was designed. The ASHA program was started in Bihar following the introduction of the NHM in 2005. Today, a grand total of more than 850,000 ASHAs are at work in India, which is very close to the target of one ASHA for every 1,000 population (Healthy Newborn Network, 2011).

One of the features of the ASHA program that distinguishes it from previous health-worker programs in India and other parts of the world was that these women were by design expected to play the role of health activists, providing a critical link between the community and public PHC system. The ASHA was to mobilize the community and work with the village health committees in building a critical awareness of health issues affecting the community and village health planning. This work was important from the perspective of making PHC programs more comprehensive. However this understanding of the functioning of the ASHAs was not adequately emphasized, and one of the key findings of this study was that the ASHAs in Bihar did not see themselves as health activists, nor did the community or other government health workers. Also, their selection and training seems to have ignored health activism, thus limiting their ability to reform the prevalent top-down selective approach to PHC and make it comprehensive.

Financial remuneration of CHWs has been an important determinant of their motivation the world over, and perhaps especially in low- and middle-income countries. In the ASHA program, the government of

India introduced a performance-based payment system for ASHAs to motivate them to achieve their objectives. While a number of studies have focused on the operational challenges faced by ASHAs (Bajpai & Dholakia, 2011; Wang, Juyal, Miner, & Fischer, 2012), our study also explored the impact of the performance-based payment system on their performance as health activists. Our study found that ASHAs did face operational challenges that impacted their ability to assist with CPHC roll-out, but remuneration also affected their understanding of their roles, which, in turn, did not facilitate CPHC either.

Research Questions and Methods

The introduction of the ASHA, a female health activist whose role included mobilizing the community to access their health entitlements, creating awareness in the community of the SDH, and engaging the community in local health planning, had immense potential to revitalize PHC and to make it more comprehensive in scope. Our overarching research question was how to strengthen the ASHAs' contribution to the implementation of CPHC. It was anticipated that this research would help us better understand the support structure and environment necessary to make the ASHA program more effective. It would also help identify gaps in the current program that need to be addressed.

The research tried to answer some key questions about the functioning and development of ASHAs:

- What are the contradictions in the stated roles of the ASHAs (as given in the NHM guidelines) and what they currently practice?
- Did the process of recruitment and training followed in Bihar enable or constrain the ASHAs from contributing to CPHC?
- How effectively did the ASHAs collaborate with the other players in the health system, the local government, and other community-based organizations?
- Do the financial arrangements supporting the ASHAs enable or constrain their role as social health activists?
- How do ASHAs and other community stakeholders perceive their role as social health activists?
- What are some of the contextual factors that affect their functioning?

This study employed a cross-sectional, mixed-methods design. Quantitative, qualitative, and participatory methods were used to measure some of the changes that ASHAs had succeeded in bringing about so as to assess their effectiveness. The research was carried out in two developmental blocks in East Champaran District, namely Adapur and Ramgarhwa.

A survey of ASHAs, *Anganwadi* workers,[1] and auxiliary nurse mid-wives (ANMs) was conducted using a structured questionnaire. The sample, derived from a stratified systematic sampling method, included 199 of the 214 ASHAs in the two blocks: 84 from Adapur block and 115 from Ramgarhwa block. Of the 309 *Anganwadi* workers, 255 were sampled, in addition to 17 of the 21 ANMs.

Key-informant interviews and focus-group discussions (FGDs) also were conducted using a structured interview schedule. Informants included members of the village *panchayat* and 15 of the 33 village headmen (*mukhiya*). Members of various community-based self-help groups (such as women's, men's, and youth groups, as well as farmers' associations) were also interviewed. The participatory methods used were Venn diagrams, line ranking, and matrix ranking.

Results and Analysis

About half the ASHAs (46%) in East Champaran District were between the ages of 26 and 30 years, and about a quarter of them (24%) were aged 31 to 35 years. Ninety percent of the ASHAs were from the Hindu community, and the remaining 10% were Muslim. All the ASHAs were married women, as this is one of the requirements of the ASHA program. Fifty-six percent of the ASHAs were from poor households, with nearly half of these falling below the poverty line and another near 10% falling in the *Antodhya* (very poor) category. However, only 6% of the ASHAs came from the scheduled caste (*Harijan* or *Dalits*), while 56% were from the other poor castes and 38% from the high-caste group. All ASHAs possessed the minimum education requirement of grade 8 certification. Twenty-six percent had completed grade 10, and 22% had completed grade 12 or its equivalent. Nineteen percent had studied beyond high school, but none had graduated from college or university. The hours worked by the ASHAs varied significantly; however, on average, an

---

1 In rural settings, the *angan* is the open place where people gather to talk, greet guests and socialize. In 1975, the government of India initiated the Integrated Child Development Service (ICDS). Under the ICDS scheme, one trained person is allotted to a population of 1,000 to bridge the gap between that population and organized health care, and to focus on the health and educational needs of children aged 0–6 years. This child development worker is referred to as an *Anganwadi* worker.

ASHA worked for 3.2 hours, 3 days a week, and directly reached out to 16 households per week.

Roles of the ASHA

Most of the ASHAs and the other stakeholders (ANMs, *Anganwadi* workers, and the members of *panchayat* community) were in agreement that the primary role and contribution of the ASHAs was in the domain of maternal and child health. Fifty-nine percent of the ASHAs felt that they were recruited to register pregnant women and 66% thought that they were to ensure that pregnant women and children were immunized against tetanus. When it came to other roles, such as the facilitation of institutional deliveries, newborn care, specific infectious-disease programs, and family planning, there were differences in perception. While 46% of the community members interviewed expected ASHAs to be involved in family planning, only 15% of ASHAs understood this to be their role. Again, while some of the ANMs and *Anganwadi* workers were of the opinion that ASHAs should promote sanitation and hygiene (47% and 34%, respectively), only 7% of ASHAs perceived it to be one of their roles.

When the ASHAs were asked to list the activities that they currently undertook, most of their responses related to maternal and child health. Fifty-nine percent were involved in registering pregnant mothers at the *Anganwadi* centre or with the ANM, 34% in immunization of children, 32% in the immunization of pregnant women, and 30% accompanied women for institutional delivery. Less than a quarter of the ASHAs said that they mobilized women for antenatal check-ups. A much smaller proportion (< 15%) was involved in some of the other activities listed under the NHM guidelines.

Roles pertaining to the SDH, such as nutrition, sanitation and hygiene, and healthy living and working conditions, were not carried out by the ASHAs. Neither were ASHAs involved in any village-level health planning with the village health and sanitation committees. These activities were not understood to be responsibilities of the ASHAs by any of the key stakeholders or the ASHAs themselves.

FGDs with the ASHAs revealed that none of them were aware of the meaning of the term "social activist" or that it was one of the roles that they were expected to play. When the question of activism was raised in the discussions, one of the ASHAs asked, "Is this some new work that is being assigned to us? We do not know anything about it since we have not received any training on it." Some ASHAs assumed that the term

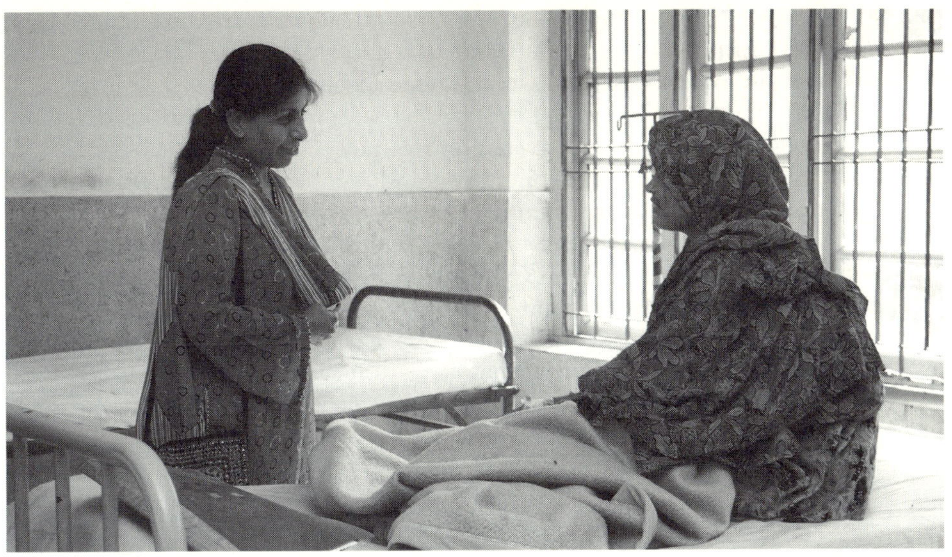

Accredited social health activist (ASHA) at work, India

referred to the fact that they were not paid a salary and they were to work with both the rich and the poor.

Recruitment and training of ASHAs

Our research revealed a significant difference between the recruitment process as envisaged in the NHM guidelines and the way in which recruitment actually took place. The village chief (known as the *mukhiya*) recruited 65% of the ASHAs in person, and the PHC medical officer recruited another 21%. The selection was based on an application made to the *mukhiya*, followed by an interview (50%) or a written test (37%). The *gram sabha* (village council), which was the prescribed authority for the selection of ASHAs, actually selected only 7%. Similar findings arose regarding the ANMs and the *Anganwadi* workers who, like the ASHAs, should have been selected by the *gram sabha* but were selected by the *mukhiya* (76% and 68%, respectively).

By the end of 2009, 78% of the ASHAs had completed the induction training, and the remaining 22% had received no training. Eighty-five percent of those who received training completed 7 days, while the remaining 15% obtained less than 7 days. The PHC medical officer trained all of them for a median time of 4 hours a day, and 98% of the ASHAs said that the predominant method of training was reading from the book (training manual). They reported learning about various diseases (66%), immunization (46%), prenatal care (58%), and basic medicines (38%) during their training. The findings of the study revealed that the 7-day induction training was inadequate for them to build the necessary competencies or develop confidence about their work. In a FGD with ANMs, one midwife stated, "ASHAs are inexperienced and need more practical training. An ASHA is unable to calculate the expected date of delivery or to make a basic assessment of women in labour." Another ANM during the discussion said that, if the ASHAs were to be useful and effective, "first all the selection of ASHAs should be done properly and then they need to be properly trained."

Support framework and collaboration of ASHAs

The participatory exercises with the ASHAs revealed that they related best to the ANMs and *Anganwadi* workers, who also were the main people who assisted them in fulfilling their roles, along with their husbands. However, in terms of importance (both voice and influence), they listed the medical officer, *mukhiya*, ANM, and *Anganwadi* worker. Other important players listed were local medical practitioners (unqualified practitioners or alternative health providers), *dais* (traditional birth attendants), and workers from NGOs. Regarding intensity of involvement or collaboration, they felt that the medical officer, PHC clerk, and *mukhiya* were distant and not very useful.

The common areas of collaboration between ASHAs, ANMs, and *Anganwadi* workers were pregnancy care and immunization. While *Anganwadi* workers supported ASHAs as coaches – 48% assisted them in identifying pregnant women and trained them about immunization – the ANMs actually taught them to give injections (44%) and provided them with medicines to treat patients (23%). ANMs also supported them by listening to the problems that they faced, giving them feedback, and also making space available to them in the primary health centre when they brought pregnant women for delivery at night. However, the ASHAs stated that they received no assistance or support from the *panchayat*, community-based organizations, or the village health and sanitation committees.

Interestingly, some FGD participants flagged a few areas in which the roles of the ANMs and *Anganwadi* workers conflicted with that of the ASHAs. ANMs were unhappy when some of the ASHAs took patients directly to the primary health or community health centre without consulting them. They complained that patients without antenatal care were being brought for deliveries and this reflected badly on the ANMs' work. One of the government health functionaries stated that "antenatal care is not a task assigned to ASHA. It is the work of the ANM. It is her fault if the ANC check-ups are not being done properly." Similarly some *Anganwadi* workers felt that the role of identifying pregnant women and registering them for ANC and immunization was theirs. They felt that the ASHAs were being given incentives for a task that was not their own. The discussions suggest that there is a lack of clarity, resulting in duplication of work. The ASHAs interviewed felt that it was meant to be a collaborative effort.

Some of the key-informant interviews revealed that ANMs and *Anganwadi* workers had an expectation that the ASHAs would split some of their earnings from incentives with them. (Note that although they are volunteers, ASHAs receive incentives.) One participant angrily explained, "ANMs have links with ASHAs. The moment that [an ANM] hears that the ASHA has received incentive money, [the ANM] has an understanding that she will be paid 50 rupees for her support."

The study also uncovered an unexpected finding: the ASHAs were organizing themselves into a union and had formed an ASHA committee to look into various aspects related to their own welfare. The ASHAs hoped that the ASHA committee would take up issues related to the timely payment of incentives and regularization of the terms of employment with the primary health centre and the government (shifting them from voluntary workers to salaried employees), and that it also would advocate for the ASHAs regarding the challenges they faced at work.

Aside from the payment of financial incentives, some of the work-related challenges that the ASHAs reported concerned transportation to the health facility when they accompanied women in labour (60%), the rude behaviour of primary health centre staff (14%), and the lack of adequate investigation and treatment facilities at the primary health centre (44%). A disaggregation of the blocks also suggests that there are variations between them. While 75% of the ASHAs from Ramgarhwa block reported that primary health centre staff members were rude to them, only 6% of the ASHAs from Adapur block reported such rudeness. When it came to investigation and treatment facilities, 46% of the ASHAs from Ramgarhwa block said that the facilities at the primary health centre were inadequate (which meant that the people were less satisfied with the services), whereas in Adapur the proportion was lower at 28%.

The study also showed that neither the *panchayat* nor the community-based organizations supported the ASHAs. The village health and sanitation committees were either nonexistent or nonfunctional; hence one of the important components of the ASHAs' support mechanism was absent in Bihar.

Financial arrangements

While the ASHA program perceives the ASHA as a volunteer village health worker, the ASHAs themselves assumed that they are regular public employees like the other workers – namely ANMs and the *Anganwadi* workers – who are paid salaries. This was also the perception of the *mukhiyas* and community members. Hence, while all the ASHAs were aware that under the current scheme they received only performance-based incentives or payments for tasks conducted, all were hoping that their payments would be regularized and that they would eventually receive a salary. The ASHAs were of the opinion that the PHC medical officer was the person who approved the payment of incentives.

There was a variation in the findings between the two development blocks examined in our study. While 82% of the ASHAs in the Adapur block reported that they had received their incentive payments either fully or partially, 75% of the ASHAs in the neighbouring block of Ramgarhwa reported that they had difficulty receiving payment. In addition, ASHAs in Ramgarhwa tended to experience delays in receiving payment; only 1% of the ASHAs from Adapur block said that their payments had been delayed, whereas more than a quarter of those from Ramgarhwa suffered delays.

The untimely or partial payment of incentives was a considerable disappointment and, as a result, 61% of the ASHAs from Adapur block and 93% from Ramgarhwa said that they considered discontinuing work as an ASHA and looking for other job opportunities. The ASHAs were united in the opinion that they were not being adequately compensated for their work and contributions. One said, "There should be a monthly fixed amount given to us rather than incentives. It will motivate us to work. How can someone be expected to work if she is not paid properly?" Another said, "If someone is not paid, her motivation to work will diminish." The study observed that the dropout rate among ASHAs was slightly higher in Ramgarhwa compared to Adapur (8% and 6%, respectively).

Contributions of ASHAs to CPHC

When asked in FGDs how their work was benefiting the community, many ASHAs said that people were going to the primary health centre and using its services to a greater extent. One of the ASHAs said, "People are now availing themselves of the services provided in the centres and they have become more functional than before." One of them also claimed, "If I do not take women to the primary health centre for delivery there will be no deliveries conducted at the centre." Some were of the opinion that they had saved many mothers from death by taking them to the health facility for delivery. In one of the discussions, an ASHA explained that "now, if there is any complication, I take the women immediately to the health facility and therefore, now-a-days, mothers are less likely to die in pregnancy."

The study did not actually measure any health or mortality indicators to validate these perceptions as doing so was beyond its scope. However, FGDs with community groups commented that the utilization of essential health services at the primary health centres had increased following the introduction of ASHAs. Many of the women agreed that ASHAs were able to motivate pregnant women to go to the nearest health facility to have an institutional delivery rather than delivering at home, which previously had been the norm. The study documented a number of cases that highlighted the role of ASHAs in increasing the institutional delivery rate. A few of the FGD participants were sceptical and attributed this increase to the cash transfers given to the mothers rather than the introduction of the ASHA. One woman said, "It looks like a game of money and nothing else." In some of the FGDs, people also reported that the number of individuals seeking tuberculosis treatment and family-planning services had also increased due to the presence of ASHAs.

Intrinsic to the ASHA scheme was that the ASHA was to identify and be seen as a facilitator, mobilizer, and activist representing her community or hamlet. FGDs with community groups found that while they felt that some of the ASHAs had mobilized the community, this function was limited largely to enabling the community to access the primary health centre facilities. As one of the participants commented, "She has brought awareness about women's health both at an individual and community level. She has succeeded in convincing many families of the importance of women delivering in an institution rather than delivering at home." Other participants felt that they had benefitted from ASHAs: "We feel that there is someone in the community who can help our pregnant women at times of crisis or in an emergency." Also, they were of the opinion that she had made their access to health care more equitable. One of the participants noted, "She is helping poor women in our community to deliver in an institution ... Because of her, more poor women are now going to the primary health centre." However, while such positive remarks did occasionally arise in FGDs, overall, most of the participants questioned the ASHAs' motivation and commitment.

While one key informant interviewed was certain that, from the Health Department's point of view, a clear message had been sent that the ASHA should not function merely as a line worker or service provider; he was quick to accept that ASHAs may not be fulfilling their stated roles as health activists. He added that the main reason for the unfulfilled role was the acute shortage of staff at the primary health centre, which pulled the ASHAs away from being "social activists" and towards being substitute health workers. He said that he had heard reports that due to the absence of ANMs, medical officers in charge were putting pressure on the ASHAs to conduct deliveries. One of the medical officers interviewed stated categorically, "ASHAs can do much for the community if properly selected like the process followed for the selection of *Anganwadi* workers."

Contextual factors that determine the effectiveness of ASHAs

A number of factors (including, among others, recruitment and selection, training, payment, and support from the *panchayat*) were compared to see if they were associated with ASHAs' effectiveness. However, this multifactor analysis did not reveal any significant association.

Discussion and Conclusion

The study shows that ASHAs in the East Champaran District of Bihar were able to contribute, to a limited extent, to the increased utilization of primary health centre services and to an increase in the number of women delivering in the health facility. Their contributions were to a large extent limited to maternal and child health and more narrowly to deliveries and immunization of both women and children. The findings from the community FGDs suggest that since the ASHAs were able to mobilize some women from poor households, this could contribute to greater equity in access and utilization of services at the primary health centre. In our study, 56% of ASHAs came from poor households. In many ways this is important because the ASHA is now in a position to ensure that the needs of the community from which she herself comes and which she now represents are addressed. However, the study also showed that the lower social-caste groups were underrepresented in the selection of ASHAs. Only 5% of the ASHAs in East Champaran were from the scheduled caste group, while their proportion in the district is substantially higher, at an estimated 15%. By referring patients and mobilizing people from their villages to actually go to the primary health centre, ASHAs inadvertently may have started to exert some pressure on the health system to make these health facilities function better.

It is unlikely that the ASHAs, left to themselves, will be able to bring about greater community participation, local village-level health planning, or promote the intersectoral coordination necessary to address the SDH. Within the NHM steering group, there is a rethinking of the feasibility of all these roles being played by a "single person." There are also a number of conflicting ideas on what the legitimate role of the ASHA should be. However, if the ASHA is to be a health activist, then community empowerment and mobilization are critical prerequisites that may have to be facilitated by other external community animators, through NGOs and other civil-society organizations. One of the reasons that the *Mitanin* program was successful in Chhattisgarh was because community mobilization – largely done through NGOs – preceded or was carried out alongside the introduction of the *Mitanins*. As a result, there was greater community ownership of social activism for health, and the *panchayats* were more involved in supporting *Mitanins* in their attempts to sustain an activist role. In the case of Bihar, this crucial element in the roll-out of the ASHA program was missing. Similarly, the absence of functional village health and sanitation committees or the active engagement of the *panchayati raj* (local self-government) in many of the villages could be critical factors hindering the ASHAs from playing a broader role necessary for CPHC. A recent review of the ASHA program by the national ASHA mentoring group also suggests that the link between the local village health and sanitation committees and the ASHAs, including their active participation in committee meetings, is important to the ASHA scheme fulfilling its purpose.

While there is sufficient evidence from the evaluation of small NGO-led projects that CHWs, such as ASHAs, can contribute effectively to CPHC and bring about positive health outcomes in communities, the challenge has been to effectively upscale to large state- or nation-wide CHW programs. This study suggests that factors critical to any large-scale ASHA program are community involvement and participation in the selection of these workers, proper training, and supportive supervision. While considerable thought and effort had been given to all these aspects in the design of the ASHA program, and the experience from the earlier Village Health Guide Scheme had been incorporated, selection and training were the major shortcomings of the Bihar ASHA roll-out. The findings that neither the community nor the *panchayat* played a major role in ASHA selection and the fact that the medical officers in charge were actually involved in the selection indicates a major deviation from the NHM guidelines. The NHM has developed excellent training material for ASHAs, and there is a considerable body of literature and many manuals on how CHWs can be trained. But often the absence of a proper training team is a major challenge in scaling up such a program. The role of the State Health Resource Centre in Chhattisgarh in curriculum development, and in identifying and developing trainers from NGOs, was vital to the success of the *Mitanin* program and appears to be a major gap in the Bihar ASHA program.

The perceptions and understanding of the community and other stakeholders (such as the ANMs or the *Anganwadi* workers) about the roles of the ASHA may be crucial in improving ASHA effectiveness. The commonly accepted understanding among all the stakeholders was that the position of the ASHA was created to facilitate institutional deliveries and to mobilize women in the community to access the maternal health and immunization services. Since ASHAs were not trained to play other roles, they slipped into functioning as maternal- and child-health workers by default. It was the coaching and assistance that they received from the ANMs and the *Anganwadi* workers that helped them to carry out these roles. Therefore, it would be important to communicate the broader social-activist roles of the ASHA to all the stakeholders. While ideally this should be done prior to ASHA selection, it would be a useful exercise even at this stage of the program. Besides bringing greater job clarity, it would also help to bring about greater collaboration and coordination between the ANMs and *Anganwadi* workers.

The financial arrangement of paying the ASHAs incentives for carrying out certain activities is also important, as the study found that

ASHAs largely fulfilled only those roles for which they were given a monetary incentive and did not actively engage in roles for which they were not given any incentives. These findings suggest that changes in the mode of payment could strengthen the ASHAs' effectiveness. Should they be paid directly by the local village government? Would a mixed-payment mechanism – salary and incentives – be more effective? These remain important questions that could and should be tested.

The study clearly shows that the role of "social activist" is hardly understood. The findings also question how effective standard training is in building activists. Do the financial arrangements present in the current NHM ASHA program encourage social activism or do they restrain ASHAs from mobilizing? Is the ASHA to be located outside the formal health system or should she be made a first-line health worker within the system?

While ASHAs can contribute towards certain aspects of CPHC and the introduction of the program under the NHM was a significant step towards a better health system in India, it is important that the program is further strengthened through better training and supportive supervision of the ASHAs, along with a broader support framework involving the community and the village councils.

ACKNOWLEDGMENTS

We wish to thank a number of individuals for their assistance during our research: Dr. Sara Bhattacharya, former professor of community medicine at the Christian Medical College Vellore, for her research mentorship; Dr. Thelma Narayan and the staff of SOCHARA who helped coordinate the Teasdale-Corti *Revitalizing Health for All* research project in Asia; and Dr. Santosh Mathew, executive director of Emmanuel Hospital Association, New Delhi. Finally, we appreciate the collaboration of the field research team based at Duncan Hospital, East Champaran in Bihar.

REFERENCES

Bajpai, N., & Dholakia, R.H. (2011). Improving the performance of accredited social health activists in India. New York, NY: Columbia University. Retrieved from: http://globalcenters.columbia.edu/files/cgc/pictures /Improving_the_Performance_of_ASHAs_in_India_CGCSA_Working _Paper_1.pdf

Dyson, T., Cassen, R., & Visaria, L. (Eds.). (2004). *Twenty-first century India: Population, economy, human development, and the environment*. New York, NY: Oxford University Press.

Healthy Newborn Network. (2011). ASHAs to be paid for providing home-based newborn care in rural India: A policy decision of the Ministry of Health. Retrieved from http://www.healthynewbornnetwork.org/resource/ashas -to-be-paid-for-providing-home-based-newborn-care-in-rural-india-a-policy -decision-of-the-ministry-of-health

International Institute for Population Sciences. (2007). *National family health survey-3 2005–2006*. Mumbai: Author.

Kumar, C. (2014). Public Lecture: The Bihar story: Resurrection of the state, inclusion and growth (Jitan Ram Manjhi). Retrieved from International Growth Centre website: http://www.theigc.org/event/public-lecture -the-bihar-story-resurrection-of-the-state-inclusion-and-growth-jitan -ram-manjhi/

Kumar, S., Ramaiah, T.J., Maru, R.M., & Bhatt, A. (1979). Repeat evaluation of the Community Health Volunteers Scheme 1979: A collaborative study. New Delhi: National Institute of Health and Family Welfare.

Leslie, C. (1989, Oct). India's community health workers scheme: A sociological analysis. *Ancient Science of Life, 9*(2), 40–53. Medline:22557674

Ministry of Women and Child Development. (2009). *Gendering human development indices: Summary report*. Government of India.

Mukherji, A., & Mukherji, A. (2012). Bihar: What went wrong? And what changed? Working Paper No. 12/107. New Delhi: National Institute of Public Finance and Policy. Retrieved from http://www.nipfp.org.in/media /medialibrary/2013/04/WP_2012_107.pdf

National Institute of Health and Family Welfare. (2015). *Committees & commissions*. National Health Committees. New Delhi: Author. Retrieved from: http://www.nhp.gov.in/miscellaneous/committees-and-commissions.

Sharma, A.N. (1995). Political economy of poverty in Bihar. *Economic and Political Weekly, 30*(41,42), 2587–602.

State Health Resource Centre. (2003 Sept). Mitanin programme: Conceptual issues and operational guidelines. Chhattisgarh, India: Author.

Timberg, T.A. (1982). Bihar backwardness: Does feudalism frustrate? *Asian Survey, 22*(5), 470–80. http://dx.doi.org/10.2307/2643873

Wang, H., Juyal, R.K., Miner, S.A., & Fischer, E. (2012). *Performance-based payment system for ASHAs in India: What does international experience tell us?* Bethesda, MD: The Vistaar Project, IntraHealth International Inc., Abt Associates Inc.

11 The Contribution of the Health Services Extension Program to Improving Coverage and Comprehensiveness of Primary Health Care Services in Southwest Ethiopia

MIRKUZIE WOLDIE, ABERA ASEFA DERESSA, AND SUDHAKAR NARAYAN MORANKAR

Background

Ethiopia is located in the Horn of Africa with an area of about 1.1 million square kilometres and an estimated population of over 90 million, 83% of which lives in rural areas (Index Mundi, 2015). It is one of the most populous countries in sub-Saharan Africa, with an annual population growth rate of 2.9% and a total fertility rate of 5.23 (Index Mundi, 2014). Politically, Ethiopia is divided into nine national regional states and two city administrative councils, which are further divided into 80 zones, 611 *woredas* (districts), and approximately 15,000 *kebeles* (villages) comprised of 5,000 urban and 10,000 rural inhabitants.

Community participation was promoted in health policymaking and implementation of health services from the beginnings of PHC under Haile Selassie to its rapid expansion after the 1974 revolution. Despite the rapid growth of PHC under Mengistu (during the Derg period, from 1974 to 1987), community participation was impacted by the protracted war and by centralized urban-based bureaucratic approaches and attitudes that failed to foster a comprehensive approach to PHC (Kloos, 1998). Considering the past gains and challenges in the process of implementing Health Sector Development Program I (1997–2000/2001), the federal government realized that necessary basic health services had not reached the people at the grassroots level as planned. In response, the government developed an innovative approach aimed at creating a healthy environment as well as healthy lifestyles by introducing a health extension package as a subcomponent of Health Sector

Development Program II (HSDP II 2002–2005). The main objective of the Health Service Extension Program (HSEP) is to improve equitable access to preventive essential health interventions through community-based health services, with a strong focus on sustained preventive health actions and increased health awareness (Federal Ministry of Health [FMOH], 2004a).

The health extension service is being provided as a package focusing on preventive health measures and targeting households, particularly women/mothers at the *kebele* level (the lowest administrative unit). The core purpose of the HSEP is to identify and provide a list of essential health services to households at the *kebele* level, thereby improving coverage and comprehensiveness of PHC services. The four major components of the package are disease prevention and control, family health service, hygiene and environmental sanitation, and health education and communication (FMOH, 2004b). These services are provided by health extension workers (HEWs), who are civil servants who receive a rapid vocational training (about a year) on 16[1] health-services packages, which are organized under the four components of the HSEP. HEWs are meant to be females who have completed at least grade 10 and are residents of the *kebele* in which they work. They are meant to complement the work of other community health workers. Community health volunteers[2] (CHVs) are voluntary health workers who are members of the community; they serve with no formal training except for irregularly provided short trainings. These HEWs (trained for about a year before deployment) offer key technical services such as immunization, family planning, and health education to the inhabitants of each *kebele*. Since the implementation of Health Sector Development Program III (2006–10), HEWs are entitled to provide basic curative services for childhood pneumonia, malaria, and diarrhea in addition to

---

1 A 17th package, behaviour-change communication, was added just after this study was conducted.

2 CHVs include voluntary community health workers of various categories. They include malaria agents, community-based reproductive health agents (CBRHA), and trained traditional birth attendants (TBAs), among others. These are trained and deployed by different nongovernmental organizations for specific services. Subsequent to this study many of the CHVs were reorganized under the heading of the "community development army," or CDA, with specific responsibilities for five households under the guidance of HEWs.

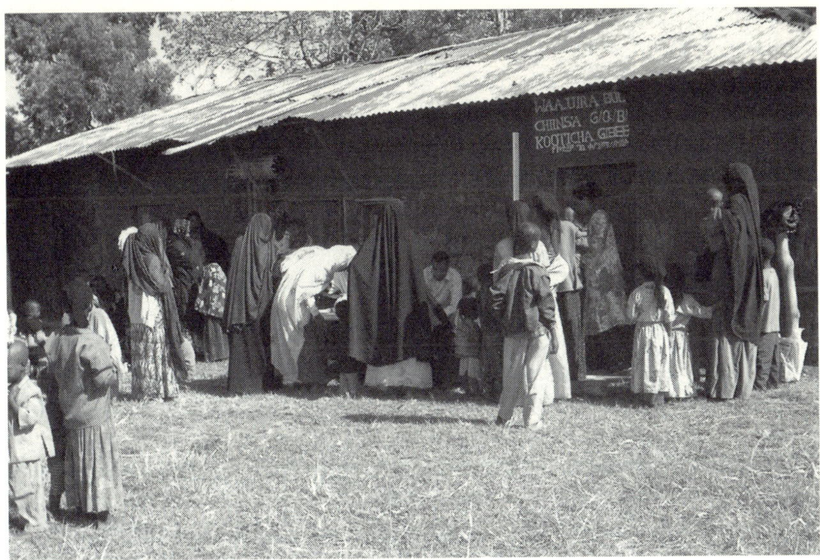

Health extension workers mobilizing women for health checks, Kooticha
Village, Ethiopia

their regular prevention activities. The plan of deploying two HEWs
and constructing and equipping a health post in each *kebele* through an
accelerated expansion of PHC facilities has been achieved, notably in
the rural areas of the country (FMOH, 2005; FMOH, 2004b).

Kebele-level health services such as the HSEP in Ethiopia have also
been observed in other countries. Such approaches, generally aimed at
community and family empowerment, are especially important in countries with restricted access to facility care or an undersupply of human
resources, as is the case in Ethiopia. To track regional and worldwide
trends of success or failure of these and other approaches, national data
are vital. Most importantly, such data should be used for appropriate action within countries and to ensure governments are accountable for the
provision of services to the poorest citizens (Rohde et al., 2008). For this
reason, the Jimma University research team set out to explore whether
introduction of the HSEP in Jimma zone has improved coverage and
comprehensiveness of PHC services delivered to the population in the
rural areas of Jimma zone, Southwest Ethiopia.

Research Questions and Methods

We collected empirical evidence that provides answers to the following two questions. First, has the recently adopted approach of the HSEP for rural health services assisted in increasing PHC coverage in Jimma zone? Second, has the HSEP enhanced community participation and intersectoral collaboration for PHC?

Data was collected in 2009 in Jimma zone, which is one of the 17 zones that make up the Oromia Regional State in Southwest Ethiopia. A cross-sectional exploratory study design employing both qualitative and quantitative methods of data collection was used. Three of the 17 rural *woredas* of Jimma zone were selected randomly. The *kebeles* in the 17 rural *woredas* of Jimma zone were at different stages with respect to introduction of the HSEP: some *kebeles* had had the HSEP years ago (since 2004), but the most recent introduction was in 2008. This created conditions for a quasi-experimental design in which the *kebeles* in the selected *woredas* were grouped by the amount of time since the HSEP had been introduced, categorized into "earliest," "medium," and "most recent." Hence, nine *kebeles* (one from each of the three strata of each of the three *woredas*) were randomly selected.

To determine the number of households to be included in the study, single population proportion formula for sample size calculation was used. The diphtheria-pertussis-tetanus–3 doses (DPT3) coverage in rural Ethiopia was 29% (Central Statistical Agency [CSA] and ORC Macro, 2006). As child health is one of the major components of the HSEP, this proportion was used as the p in the sample size calculation. After multiplying with a factor of 2 for design effect due to the multistage sampling process, and adding 10% nonresponse rate, the final sample size was 695. The total sample of households was then proportionally distributed to the nine *kebeles*. Finally, the households from each *kebele* were selected using systematic sampling.

Focus-group discussions were conducted with 16 HEWs and nine community health volunteers (CHVs), nine chairpersons and members of the *kebele* health committees (KHCs), and agricultural development agents[3] in the *kebeles*. In-depth interviews were conducted with three

---

3 Agricultural development agents are formally trained (at least grade 10 complete) male or female cadres deployed by the government to serve the community at the grassroots to improve agricultural productivity. They are the agriculture-sector equivalents of the HEWs.

woreda HSEP supervisors and one zonal HSEP supervisor. All focus-group discussions and in-depth interviews were audio recorded and supplementary notes were taken. The tape-recorded qualitative data were translated and transcribed word for word, followed by thematic coding, mapping, and interpretation to answer the research questions.

Data were collected through review of relevant records at the health posts, *woreda* health offices, and the Jimma Zonal Health Department. Face-to-face interviews of the female head in the sampled households were conducted using a structured questionnaire. To assess vaccination status, data was obtained only for children in possession of a vaccination card during the time of interview.

Coverage of PHC services was measured through the availability of health posts, number of HEWs per *kebele*, distance to the nearest health post, DPT3 and measles vaccination coverage, sources of health information, place of delivery, delivery attendance by a skilled person, knowledge about malaria, insecticide-treated net use, and other service indicators.

Quantitative data were cleaned and entered into *SPSS* version 14 to obtain summary figures and percentages. Pearson's Chi-Square Test of association was applied to look for differences in the coverage of PHC services among the three categories of *kebeles*. The study protocol was approved by the ethical review committee of Jimma University. Each of the health managers received a letter from the Research and Publication Office of Jimma University requesting his or her participation or that of a designate from their offices. The importance of accessing relevant records was also mentioned in the letter to the health managers. Written consent was obtained from each of the respondents. Respondents' right to refuse to respond to any of the questions or to refuse to participate was respected. Finally, all data accessed were kept confidential and remained so throughout the project period and thereafter.

Results and Analysis

Characteristics of the respondents

The respondents were almost equally distributed among the three *woredas*. The nine *kebeles* from these three *woredas* were grouped into three categories indicating the time of introduction of the HSEP: specifically, "most recent" (implemented less than one year at the time of our study); "medium" (running one to three years at the time of our study); and, "earliest" (where the program had been up and running three or more years before our study began).

A total of 683 households were included in this study giving a response rate of 98.3% (see Table 11.1). A majority of the women interviewed were married, of childbearing age, ethnically Oromos, and Muslim. Most reported being unable to read and write while, almost all of those who were literate and had some formal education had completed only grade 8.

As may be expected, most of the households earned their livelihood from farming. More than one-fourth of the households had annual expenses of 1,500 Ethiopian birrs (US$150, at the time of the study). On the other hand, the mean annual spending and income of the households were 3,907.94 and 9,977.18 Ethiopian birrs (US$391 and US$998), respectively.

Availability and use of health posts and health extension workers

Within the 17 rural *woredas* of the Jimma zone there are a total of 510 rural *kebeles*. The average number of rural *kebeles* in a *woreda* is 30, with a minimum of 14 in Gumayi *woreda* and a maximum of 53 in Dedo *woreda*. As demonstrated in Table 11.2, nearly 94% of the rural *kebeles* in the zone have two HEWs per *kebele*. Except for Gera and Tiro Afeta *woredas*, none of the *woredas* have more than three *kebeles* with less than one HEW.

A look at the coverage of the rural *kebeles* with health posts reveals that nearly 65% of the *kebeles* had a functional health post during the time of data collection. However, nearly one-third of the rural *kebeles* were in the process of constructing health posts, while 4% did not have any at all (Table 11.2).

Nearly 90% of the total 683 survey respondents claimed it took less than an hour to reach the health post in their *kebele* by foot (see Table 11.3). The remainder reported that it took them more than an hour. Respondents with access to HSEP programs that had come into effect recently or during the three years prior to our study had the shortest amount of travel time.

Survey participants were asked whether they can use the health post in their *kebele* any time they need. More than 96% of the respondents answered this question. More than half said that they can "always" use it any time if the need arises, while nearly 40% of them replied "sometimes" and the remaining said "never." The possibility of using the health post was significantly different among the three categories of *kebeles*, again implying association with time of introduction of the HSEP (p = 0.008), this time with the more recently implemented HSEP

Table 11.1 Origin and characteristics of the respondents, Jimma zone

Variables	Number (%)	Variables	Number (%)
Age		Grade attained	
15–49	592 (86.7)	1–8	99 (88.4)
> 49	91 (13.3)	9–10	10 (8.9)
Woreda		11–12	3 (2.7)
Mana	240 (35.2)	Occupation	
Kersa	227 (33.2)	Farmer	530 (77.6)
Shebe sombo	216 (31.6)	Trader	78 (11.4)
Kebele category (when HSEP was introduced)		Housewife	38 (5.6)
Recent (< 1 year)	244 (35.7)	Other**	37 (5.4)
Medium (1–3 years)	235 (34.4)	Family size	
Earliest (> 3 years)	204 (29.9)	< 5	357 (52.3)
Marital status		5–9	291 (42.6)
Married	609 (89.1)	> 9	35 (5.1)
Widowed	43 (6.3)	Annual income ($)*** (n = 663)	
Divorced	23 (3.4)	< 408	166 (25.0)
Never married	8 (1.2)	408–780	170 (25.7)
Ethnicity		780.1–1266.0	163 (24.6)
Oromo	545 (79.8)	> 1266.0	164 (24.7)
Amhara	57 (8.3)	Annual expenditure ($) (n = 678)	
Yem	55 (8.2)	< 150	179 (26.4)
Kefa	26 (3.7)	150–300	231 (34.0)
Religion		300.1–500.0	138 (20.4)
Muslim	535 (78.3)	> 500	130 (19.2)
Orthodox	131 (19.2)		
Protestant	17 (2.5)		
Educational status			
Unable to read and write	519 (76.0)		
No formal education*	52 (7.6)		
Have formal education	112 (16.4)		

*Able to read and write but have no formal education.

**Other includes government employees and daily labourers.

***1 USD = 10 Ethiopian birrs, roughly (at the time of the study).

programs performing worst. However, the fact that health posts were the first place to seek help during illness was not shown to have statistically significant association with the time of introduction of the HSEP into the *kebeles* (p = 0.053) (Table 11.3).

As one male CHV in the *kebele* of Doyo Tollu reported,

Before the arrival of health extension workers, people used to walk one to two hours to visit a health center or clinic. The nearest clinic takes one

Table 11.2 Availability of health extension workers (HEWs) and health posts in rural *kebeles* of Jimma zone, Southwest Ethiopia, May 2009

No.	Woreda	Total number of rural Kebeles	Availability of HEWs in the kebeles			Number of kebeles with health posts		
			Two	One	None	Available	Under construction	Not available
1	Chora Botor	30	28	2		24	6	
2	Dedo	53	52	1		20	26	7
3	Gera	29	21	8		29	0	
4	Gomma	36	34	1	1	16	14	6
5	Gumayi	14	13	1		10	4	
6	Limmu Kossa	40	40	0		24	16	
7	Limmu Seka	37	36	1		35	2	
8	Manna	24	23	1		13	11	
9	Nono Benja	19	16	3		15	2	2
10	Omo Nada	39	37	2		30	9	
11	Kersa	30	30	0		18	12	
12	Setemma	21	20	1		8	13	
13	Seka Chokorsa	36	36	0		15	21	
14	Shebe Sombo	20	19	1		14	4	2
15	Sigimo	19	18	1		16	3	
16	Sokoru	36	33	3		21	11	4
17	Tiro Afeta	27	22	5		19	8	
	Total	510	478 (93.7%)	31 (6.1%)	1 (0.2%)	327 (64.1%)	162 (31.8%)	21 (4.1%)

Table 11.3 Time of introduction of the HSEP with availability and use of the health posts in rural *kebeles* of Jimma zone, Southwest Ethiopia

Variables	Category of *kebeles*			
	Most recent	Medium	Earliest	
	No. (%)	No. (%)	No. (%)	p-value
HP* is available				
Yes	233 (95.5)	226 (96.2)	201 (98.5)	0.184
No	11 (4.5)	9 (3.8)	3 (1.5)	
Walking distance to the HP				
< 1 hour	213 (91.4)	189 (83.3)	186 (92.5)	0.003
> 1 hour	20 (8.6)	38 (16.7)	15 (7.5)	
Able to use the HP any time				
Always	112 (48.1)	123 (54.9)	114 (56.7)	0.008
Sometimes	99 (42.5)	87 (38.8)	84 (41.8)	
Never	22 (9.4)	14 (6.3)	3 (1.5)	
Place of first help				
HEWs	107 (43.9)	112 (50.0)	15 (6.1)	0.053
Other health professionals	112 (47.7)	109 (46.3)	14 (6.0)	
Nonhealth professionals	118 (57.9)	78 38.2)	8 (3.9)	

*HP = health post

hour to reach from our village. Now, since the arrival of these extension health workers and after we have advocated the activities of these workers, the community has been getting good services from them. Now our community has accepted them very well. The community has been involved on a voluntary basis in activities like environmental protection without being forced... Bed net use has increased in our kebele more than ever before.

Coverage of primary health care

The proportion of children who received earlier vaccination doses was higher than that given at a later age. One in 10 households had at least one child (0–23 months old) with diarrhea during the two weeks preceding the survey. More than one in four of the children were given nothing to drink during the diarrheal attack, while about 30% received somewhat less than the usual. About half of the mothers did not seek help from any source for the diarrheal episode. The majority (over 70%) sought treatment for the diarrheal attack only one or two days after it started. Neither the magnitude of child health problems nor the utilization of child health services showed significant difference with the time of introduction of the HSEP (p > 0.05).

An HEW from the Kersa-Tolikerso *kebele* confirmed their assigned duties as per Ministry of Health guidelines:

> We do have a program/schedule for all. Two days a week we provide health services at the health post. The remaining three days of work take place in the community; we conduct house-to-house visits. We provide health services on 16 packages. We provide services for malaria, pregnant women, environmental sanitation, personal hygiene, and others. On top of this, we do have regularly scheduled meetings with the kebele council once a week to report our progress, plan for the next get-together, discuss activities conducted and solve problems, if any, jointly.

Improvements were made in take-up of immunization, family planning, and ANC services through regular meetings, as one female CHV from Shebe *kebele* explained: "We have regular meetings. It depends on religious backgrounds. For Christians we visit churches every Sunday, but for Muslims we go every Wednesday to Mosques."

Of the 683 households, a slight majority had private pit latrines with shade, while the remaining households dispose excreta in private pit latrines without shading or on the open field. Handwashing after defecation showed no significant difference among the households in the different categories of *kebeles*; however, handwashing before main meals showed a statistically significant difference among the different categories of the *kebeles* (p = 0.011). Handwashing "always" after defecation or before meals was practised by only a minority of respondents, with a sizeable number "never" washing hands (see Table 11.4). A female CHV of Yebbu *kebele* added that,

> as per my kebele... we have been convincing households so that they keep their environment clean and consequently great changes have been registered. We influence the community to own latrines and to make their latrines standardized, putting a cover on the pit, making water and soap available and washing hands after use.

An unfavourable finding with regard to environmental health in this survey was that the majority of households dispose of refuse on the open field. The remaining households dispose of garbage in a pit in the house yard or burn it. The way the households disposed of garbage did

Table 11.4 Association of time of introduction of the HSEP with environmental and personal-hygiene practices of households in rural *kebeles*, Jimma zone

Variables	Category of *kebele*				
	Most recent	Medium	Earliest		
	No. (%)	No. (%)	No. (%)	Total	p-value
Excreta disposal					
Open field	33 (47.2)	26 (37.1)	11 (15.7)	70	0.003
Private pit latrine without shading	77 (31.6)	99 (40.6)	68 (27.8)	244	
Private pit latrine with shading	134 (36.3)	110 (29.8)	125 (33.9)	369	
Place of garbage disposal					
Open field	174 (37.3)	146 (31.2)	147 (31.5)	467	0.114
Hole in the house yard	61 (33.3)	76 (41.5)	46 (25.2)	183	
Burn/bury	9 (27.3)	13 (39.4)	11 (33.3)	33	
Handwashing with soap after defecation					
Yes, always	74 (32.4)	87 (38.2)	67 (29.4)	228	0.291
Yes, sometimes	141 (38.6)	120 (32.9)	104 (28.5)	365	
Not at all	29 (32.2)	28 (31.1)	33 (36.7)	90	
Handwashing with soap before main meal					
Yes, always	73 (30.3)	103 (42.7)	65 (27.0)	241	0.011
Yes, sometimes	148 (39.9)	109 (29.4)	114 (30.7)	371	
Not at all	23 (32.4)	23 (32.4)	25 (35.2)	71	
Contribution of HEWs to the above practices					
Excellent	8 (12.3)	23 (35.4)	34 (52.3)	65	0.000
Very good	97 (37.3)	103 (39.6)	60 (23.1)	260	
Good	97 (37.2)	81 (31.0)	83 (31.8)	261	
Poor	28 (38.9)	20 (27.8)	24 (33.3)	72	
Very poor	14 (56.0)	8 (32.0)	3 (12.0)	25	

not demonstrate significant difference among the households from the different categories of *kebeles* (p = 0.114).

Finally, households were given the chance to rate the contribution of the HEWs to their environmental and personal-hygiene practices. The majority rated the contribution of the HEWs as "good" or "very good." Nonetheless, nearly 15% of households said their contribution was "poor/very poor," and the remaining 10% rated them as "excellent." The rate given to the contribution of the HEWs for the environmental and personal-hygiene practices of the households had statistically significant differences among the households from the three categories of the *kebeles* (p = 0.000) (see Table 11.4).

About 60% of the 683 respondents reported having used a contraceptive method to avoid or delay pregnancy. Interestingly, the initial sources of information for the majority of women using contraceptives were HEWs (65%), followed by radio (29%). Other sources included the community-based reproductive-health agent (CBRHA),[4] health facilities, and friends/neighbours. Nonetheless, of the 683 households surveyed, 300 had women who had been pregnant during the three years preceding the survey. Though more than a quarter of these women did not receive ANC during their most recent pregnancy, the majority (more than 70%) did have at least one ANC visit. More than 90% of the deliveries occurred at home. There was statistically significant difference with the categories of the *kebeles* ($p < 0.05$) regarding the fact that the health post was the main source of family-planning information and the possibility that the health post was the place where women received ANC.

Community participation and intersectoral collaboration

Members of the Kebele Health Committees (KHCs) commented that when the HSEP was initially introduced, community members did not trust the HEWs as trained personnel. However, following HEW efforts to train every household on the 16 packages, members of the community began to accept them. The HEW strategy was to identify "model families" who were educated about these packages and would be expected to practice what they learned. In turn, these model families were expected to pass on their new knowledge and practices to their neighbours. KHCs were also found to be key players in organizing community mobilization activities based around these packages.

Our study revealed that HEWs work with almost all social, cultural, religious, and administrative structures available in the *kebele*. The HEWs are using religious leaders to encourage individuals and families in the *kebeles* to make use of available modern health facilities. Schools and agricultural-development agents are important parties who work with the HEWs to improve community participation at the grassroots level. CHVs are also playing a very important role in implementing the HSEP by closely working with HEWs free of cost. Supplies and technical support provided by HEWs to CHVs were reported to be commendable.

---

4 CBRHAs are voluntary community health workers trained and deployed by nongovernmental organizations to distribute family-planning methods to increase access to contraceptives.

Kebele councils and *kebele* health committees are actively involved in supporting HEWs' activities. HEWs are also receiving technical and managerial support from supervisors at the health centres and the *woreda* health offices. However, shortages of drugs and other medical supplies are sometimes encountered, resulting in failure to achieve planned activities. One of the male KHC members of Yebbu *kebele* noted,

> As for our kebele we, the KHC, do a lot so that our community is well equipped about health by educating the community to have know-how and apply the 16 packages. For this we each are working on the sites we are assigned in the kebele. It is the committee that follows and reports when new diseases occur and mobilises the community to meet on health education for behavior change. Now-a-days we are working on health activities like facilitation of latrine ownership and its sanitation, FP, children's personal hygiene and environmental sanitation and the like… together with the HEWs.

Except for school-based activities and limited work with agricultural-development agents, HEWs are not much engaged in ISA for health. Supervisors from the zonal and *woreda* levels reported that intersectoral collaboration for health is nonexistent at higher levels.

Discussion and Conclusion

The physical presence of health posts in the study *kebeles* was not meeting the government's forecast to provide 100% coverage. Only 64% of the *kebeles* had functional health posts, although other health posts were being constructed in Jimma zone. Almost all of the *kebeles* in the zone already had two HEWs assigned, stationing themselves in the *kebele* administration office and schools. However, the HEWs rated the health services they provided to be between "good" and "moderate" along a scale of "excellent" to "very poor." Major reasons given for this somewhat low ranking were deep-rooted beliefs and misconceptions held by the communities, hindering the uptake of family planning and immunization services. Furthermore, members of the community failed to attend health-education sessions, to volunteer to become a model family, to dig pits for waste disposal, and so on.

Looking at specific health services, the vaccination status of children as measured by DPT3 was 67.9%. This coverage is well below the 76.8% reported on the Ministry of Health's 2005/06 health and health-related indicators. It is even lower than the pentavalent coverage

Figure 11.1 Interaction of health extension workers with governmental
and community-based structures

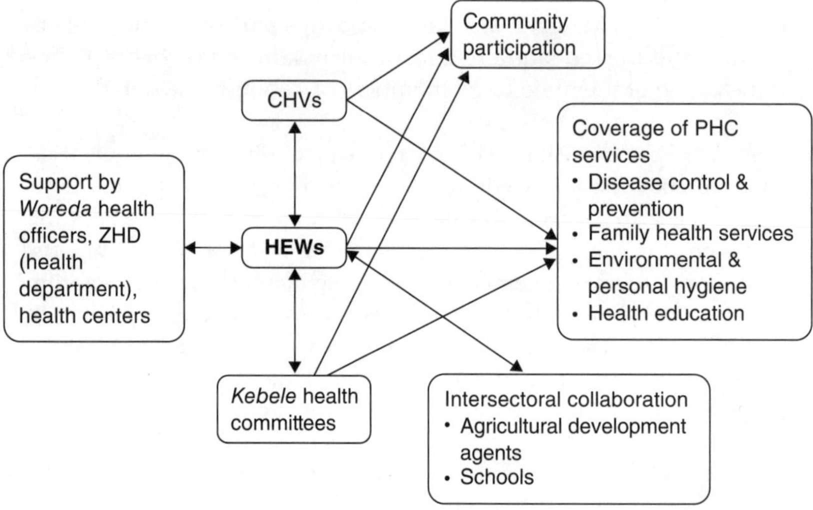

(81.6%) reported for the years 2008/09 (FMOH, 2008). Our study and
the latest figures from the Ministry of Health's Extended Program of
Immunization demonstrate that Ethiopia in general and the study area
in particular have lower rates of immunization than countries that have
selective PHC in place (Rohde et al., 2008). However, this lower coverage is still more than twice the rate than that reported by the 2005
Ethiopian Demographic and Health Survey for both the Oromia region (28.5%) and the country as a whole (31.9%) (CSA and ORC Macro,
2006). Immunization rates can therefore be said to be comparatively
high in the Jimma zone region.

The implementation of the Reach Every District approach[5] in Africa
was credited with increasing regional DPT3 coverage from 54% prior to
its 2002 implementation to 66% in 2004 (Sambo, 2006). Similarly, if the
finding of the 2005 Ethiopian Demographic and Health Survey (28.5%) is

---

5 The Reach Every District approach was developed and introduced in 2002 by WHO,
   UNICEF, and the GAVI Alliance to improve immunization systems in areas with low
   coverage. The approach outlines five operational activities aimed at improving coverage in local *woredas*. *Global Immunization Vision and Strategy 2006–2015* (Geneva: WHO
   &UNICEF, 2005).

taken as the baseline, the introduction of the HSEP may have contributed substantially to the current level of 67.9% in the *kebeles* of Jimma zone.

Focusing on where the services were obtained, seven out of 10 women who claimed to have a family planning service nearby identified the health post as the place of service. The initial sources of information for the majority of the women (65.4%) using contraceptives were the HEWs, followed by radio (28.7%).

In the study *kebeles*, only 10.2% of households dispose of excreta on the open field; the remaining use pit latrine with or without shading. This is quite an encouraging finding in light of the national (62.0%) and rural (70.0%) proportion of households not using latrine facilities (CSA and ORC Macro, 2006). Similarly, only 13.2% and 10.4% of the households reported that their members do not practice handwashing with soap after using the latrine and before main meals, respectively, while the remaining majority do so. A study of a rural school in Ethiopia showed that most students practiced handwashing before meals, but only 36.2% of them used soap. Similarly, although 76.7% of students reported that washing hands after defecation was important, only 14.8% reported actually following this practice (Vivas et al., 2010).

It has been frequently claimed that "active community participation is essential for effective community interventions such as those for maternal, newborn, and child health and environment-related diseases" (Viswanathan et al., 2009). In Ethiopia, from the beginnings of PHC under the Selassie regime to its rapid expansion after the 1974 revolution, community participation was promoted through health policy and implementation as well as through the use of health services (Kloos, 1998). However, palpable changes in community empowerment were not realized until recently, when the HSEP was introduced. This study revealed that HEWs work with almost all social, cultural, religious, and administrative structures available in the *kebele*.

HEWs are using religious leaders to initiate individuals and families in the *kebeles* to make use of available modern health facilities. Schools and agricultural-development agents are important parties who work with HEWs at the grassroots level to improve community participation. Supplies and technical support provided by HEWs to CHVs (whether they be TBAs or malaria agents) are significant. Female CHVs have created space for women in the *kebele* to share personal information about women's reproductive health.

Community members did not initially trust the HEWs as trained personnel, regarding them only as laywomen from the *kebele*. That is why a study that assessed the sustainability of HSEP recommended providing "sufficient orientation to communities regarding the significance of improved health practices and the role of CHVs" (Amare, 2009).

Although "intersectoral action linking health and development including that for better water, sanitation, nutrition, food security, and HIV control" (Lawn et al., 2008) has been recommended since the Declaration of Alma-Ata, its implementation has proved to be difficult in most settings (Viswanathan et al., 2009). This was also observed by HEWs themselves in the Jimma zone, even after the introduction of the HSEP. Supervisors at the zonal and *woreda* levels reported that intersectoral collaboration is weak at higher levels. However, they said that schools and agricultural development agents in the *kebeles* are collaborating with the HEWs in health-related activities.

Findings from this study were shared with community representatives, government officials, and NGOs on several occasions. Community members and government officials willingly took part in data provision. Interest in uptake of the findings was discernable, although no follow-up study has been undertaken to track uptake and changes. What is known is that HSEP is being scaled up to urban areas of the country. The difference between the cadres in the rural and urban health posts is that the urban cadres are already trained nurses who received special training to work as health extension professionals. In addition, HEWs in rural settings are becoming more involved in basic curative services while implementing what is known as integrated community case management of childhood illnesses (a program being piloted in several parts of the country, including the Jimma zone).

Findings in this study showed that institutionalizing *kebele* health service by employing civil servants at the village level has contributed significantly to improved coverage and comprehensiveness of PHC, as was demonstrated by the following core findings:

- The distribution of HEWs and availability of health posts throughout the Jimma zone have improved significantly since the introduction of HSEP. There are only a few *kebeles* without a health post and health extension workers, and in these cases, the *kebeles* at least have HEWs and a health post under construction.
- Access and coverage of maternal and child health services (family planning, ANC, vaccination), environmental and personal hygiene, disease prevention and control measures, as well as health information have significantly improved since the introduction of the HSEP.

However, behaviour change in the use of family-planning methods, institutional and skilled delivery, management of childhood diarrhea, and malaria prevention and control did not show much change, even in the *kebeles* where the HSEP was introduced early on, more than three years prior to our study.
* HEWs worked with almost all social, cultural, religious, and administrative structures available in the *kebele*. However, there is little evidence of ISA for health, either at the *kebele* or higher administrative levels.

Despite notable gains and progress in the PHC program, challenges to CPHC were observed. The roll-out of health posts and subsequently of health workers succeeded in improving delivery of PHC services in the rural areas of Jimma zone, although the number of functional health posts in the zone was below the government's target. While HEWs typically struggled at first for acceptance in the community, most reported eventually gaining their community's trust. But intersectoral action, needed to make the program more comprehensive, proved difficult in most settings. Community participation was also lacklustre. HEWs attributed this to misconceptions held by the communities that hindered their uptake of family-planning and immunization services. Members of the community shunned not only health-education sessions, but also volunteering to become a model family and digging pits for waste disposal. In sum, there clearly remain extensive challenges to expanding the Health Services Extension Program to become more comprehensive.

ACKNOWLEDGMENTS

We are grateful to the study participants and health managers who were very helpful during the conduct of the data collection. We also would like to thank Jimma University for the cooperation we received throughout this project.

REFERENCES

Amare, Y. (2009). Non-financial incentives for voluntary community health workers: A qualitative study. Working paper no. 1: The last ten kilometers project. Addis Ababa, Ethiopia: JSI Research & Training Institute, Inc.

Central Statistical Agency and ORC Macro. (2006). *Ethiopia demographic and health survey 2005*. Addis Ababa, Ethiopia, and Calverton, Maryland, USA: Author.

Federal Ministry of Health. (2004a). *An overview of Health Extension Package*. Addis Ababa, Ethiopia: Author.

Federal Ministry of Health (2004b). Accelerated expansion of primary health care coverage of Ethiopia: 2005–2009. Addis Ababa, Ethiopia.

Federal Ministry of Health. (2005). *Health sector strategic plan (HSDP III 2005/6/ –2009/10)*. Addis Ababa, Ethiopia: Author.

Federal Ministry of Health (2008). *Health and health related indicators, 2008/09*. Addis Ababa, Ethiopia.

Index Mundi (2014 and 2015). *Ethiopia*. Retrieved from http://www .indexmundi.com/ethiopia/

Kloos, H. (1998, Feb–Mar). Primary health care in Ethiopia under three political systems: Community participation in a war-torn society. *Social Science & Medicine, 46*(4–5), 505–22. http://dx.doi.org/10.1016/S0277 -9536(97)00194-9 Medline:9460830

Lawn, J. E., Rohde, J., Rifkin, S., Were, M., Paul, V.K., Chopra, M. (2008). Alma-Ata 30 years on: Revolutionary, relevant, and time to revitalize. *The Lancet, 372*, 917–27. doi: 10.1016/S0140-6736(08)61402-6

Rohde, J., Cousens, S., Chopra, M., Tangcharoensathien, V., Black, R., Bhutta, Z.A., &Lawn, J.E. (2008, Sep13). 30 years after Alma-Ata: Has primary health care worked in countries? *The Lancet, 372*(9642), 950–61. http://dx .doi.org/10.1016/S0140-6736(08)61405-1 Medline:18790318

Sambo, L. (2006). *Revitalizing health services using the primary health care approach in the African region. International Hospital Federation Reference Book 2006/2007.* London, UK: Pro-Brook Publishing Limited.

Viswanathan, M., Kraschnewski, J., Nishikawa, B., Morgan, L.C., Thieda, P., Honeycutt, A., &Jonas, D. (2009). *Outcomes of community health worker interventions.*

Vivas, A.P., Gelaye, B., Aboset, N., Kumie, A., Berhane, Y., &Williams, M.A. (2010, Jun). Knowledge, attitudes and practices (KAP) of hygiene among school children in Angolela, Ethiopia. *Journal of Preventive Medicine and Hygiene, 51*(2), 73–9. Medline:21155409

12 The Contribution of Health Extension Workers in Improving the Utilization of Maternal Health Services in Rural Areas of Tigray, Ethiopia

ARAYA ABRHA MEDHANYIE, MARK SPIGT,
YOHANNES TEWELDE KIFLE, NIKKI SCHAAY,
DAVID SANDERS, ROMAN BLANCO,
GEERT-JAN DINANT, AND YEMANE BERHANE

Background

Ethiopia, like many resource-constrained countries, has over the past couple of decades been training and deploying different categories of volunteer community health workers (CHWs), such as trained traditional birth attendants (TBAs), community-based reproductive-health agents, and community health agents. However, in 2003, to accelerate the expansion of primary health care (PHC) coverage and to ensure equitable access to health services, the government of Ethiopia started deploying a new cadre of specially trained community-based health workers called health extension workers (HEWs). Apart from the requirement of having completed high school and undergone one year of comprehensive training prior to being deployed, the HEWs are also distinct from the volunteer CHWs in that they are employed by the Ministry of Health and are paid a monthly salary.

This initiative, with the HEWs as its backbone, is known as the Health Extension Program (HEP).[1] Modelled on the country's agricultural extension worker program and designed with the concept and principles

---

1 Ethiopia variously refers to this program as "Health Services Extension Program" (HSEP), the term used in Chapter 11, and as the "Health Extension Program" (HEP), the term used in this chapter. They are the same program.

of comprehensive primary health care (CPHC) in mind (Federal Ministry of Health of Ethiopia, 2005, 2007, 2010; Datiko & Lindtjørn, 2009), the HEP recognized the important role that HEWs can play in working in collaboration with other sectors to address some of the socioeconomic determinants of ill-health within communities.

By 2010, approximately 34,000 HEWs were trained and deployed throughout the country. Maternal health is one of their key areas of responsibility. With the aim of reducing maternal mortality, HEWs are trained to provide care to pregnant mothers throughout pregnancy, birth, and the postnatal period. HEWs inform pregnant mothers on safe motherhood when they provide antenatal care (ANC), birth, and postnatal care (PNC). HEWs also provide family-planning services and are trained to educate women on the use of iodized salt and HIV testing.

However, since the implementation of the HEP, few studies have published findings on the effectiveness of HEWs (Koblinsky et al., 2010). Although these studies have shown HEWs' effectiveness in improving utilization of family-planning and immunization services, none of them investigated the role of HEWs in improving utilization of comprehensive maternal health services.

Research Questions and Methods

This study sought to determine the extent to which the specially trained HEWs have contributed to improving utilization of maternal health services by rural women in Ethiopia.

The study was conducted in Tigray, the northernmost regional state of Ethiopia. The 2007 Ethiopian census showed the population of the region to be 4.3 million, of which 80% lived in rural areas and 51% were female (Central Statistical Agency of Ethiopia, 2008). The poor health status of Tigray's population is comparable to the rest of the country, showing a relatively high infant mortality rate (67/1,000), low institutional delivery (8.6%), high HIV prevalence (2.7%), and low family-planning utilization (16.5%) (Central Statistical Agency of Ethiopia, 2006).

Three rural districts in Tigray were purposively selected as the study site. Within each of these districts, three *kebeles* (villages), each with a functional health post and HEWs, were purposively selected as the data-collection sites.

Between August and November 2009, a cross-sectional survey was undertaken in the nine *kebeles*. Data was collected by six data collectors using a questionnaire developed and administered in the local language, Tigrigna. The following variables were used to ascertain the interviewee's utilization of maternal health services:

1 Family planning: whether the woman has been using contraceptives during the interview period (current utilization) or whether the woman has ever used contraceptives in her lifetime (total utilization).
2 Antenatal care (ANC): whether the woman attended a health facility for ANC at least once in her last successful pregnancy.
3 Health-facility delivery: whether the woman, for her youngest child, gave birth at a health facility.
4 Postnatal care (PNC): whether a health professional or CHW visited the woman at her home within 24 hours of the birth of her youngest child.
5 HIV testing: whether the woman had ever had an HIV test by the time of interview.
6 Use of iodized salt: whether iodized cooking salt (with 15 parts per million based on salt-testing kits) was found in the woman's house. This was considered as a maternal-health service because educating women on the use of iodized salt and distributing subsidized iodized salt are among the tasks of HEWs.

Using the HEWs' log books – which each have a list of households in their *kebele* – and a process of systematic random sampling, women with under-5 children from the nine selected *kebeles* who were willing and healthy enough to be interviewed were identified to participate in the survey. When a woman selected for an interview was not available, a neighbouring woman was interviewed. A total of 726 women were interviewed, and data from 725 women were included in the analysis, with one questionnaire being unusable because of its incompleteness.

In addition, we measured several other variables such as age, educational status, marital status, religion, year of enrolment in the HEP, household status in relation to working towards graduation or having graduated as a "model family," and participation in government or community-initiated income-generating activities (IGAs). These IGAs include irrigation schemes, microfinance credit, cattle rearing, poultry production, and bee keeping.

A "model family" is by definition a family that has or is receiving health education and basic health services from their local HEW about the prevention and control of disease (e.g., TB, HIV/AIDS, and malaria);

family health (maternal and child health, immunization, and nutrition); and hygiene and environmental sanitation (e.g., excreta disposal) – themes and topics that have been prioritized by the HEP and fall within the HEP "package" of services offered by HEWs.

Frequencies of utilization of specific maternal health services were then calculated. To estimate changes in the utilization of maternal health services over the years, we compared our findings with findings of the Ethiopian Demographic Health Survey (EDHS) 2005. The EDHS 2005 was a nationally representative survey of 14,070 women aged 15 to 49 years. The data collection for this survey was conducted from April 27 to August 30, 2005.

To investigate which factors were associated with good utilization of maternal health services, we used logistic regression. To calculate adjusted odds ratios (AOR), we included all independent variables in one model. The dependent variable was computed by combining the six outcome variables. Using the mean (3.01) as a cut-off point, we categorized utilization of maternal health services into two categories. Women who had used four or more maternal health services were defined as having good utilization, while those who had used fewer than four were considered as having poor utilization. Women's responses to questions on religion, marital status, and occupation were virtually the same. Therefore, these variables were not used in the analysis.

The study was conducted in consultation with the Tigray Regional Health Bureau and approved by the ethics committee at the College of Health Sciences of Mekelle University, Ethiopia.

Results and Analysis

Respondents' characteristics

The mean age of the 725 study participants was 31.4 years, and almost all (99.9%) were orthodox Christians. The mean number of children per woman was 4.15. The majority of participants (86%) were involved in at least one IGA, with microfinance credit and the safety-net programs being the most reported IGAs.

Utilization of maternal health services

More than half (67%) of the women had used contraceptives, while 38% were current users. An ANC visit at health facility was reported by

85%. However, less than half (48%) had the World Health Organization (WHO)–recommended four or more ANC visits. A small number (5%) said that they gave birth at the health facility. A similar percentage (5%) had PNC check-ups. More than three quarters (85%) had been tested for HIV. Iodized salt of greater than 15 ppm was found in only 13% of the women's households.

The role of HEWs in improving the utilization of maternal health services is greatest in relation to family planning and ANC. With respect to advice on family planning, 72% of the mothers reported having received information on this topic from the HEW. Forty-four percent of the mothers reported having been visited before delivery by HEWs. However, postnatal care and especially assistance during delivery are areas in which HEWs provide less support. The majority of the women (81%) delivered their babies with the help of relatives or friends, and only 7% were assisted by the HEW. Trained traditional birth attendants were, at 20%, more likely than HEWs to assist births.

Women's utilization of primary care facilities for maternal health services

Health posts were rarely used by women for delivery services and PNC check-ups. Only 1% of the study participants gave birth at health posts. A similar percentage had had PNC check-ups for their babies at health posts. The utilization of health posts for family planning and ANC by women was relatively higher than for delivery. About 21% of the study participants had obtained contraceptives from the health posts. It seemed that women preferred the health centre to the health post for ANC follow-up (61% versus 23%).

Compared to EDHS 2005 (Table 12.1), there is an increase in the percentage of women who have used family planning, ANC, and HIV testing. However, we observed no positive changes in the percentage of women who have used health-facility delivery and iodized salt.

Calculated AOR through logistic regression analysis showed that women who were able to read and write (AOR 1.85; CI 1.22–2.80), listened to a radio (AOR 1.45; CI 1.05–2.02), had good participation in IGAs (AOR 1.43; CI 1.03–2.00), and had been working towards graduation or had graduated as model family (AOR 2.13; CI 1.40–3.23) had good utilization of maternal health services. However variables, including place of residence, age, and year of enrolment, did not show any significant association with good utilization of maternal health services.

Table 12.1 Comparison of findings of our study with findings of the 2005 EDHS for Tigray region and Ethiopia

Access to maternal health services	National EDHS 2005 (%)	Regional Tigray EDHS 2005 (%)	Our study 2009 (%)
Family planning: current users	14.7	16.5	41.8
Antenatal care	27.6	35.3	84.6
Delivery at health facility	5.3	6.1	4.7
Postnatal check up	5.5	8.2	5.3
HIV (ever tested)	4.0	3.2	85.4
Iodized salt (> 15 ppm)	19.9	28.0	13.2

Discussion

Since the introduction of the HEP in 2003 and deployment of HEWs, there has been an increase in the percentage of women who have used family planning, ANC, and HIV testing. However, the HEWs' deployment and work have not shown to have improved the utilization of health facilities for delivery, postnatal check-up, and use of iodized salt.

Our findings in relation to family planning are in agreement with other studies conducted in Ethiopia (Kitaw, Ye-Ebiyo, Said, Desta, & Teklehaimanot, 2007; Abraha & Nigatu, 2009), which similarly showed that HEWs have improved women's access to family planning. A study conducted in the southern part of Ethiopia found that women who were able to read and write are more likely to access maternal health services, similar to our findings. This study also showed, similar to our findings on ANC, that the percentage of women who had at least one ANC visit has increased considerably (Ergano, Getachew, Seyum, & Negash, 2012). Nevertheless our study showed the percentage of women who had four or more ANC visits as recommended by WHO was still low (48%). A concerted effort by HEWs and volunteer CHWs is necessary to educate women about the importance of having four and more ANC visits.

Another important achievement observed in our study is the increase in HIV testing. A study on antiretroviral treatment in Ethiopia depicted a similar substantial expansion of access to HIV counselling and testing in Ethiopia (Assefa, Jerene, Lulseged, Ooms, & Van Damme, 2009). This increase might not be totally attributed to HEWs, because nongovernmental organizations (NGOs) and other stakeholders also play a crucial role in HIV testing and education through different approaches, such as campaigns. HIV programs are highly supported by NGOs and other stakeholders. However, the positive role of HEWs in improving HIV testing and prevention in rural areas is undisputable. In reality, in rural *kebeles* in Ethiopia, HIV testing and education on HIV prevention is carried out primarily by HEWs. Even HEWs who are not trained for HIV testing organize and coordinate the campaigns for HIV testing using HIV test kits. Practically all the health activities including campaigns at rural *kebeles* in Ethiopia are undertaken and organized by HEWs.

The HEWs did not succeed in improving utilization of health-facility delivery, PNC check-up, and use of iodized salt. This finding calls for urgent intervention in the HEP. Innovative approaches are needed to improve HEW effectiveness in relation to these services. Similar to our study, another study also showed no progress in skilled birth assistance and PNC coverage in Ethiopia since 1998 (Abraha & Nigatu, 2009). Contrary to the findings of a cross-sectional study of 60 households in the Tigray region that was conducted at the earlier stages of HEP implementation, our study revealed the percentage of women who were assisted during births by trained TBAs is much higher than those assisted by HEWs (Negusse, McAuliffe, & MacLachlan, 2007). This difference might be due to the fact that the number of TBAs in a *kebele* is higher than the number of HEWs. It also might be that TBAs are tried and tested by women and seen to be experienced in conducting deliveries; perhaps they are closer and more accessible to village women. However, low competency of (and confidence in) HEWs in assisting births, less favourable working conditions at the health posts, heavy workloads, and long walking distances at night to assist with home births also might explain the low performance of HEWs in assisting with births (Teklehaimanot et al., 2007).

Although further research is needed to study HEWs' performance in birth assistance, we propose several reasons for the present findings of their low participation in this role. First, health-facility delivery is demanding in relation to cost, skill, and competency. It requires that HEWs have the necessary skills and that communities have accessible and well-supplied facilities in place.

Second, encouraging this behavioural change is time-consuming work (Wahed, 2009a; Wahed 2009b; Campbell & Graham, 2006). Women's preference for giving birth at home is a deeply embedded cultural belief. Women may believe that it is appropriate to go to a health facility for birth assistance and check-up only if there are visible complications during birth (Wahed, 2009b). Other determinants, such as women's age, education, income, number of children, and health-seeking behaviour, could also influence women's preference for delivering with trained TBAs (Ergano et al., 2012). Thus, focused birth preparedness by pregnant women is necessary for women to give birth at health facilities or assisted by health professionals. It is advisable for HEWs and other CHWs to carry out effective discussions on birth preparedness with pregnant women when they conduct home-based ANC visits.

Third, health posts are not well-equipped for providing delivery service, which is a disincentive for women to use these facilities. Almost all health posts are a single room only, with no waiting area, water source, or electricity. Hence a strong referral system should be established between health posts and health centres (which are better equipped for birth deliveries) until health posts meet the necessary standards for delivery service.

Fourth, the low performance of HEWs in assisting births also relates to how HEWs are perceived by the community. The community may regard HEWs as less competent to assist births. Unpublished reports from Tigray's Regional Health Bureau on the HEP indicate that the community perceives the main tasks of HEWs to be health education, sanitation, and personal hygiene (e.g., HEWs were associated with latrine construction). For all these reasons, and considering the present workload of HEWs as well as the poor conditions of health posts, it may be unrealistic to expect greater involvement in birth assistance by HEWs or that women would choose to give birth at health posts (Teklehaimanot et al., 2007; Wahed, 2009a; Wahed, 2009b; Campbell & Graham, 2006; Dudley, Hviding, & Paulsen, 2009).

The 1978 Alma-Ata Declaration on Primary Health Care (World Health Organization, 1978), and subsequent reviews of PHC reforms, call for intersectoral collaboration to address socioeconomic determinants of community health, in which ensuring universal access to health services is one element (World Health Organization, 2008a; World Health Organization, 2008b). In consideration of these other social determinants of women's health, this study looked at whether participating in IGAs was associated with utilization of maternal health services. Logistic regression analysis revealed that women who have been participating in three or more IGAs were 1.72 times more likely to have good utilization of comprehensive maternal health services. The regression analysis also demonstrated that women who were literate, listened to the radio, and had been working towards graduation or graduated as model families for the HEP were more likely to have good utilization of maternal health services. Hence these potential social factors could be targets for future intervention and support, as a means of increasing health-care utilization. Year of enrolment in the HEP was not associated with good utilization of maternal health services. This may be due to the effect of diffusion of the intervention. Households that were enrolled later in the program may have had opportunities to learn from households that were enrolled earlier and to share experience regarding positive health behaviours and information.

Conclusions

This study has shown that HEWs have brought essential maternal health care closer to the rural population in Ethiopia. Nevertheless, their success does not apply to all components of maternal health services: HEWs brought improvement in utilization of family planning, ANC, and HIV testing but not in assisting births. The perception that HEWs may be less competent in assisting births, the huge workload they already have, poorly equipped health posts, and strong cultural beliefs supporting home births make it unreasonable at present to expect substantial change in where and how women give birth. These challenging factors call for innovative strategies to support the efforts of HEWs in identifying risky pregnancies and birth preparedness, as well as in increasing referrals to health centres where midwives and better facilities for assisting births are available.

ACKNOWLEDGMENTS

We wish to acknowledge the support given by the facilitators of the project, most notably the University of Ottawa and the University of the Western Cape. We also would like to thank Mr. Awala Equar for his participation in design and data collection. We are grateful to all those who participated in this study. Some material in this chapter previously appeared in Medhanyie, A., Spigt, M., Kifle, Y., Schaay, N., Sanders, D., Blanco, R., Geertlan, D., & Berhane, Y. (2012) The role of health extension workers in improving utilization of maternal health services in rural areas in Ethiopia: A cross-sectional study. *BMC Health Services Research, 12*, 352.

REFERENCES

Abraha, M.W., & Nigatu, T.H. (2009, Dec13). Modeling trends of health and health related indicators in Ethiopia (1995–2008): A time-series study. *Health Research Policy and Systems*, 7(1), 29–46. http://dx.doi.org/10.1186/1478 -4505-7-29 Medline:20003381

Assefa, Y., Jerene, D., Lulseged, S., Ooms, G., & Van Damme, W. (2009, Apr28). Rapid scale-up of antiretroviral treatment in Ethiopia: Successes and system-wide effects. *PLoS Medicine*, 6(4), e1000056. http://dx.doi.org /10.1371/journal.pmed.1000056 Medline:19399154

Campbell, O.M., Graham, W.J., & *Lancet* Maternal Survival Series steering group. (2006, Oct7). Strategies for reducing maternal mortality: Getting on with what works. *Lancet*, 368(9543), 1284–99. http://dx.doi.org/10.1016 /S0140-6736(06)69381-1 Medline:17027735

Central Statistical Agency of Ethiopia. (2008). *Ethiopia national census: First draft report 2007*. Addis Ababa: Author.

Central Statistical Agency of Ethiopia and ORC Macro. (2006). *Ethiopia demographic and health survey 2005*. Addis Ababa, Ethiopia, and Calverton, Maryland: Author.

Datiko, D.G., & Lindtjørn, B. (2009). Health extension workers improve tuberculosis case detection and treatment success in southern Ethiopia: A community randomized trial. *PLoS One*, 4(5), e5443. http://dx.doi.org /10.1371/journal.pone.0005443 Medline:19424460

Dudley, L., Hviding, K., & Paulsen, E. (2009). The effectiveness of policies promoting facility-based deliveries in reducing maternal and infant morbidity and mortality in low and middle-income countries. *Cochrane Database of Systematic Reviews, 3*, 1–10Art. No. CD007918.

Ergano, K., Getachew, M., Seyum, D., & Negash, K. (2012). Determinants of community based maternal health care service utilization in South Omo pastoral areas of Ethiopia. *Journal of Medicine and Medical Sciences*, 3(2), 112–21.

Federal Ministry of Health of Ethiopia. (2005). *Essential Health Services Package for Ethiopia*. Addis Ababa: Author.

Federal Ministry of Health of Ethiopia. (2007). *Health Extension Program in Ethiopia: Profile*. Addis Ababa: Health Extension and Education Center.

Federal Ministry of Health of Ethiopia. (2010). *Health Sector Development Programme III*. Addis Ababa: Annual Performance Report, Ministry of Health.

Kitaw, Y., Ye-Ebiyo, Y., Said, A., Desta, H., & Teklehaimanot, A. (2007). Assessment of the training of the first intake of health extension workers. *Ethiopian Journal of Health Development*, 21(3), 232–9.

Koblinsky, M., Tain, F., Gaym, A., Karim, A., Carnell, M., & Tesfaye, S. (2010). Responding to the maternal care challenge: The Ethiopian Health Extension Program. *Ethiopian Journal of Health Development, 24*(1), 105–9. http://dx.doi.org/10.4314/ejhd.v24i1.62951

Negusse, H., McAuliffe, E., & MacLachlan, M. (2007, Aug24). Initial community perspectives on the Health Service Extension Programme in Welkait, Ethiopia. *Human Resources for Health, 5*(1), 21. http://dx.doi.org/10.1186/1478-4491-5-21 Medline:17718900

Teklehaimanot, A., Kitaw, Y., Girma, S., Seyoum, S., Desta, S., &Ye-Ebiyo, Y. (2007). Study of working conditions of health extension workers in Ethiopia. *Ethiopian Journal of Health Development, 21*(3), 246–59.

Wahed, T. (2009a). *Healthcare and cultural practices during pregnancy and childbirth in Korail, a slum in Dhaka, Bangladesh.* Manoshi Research Brief. Dhaka, Bangladesh: ICDDR and BRAC, 1–5.

Wahed, T. (2009b*). Beyond the inception phase of the birthing centers: Acceptance within the community.* Manoshi Research Brief. Dhaka, Bangladesh: ICDDR and BRAC, 1–4.

World Health Organization. (1978). *United Nations Children's Fund: Report of the International Conference on Primary Health Care.* Alma Ata, Former USSR.

World Health Organization. (2008a*). Report on the review of primary health care in the African region.* Brazzaville, Republic of Congo: WHO Regional Office for Africa.

World Health Organization. (2008b). *World health report 2008. Primary health care: Now more than ever.* Geneva: Author.

SECTION FOUR

Governance and Intersectoral Action

It has long been recognized that improved health equity requires changes in policies that affect SDH. Although aligning it primarily with traditional PHC concerns (such as education, sanitation, and safe water), the Alma-Ata Declaration recognized the importance of intersectoral action for health (IAH). IAH (and related terms, such as "healthy public policy" and more recently "health in all policies" or HiAP) underscores the importance of health systems engaging with other government (state) and nonstate (private) sectors to improve the conditions that shape health opportunities. Governance describes the processes by which these engagements occur, such as institutional rules or mandates of decision making and various means by which "stakeholders" – those with knowledge, resources, or interests in the decision-making – are able to participate. Evidence of health-system work in IAH and its governance mechanisms was found in only some of the projects:

Our funded team in **Brazil** examined health-care coordination and the challenges of implementing access across the full range of services within a comprehensive system of primary health care. Brazil recognized the right to health as a constitutional right in 1988, and the effective coordination of care is generally considered a means of ensuring respect for the right to health and a comprehensive approach to PHC. The current CPHC model in Brazil – originally the *Programa Saúde da Família* (the Family Health Program) and now known as *Estratégia Saúde da Família* (the Family Health Strategy) – extends health-care coverage to 50% of Brazil's population of 90 million people with 32,000 family health teams and 240,000 CHWs. Brazil's family health teams have become a model for CPHC reform across Latin America and in much of

Africa, and have been the subject of several studies, as our Brazil team's chapter indicates. Our Brazil team's study did not focus on the Family Health Strategy itself so much as on the link between the primary level of care (the family health teams) and secondary and tertiary levels of care, and the extent to which this link strengthened the family health teams in their work. The study's concern was with the important topic of CPHC governance with respect to access across all levels of care, such access being an important component of PHC reform even since the days of the Alma-Ata Declaration. Four municipalities (the governance level responsible for the family health teams and for clinics and hospitals) were studied to determine how integrated the health system had become and which factors allowed for better integration and access across all care levels. The most successful actions used a combination of system-integration strategies that included investments in decentralized and computerized regulation systems, waiting-list monitoring, an increased supply of the municipalities' own financed services, and the introduction of clinical guidelines and e-records. The research team found that those municipalities suffering from "organizational fragmentation" were unable to improve accessibility issues (e.g., by enabling family health teams to perform their intended role as the gateways to the health-care system). It also found that most physicians and nurses working in the family health teams did not believe that they enjoyed the same public esteem as specialists. Improving the visibility and importance of these teams was considered vital to sustaining and strengthening CPHC within the country's overall health system.

In **Argentina**, the research team undertook a unique approach to its study, focusing on a detailed historic analysis of competing models of PHC in two different geographic settings: one, a "shanty town" neighbourhood in Buenos Aires; the other, a set of rural industrial communities in a northern province. Both cases were selected for having undergone different periods of health- and political-policy change. The rural communities were seen as following a "sanitarian" approach to PHC, influenced by the Rockefeller Foundation's successful anti-malarial programs. The shanty town case followed a more European public-health model, with an emphasis on sanitation, housing, and potable-water supply. In both cases, implementation of the PHC programs were subjected to profound political swings, sometimes leading to violent interventions by the state, such as efforts to eradicate the shanty town and destroy its health facilities. The study concludes, in part, that an initial failure to clearly define a PHC framework for

Argentina led to a complex of implementation typologies, elements of which could be seen in both historic cases, and none of which fully reflect the comprehensive vision of Alma-Ata. At the same time, the research team found several examples of "good practice" that they consider to be "seeds of the future" for more comprehensive PHC.

Finally, the case of Guarjila, **El Salvador**, provides an exemplary model of community governance and intersectoral action. Although its success was made possible only through financial and technical resources from sympathetic international donors and NGOs, this support was always channeled through formal community structures that allowed for local-level self-determination and authority. The community essentially self-governed and self-implemented a large suite of health, education, sanitation, and rehabilitation programs, representing the most comprehensive PHC implementation among all our study sites. The success of the Guarjila program has since become the model for PHC reform within the country, which nonetheless faces challenges associated with insufficient financing and persisting violence as legacies of its long civil war. The comprehensiveness of PHC in Guarjila may also be somewhat unique as a "global" model, given its unique history as, first, encompassing a very small community and, second, arising in a difficult context of adversity following the armed Salvadorian conflict, which was characterized by militarization and institutionalized repression, displacement, and migration. Although it would thus be difficult to claim Guarjila to be a transferable model of CPHC reform, its experience provides lessons in how a combination of international solidarity and community empowerment can yield substantive gains in health and in its social determinants.

Two of our projects in which governance and international action for health were prominent were unable to contribute chapters to this book. Their research reports nonetheless highlight some important lessons for CPHC, which are summarized below:

1. Victorian Aboriginal Health Service (VAHS)[1]

The VAHS approach to CPHC was captured through a historical review of the organization. The southeastern seaboard of Australia,

---

1 The researchers on this project who prepared this summary were Bronwyn Fredericks, Joanne Luke, and Alan Brown.

which includes the state of Victoria, was colonized early in the history of Australia and, as a result, the Aboriginal people of this region were among the most heavily impacted. Aboriginal people in Victoria have been subject to policies of protection, segregation, and assimilation, all of which denied communities access to their culture, traditions, knowledge, and lands.

The VAHS was established in 1973 in the Melbourne suburb of Fitzroy. The location was strategic, as almost half of Australia's Aboriginal population lives in Melbourne. It was established as a direct response to the poor health conditions of the Aboriginal people, which were largely the result of racism and a self-perpetuating cycle of poverty. The health problems were numerous, with high levels of respiratory, infectious, liver, and heart problems, as well as sexually transmitted infections. Alcohol abuse was also a serious problem. Community leaders decided to seek solutions to their own health needs and to empower the community to change its social conditions. Since this time, VAHS has been offering CPHC services to the Australian Aboriginal population residing in the region or visiting Melbourne. The population serviced is very diverse, representing many nations and language groups.

As the first Aboriginal health service in Victoria, VAHS was responsible for providing emerging health services with leadership, support, and – most important – a working model of a community-controlled health service that could be transposed to regional communities. VAHS was initiated and is controlled and operated by Aboriginal people to deliver holistic, comprehensive, and culturally appropriate PHC to the Aboriginal community. Our research demonstrated the importance of addressing the poor health and well-being of Aboriginal people together with a continuum of activism for the rights of Aboriginal people. Our research also found that Aboriginal community control, self-management, rights, advocacy, social inclusion, access, and equity have been central in all of VAHS's activities.

As a good example of how intersectoral actions came into play, VAHS was concerned by how Aboriginal people were discriminated against in their contacts with the justice system, including contact with police and custody settings, and the way in which their treatment affected their health. There were numerous complaints of police brutality. As a response, VAHS joined with the Victorian Aboriginal Legal Service and other community members to gather and record evidence of alleged assaults. This included documenting the police officers involved, taking medical and photo records of injuries, and ensuring that appropriate actions were taken. Not only did VAHS empower and support the community in seeking justice, it also played a role in lobbying for better relationships between police and Aboriginal people. VAHS also played a vital role in advocating that their community members call upon their rights. Working closely with Australian social and welfare services, VAHS sought to make these services aware of their rights, such as sickness benefits and unemployment benefits. VAHS has become strongly respected by the Victorian community and became a role model for other Aboriginal communities wanting their own health services.

The project revealed that Aboriginal people have been one of the driving forces behind the CPHC agenda in Australia; activist activities were evidence of the will and determination of Aboriginal people to change their health status and the factors that impact health statuses. VAHS has played a vital role in securing CPHC for the Fitzroy Aboriginal community and has proven to be a strong example of an Aboriginal community-controlled health service.

2. Models of PHC Governance in Pakistan[2]

Three models of PHC governance were studied by the team in Pakistan to see if one was more suited to CPHC. To a varying extent, all three models had CHWs working collaboratively with individuals on sanitation, literacy, and income-generation projects to develop joint activities, embracing the intersectoral action on SDH implicit in the Alma-Ata Declaration. More specifically, the study was interested in determining which model would be more conducive to the community's engagement with the health-care system and sustained actions on SDH. The first model was "top down" (institution-led), in which activities were fully developed and managed by the NGO. The second model was more "bottom up" (community-led), in which activities and financing were largely determined by the local community with minimal NGO involvement. The third model was more of a mixed affair (copartnership), involving equally, if differently, the lead NGO and the local community.

Researchers found that the community-led model (used in a slum area of 7,000 people) was effective; it benefitted the community by

---

2 The researchers on this project who prepared this summary were Parvez Nayani, Agha Ajmal, and Yousuf Memon.

increasing knowledge about health issues and their cause and prevention. The model saw the community members make decisions about their health and begin to frame the type of PHC program needed. A monitoring and evaluation system was put in place through the active participation of the community. The institution-led model (serving a slum community of 60,000) worked in a similar manner as the community-led model had, except that community participation was passive. The field team put in charge of delivering PHC made all the decisions regarding its establishment and management. Self-reliance and empowerment were not high. The monitoring system simply recorded morbidity and mortality. The copartnership model (used in a site with an estimated population of 85,000) proved not only sustainable, with the community developing a sense of ownership over the project and maintaining both its PHC and its SDH activities; it was also more effective in generating and sustaining intersectoral action (as well as community participation) than the two other models.

The Pakistan study captures a somewhat novel finding: that the copartnership model was more effective and comprehensive than the community-led model. This was not the research team's original hypothesis, which had been that the model driven by the community would outperform the other two – an assumption frequently encountered in the literature that underscores the importance of community-led health initiatives. Without overstating the significance of the Pakistan finding, it is probable that the copartnership model was more effective precisely because it combined the strengths of the institution-led model (notably sustained and predictable resources, and useful "expert" knowledge) alongside those of the community-led model (mobilized citizenry, strong local knowledge, and sense of ownership). Researchers on this study concluded that the copartnership model exhibited a number of advantages over the other two, including more emphasis on social development, capacity building, self-reliance, and community empowerment. The partnership process between institution and community was consultative and collaborative, and the program delivered and addressed both health and development goals.

13 Health-Care Coordination: Building Comprehensive Primary Health Care in Brazil

PATTY FIDELIS DE ALMEIDA, LÍGIA GIOVANELLA, AND BERARDO AUGUSTO NUNAN

Background

For the first time in Brazil's history, the 1988 federal constitution enshrined health as a citizen's right to be guaranteed by the state through economic and social policies designed to reduce the risk of disease and disorders and grant access to health care and services capable of ensuring the well-being of the population. The creation of a universal public system financed with tax revenue was directly related to the struggles of social movements for a return to democracy and for the exercise of full civil rights. To guarantee this constitutional universal right to health, the Unified Health System (*Sistema Único de Saúde*, SUS) was created in 1988 by integrating medical care provided by social security with other public health services under the management of the Ministry of Health. The SUS is a national health system with universal access that is funded by tax revenue and is based on the following principles: i) health as a universal right and the responsibility of the state, meaning universal access to health services for all citizens, regardless of income, social class, ethnicity, occupation, or tax contribution; ii) decentralization for states and municipalities, with shared responsibilities among different spheres of government; and iii) citizen participation.

The process of implementing a national health system in Brazil, however, has been long and tortuous. There have been many stumbling blocks, starting with the unfavourable international climate of the 1990s. In 1993, the World Bank's World Development Report, *Investing in Health*, declared that only in some situations was health a public responsibility. Meanwhile, efforts to mitigate the effects of fiscal-adjustment policies focused on poverty relief. The lesson learned was that we must universalize packages of selective programs focused on the poorest population groups.

It was in that context (which was, at best, politically unfavourable) that Brazil undertook the task – by way of primary health care (PHC) – of changing the curative medical model of health care that had been firmly consolidated during the military dictatorship. It must be said that the early initiatives were modest at best. In 1994, the Ministry of Health set up the Family Health Program (*Programa Saúde da Família*, PSF) as merely one more selective program targeting at-risk populations. Health-care teams, purportedly comprising a "general" practitioner, a nurse, a nursing assistant, and community health workers (CHWs), were responsible for the care of 3,000 to 4,000 people in a specific catchment area. After its initial implementation and over the next several years, the program did not develop much. By 1999, there were little more than 4,300 teams covering 14.7% of the population, generally in small municipalities.

In 1998, financial incentives in the form of per capita payments, transferred directly to municipalities from the federal government, fostered expansion of the PSF and, as this spread nationwide, the "basic PHC package" grew and demonstrated its potential to establish new forms of health care. Studies have shown, for instance, that for every 10% increase in population coverage by the PSF, there was a mean 4.6% reduction in the infant mortality rate (Macinko, Guanais, & Souza, 2006; Macinko, Souza, Guanais, & Simões, 2007). By 2015, 21 years after the first family health teams were introduced, the figures were impressive: 32,000 teams, 248,000 CHWs, and coverage extended to 101 million Brazilians (53% of the population). The challenges of implementation are proportionate to Brazil's vast size.

Our once modest PSF is now known as the Family Health Strategy (*Estratégia Saúde da Família*, ESF). The name unequivocally distances the ESF from selective programs and underscores the potential of a "strong PHC" to create new forms of care with better health outcomes, and to do so in a more ethical manner.

To assess the implementation of the ESF in this study, we set out to determine the characteristics that might distinguish it from selective PHC proposals and then leverage its ability to transform the Brazilian health-care model. Health-care coordination is a fundamental issue. In the Latin American context, where historically differing conceptions of PHC compete, experts recently agreed that two goals of PHC are to achieve coordination among different levels of care and to influence the social determinants of health through intersectoral collaboration

(Haggerty, Yavich, & Báscolo, 2009). The experts also acknowledged that these elements are essential for developing a comprehensive approach. Care coordination is crucial to guarantee comprehensive care and reduce inequalities in access to health services, which is one of the desired outcomes of CPHC (Labonté et al., 2009).

Research Questions and Methods

Coordination among levels of health care can be defined as the organization among different health services related to a specific intervention so that, regardless of where these services are provided, they are synchronized so as to achieve a common goal (Boerma, 2007; Terraza Núñez, Vargas Lorenzo, & Vázquez Navarrete, 2006; Haggerty et al., 2003; Starfield, 2002). This is dependent on an integrated network of health-care providers that enables users to continuously benefit from different health interventions that are appropriate to their needs and compatible with their personal expectations. Therefore, care coordination among levels of care is an organizational element of health care that is reflected in users' perceptions of the continuity of care (Haggerty et al., 2003).

In the context of the global health research initiative *Revitalizing Health for All* (*RHFA*), this study's goal was to describe and analyse the development of care-coordination strategies and tools in Brazilian municipalities that were successful in implementing the ESF on two fronts: strengthening PHC and integrating levels of care. This study was based on two premises. The first was the assumption that PHC services, given their characteristics, would be the most appropriate for assuming the responsibility of coordinating users' clinical pathways in most cases and guaranteeing the right to access health services. Therefore, strong PHC is necessary to mobilize support and resources. Thus, our first question was, what are Brazilian municipalities' initiatives to strengthen the ESF? The second premise was that integration of the network of health services is a necessary element of care coordination. Therefore, the study set out to investigate the following: What strategies and tools have large urban areas developed to integrate the ESF with higher levels of care in the health-care system?

In a national research project funded by the Department of Primary Care under the Brazilian Ministry of Health, four large urban areas (Giovanella et al., 2009) with high rates of the population covered by family health teams were selected as case studies (Aracaju, Belo Horizonte, Florianópolis, and Vitória) (Table 13.1). The methodology used in these

Table 13.1 Number of physicians, nurses, community health workers, nursing assistants, families, and administrators interviewed by municipality

Respondents	Aracaju	Belo Horizonte	Florianópolis	Vitória	Total
Physicians	56	72	61	35	224
Nurses	66	75	70	50	261
Community health workers	150	170	140	127	587
Nursing assistants	60	89	72	43	264
Families	800	900	789	822	3311
Administrators/managers/ representatives of professional organizations	19	22	18	18	77

(Giovanella et. al., 2009)

case studies was qualitative as well as quantitative, using semistructured interviews with administrators and surveys with health professionals and enrolled families conducted in 2008 as information sources.

Results and Analysis

Strengthening primary health care

The study is based on the premise that PHC services, given their characteristics, would be most appropriate, in the majority of cases, for assuming the responsibility of coordinating users' clinical pathways. However, only strengthened PHC, capable of mobilizing the necessary support and political, economic, financial, and human resources, can be responsible for the coordination of care. According to Starfield, Shi, & Macinko (2005), coordination is positively associated with PHC strength. Indeed, measures to strengthen PHC represent the most important set of pro-coordination reforms.

According to the vast majority of the physicians and nurses in the cities surveyed, the family health clinic (*unidade de saúde da família*, USF) is the first service sought when medical care is needed. In Aracaju, Belo Horizonte, and Vitória, approximately 70% of families indicated that they use the USF regularly. However, in three of the cities, the USF was not the service sought by more than half the families during recent bouts of illness (Table 13.2).

The study's results show that the municipalities researched had measures in place aimed at strengthening PHC and integrating it into the Brazilian SUS. The most successful initiatives were those designed to

Table 13.2 Indicators of the consolidation of the PHC gatekeeper role according to professionals and users, *Estratégia Saúde da Família*, four large urban areas, Brazil

Gateway	Aracaju	Belo Horizonte	Florianópolis	Vitória
% of physicians and/or nurses who strongly agree/agree that people turn to the USF first when in need of health care	92.5	89.2	87.2	83.0
% of families that seek the same health service for medical care or for prevention	76.4	85.0	73.8	75.6
% of families* who name the USF as the service they regularly seek	69.6	74.4	50.3	69.1
Health services used by families with members who fell ill in the past 30 days				
USF	41.1	52.4	31.8	47.0
Emergency service	29.0	15.3	28.0	8.1
Private health services	20.6	18.6	23.3	17.7
Hospital outpatient department	5.1	7.3	2.6	20.2
Polyclinic	–	4.4	9.5	2.5
Other	4.2	2.0	4.8	4.5

* Of families that indicated that they have a regular source of care (Giovanella et al., 2009)

improve accessibility; consolidate the gatekeeper role; improve resolution rates of health problems; and link public health, health surveillance, and health-care services together. The more it was understood that the ESF must coordinate clinical pathways within the health-care system, the more measures were introduced to expand and strengthen it, corroborating the hypothesis that only strong PHC would be able to fulfil the task of coordinating care (Almeida, Giovanella, Mendonça, & Escorel, 2010).

The general consensus is that the desired resolution rate of PHC services is 85%; that is, it is hoped that integrated health-care networks with primary care units (*unidades básicas de saúde*, UBSs) serving as gateways are able to resolve the vast majority of health problems without having to refer patients to specialists. In the four municipalities, about 60% of those surveyed reported having resolved their health problems without needing to be referred to a specialist (Table 13.3). In the cases studied, the main measures designed to increase the rate of resolution in PHC included expanding the exams that are performed directly by family physicians without referrals, collecting material for diagnostic tests, and improving the availability of medicine in the UBS.

The families stated that there was an improvement in PHC services after the implementation of the ESF. In Vitória, 51% believe that

Table 13.3 Resolution and assessment of improvement in care according to users, *Estratégia Saúde da Família*, four large urban areas, Brazil

Resolution by the *Estratégia Saúde da Família*	Aracaju	Belo Horizonte	Florianópolis	Vitória
Families' assessment of need for referral to a specialist				
Managed to resolve the health problem at this appointment	60.4	60.5	56.9	61.6
Needed to go to a specialist	35.9	32.5	39.9	37.5
Families' assessment of improvement in care since introduction of the *Estratégia Saúde da Família*				
Improved greatly	26.6	32.9	22.4	51.3
Improved slightly	44.5	40.1	33.5	28.2
Same	15.1	15.2	17.5	12.7
Worse	5.1	2.8	2.3	2.3
Do not know/did not answer	8.7	9.0	24.3	5.5

(Giovanella et al., 2009)

health care has improved significantly since the introduction of the ESF (Table 13.3).

Nonetheless, challenges remain for care in terms of meeting spontaneous and expected demand with higher resolution rates and ensuring that the USFs become a regularly used service. The barriers to accessing timely care in PHC services are a significant shortcoming in Latin American health systems and are aggravated by health-centre opening hours that are incompatible with people's working days, long waiting lists, low rates for resolution of health problems, and difficulties coordinating with specialized care. These factors may be related to the fact that a substantial number of users who have recently been ill have sought care at emergency services (Table 13.2) (Almeida et al., 2010).

PHC's professionals must be valued if PHC is to be strengthened. The assessment of physicians and nurses shows that it is urgent that local and national strategies be intensified in order to give visibility to the work of the ESF's professionals and increase their public esteem. PHC workers lack credibility and recognition, which constitutes an obstacle to care coordination at the PHC level (Table 13.4).

Integrating among levels of care

A fundamental characteristic of comprehensive PHC is the proper integration of PHC services into the health-care network to guarantee

Table 13.4 Perception of professional recognition, *Estratégia Saúde da Família,*
four large urban areas, Brazil

Professional recognition of ESF personnel	Aracaju	Belo Horizonte	Florianópolis	Vitória
% of physicians/nurses who strongly agree/agree that ESF personnel enjoy the same public esteem as specialists	22.0	13.0	29.4	14.6

(Giovanella et al., 2009)

Table 13.5 Position of the *Estratégia Saúde da Família* within the health-care network according
to administrators, four large urban areas, Brazil

Indicators	Aracaju	Belo Horizonte	Florianópolis	Vitória
		Administrators		
Preferred gateway of administrators	ESF	ESF	ESF	ESF
Medical professionals with basic specialties as support for ESF teams	Yes	Yes	Yes	Yes
Care strategies for spontaneous demand	Daily acceptance of patients and medical care	Daily acceptance of patients and medical care	Weekly acceptance of patients and medical care	Daily acceptance of patients and medical care
Regionalization of polyclinics/specialty centres	Partial	Yes	Yes	Yes

(Giovanella et al., 2009)

access to more complex levels of care. The primary characteristic of selective PHC is the restriction of the basket of services to only some low-cost services at the first level of care, without guaranteeing access to more complex services in line with individual and collective health needs, thereby deepening social inequality.

The findings of the case studies point to advances in the integration of family health into the health-care network, thereby strengthening PHC services as a regularly sought first point of contact and the preferred gateway to the health-care system (Table 13.5).

Measures aimed at integrating PHC with other services within the health system include investing in decentralized IT systems to enable oversight at health centres, organizing flows to specialized care so that access is by ESF physician referral only, monitoring waiting lists,

Table 13.6 Access to specialist (secondary care) according to users and professionals, *Estratégia Saúde da Família*, four large urban areas, Brazil, 2008

Access to specialist	Aracaju	Belo Horizonte	Florianópolis	Vitória
Main access to specialist reported by users referred in the past 12 months				
Appointment with specialist made by ESF	43.2	66.7	40.1	62.7
User approached specialist on own initiative with no referral	25.7	19.4	15.0	19.4
% of physicians/nurses who reported that there are always/almost always periodic assessments to determine the need for referral to other levels of care	26.3	25.9	19.8	11.8
% of physicians who always/almost always schedule other services				
Specialized care services	42.9	80.6	47.6	71.5
Diagnosis and treatment support services	37.5	55.5	42.7	42.9
Maternity	57.2	86.1	75.4	74.3

(Giovanella et al., 2009)

increasing the availability of municipalities' own specialized services, introducing clinical protocols agreed upon between PHC and specialized service workers, and implementing e-records (Tables 13.6 and 13.7).

Nevertheless, the process of integration with the health-care system is incomplete due to both a lack of regulation and of formal flows to inpatient care. Systematically evaluating referrals from USFs could improve their effectiveness and promote sounder use of specialized resources. Another difficulty identified was the insufficient supply of specialized care, aggravated by poor integration among providers at different levels of government (Almeida et al., 2010). The virtual absence of counterreferrals also lessens the likelihood of care coordination by PHC teams (Table 13.8).

Discussion and Conclusion

We can say that there is concern over establishing mechanisms to integrate and strengthen PHC within the Brazilian health-care system, SUS, in the four cities. The results of each case study indicate varying success in terms of implementing tools to achieve integrated networks and initiatives to strengthen PHC, although their paths have been similar. The triangulation of methods and data from different sources has allowed

Table 13.7 Wait time for specialized procedures according to users, *Estratégia Saúde da Família*, four large urban areas, Brazil

Wait time for specialized procedures	Aracaju	Belo Horizonte	Florianópolis	Vitória
User estimates of wait time for specialized care				
Up to 30 days	59.5	58.1	43.9	76.5
3 months or more	9.2	17.0	16.0	10.8
User estimates of wait time for exams performed				
0 to 7 days	18.0	53.6	19.0	50.4
Up to 30 days	68.4	89.4	57.7	90.6

(Giovanella et al., 2009)

Table 13.8 Continuity of information, *Estratégia Saúde da Família*, four large urban areas, Brazil

Clinical records	Aracaju	Belo Horizonte	Florianópolis	Vitória
% of doctors who provide written information always/almost always when referring a patient	76.8	95.8	93.4	100.0
% of doctors who receive counterreferrals always/almost always after user appointment with specialist	5.4	2.8	11.5	11.4

(Giovanella et al., 2009)

us to respond to the research questions and identify the measures and strategies now understood to potentially improve PHC coordination.

In this study, our goal was not to measure or evaluate care coordination in itself but rather to describe and analyse the factors that contribute to achieving greater coordination among health-care services and interventions so that they are synchronized and have a common goal, regardless of where they are provided. Therefore, we have attempted to develop a model of important factors that facilitate analysis of the components that affect PHC coordination, although in the future there is room to incorporate other important factors into the model.

PHC has been strengthened and better integrated into the health system, although it does not yet coordinate the entire cycle of care. The difficulties that were encountered that possibly affect care synchronization include insufficient communication and ties among providers, difficulties in the supply of specialized care, no clear protocol for flows to hospital care, lack of a culture of collaboration among different levels of care, PHC workers' low professional and social prestige, and challenges that persist regarding the consolidation of the ESF's gateway role. Establishing common goals so that health care becomes patient-centred and is organized according to users' personal expectations and health needs is part of the concept of coordination and highlights certain steps that should be taken.

This study also sought to contribute to greater theoretical and practical knowledge in the field of care coordination, given that it is an aspect of Latin American health systems that remains underdeveloped and is now understood as essential for providing comprehensive health care and for guaranteeing the right to access quality health services. Furthermore, we aimed to identify and disseminate successful practices, which, taking into account specific local conditions, can contribute to building more just and equitable health-care systems that are of higher quality and are responsive to the health needs of our region's population.

An important part of *RHFA* was the opportunity and the incentive to develop knowledge-transfer strategies. The discussion of the results with the research subjects in each city of our study laid the groundwork for recommendations for health administrators that could improve access and guarantee the right to health. The comparative analysis of the four cities enabled us to identify good practices – solutions for common problems – that were shared during the presentations. At the same time, discussions with the research subjects allowed the research team to improve upon their analyses and delve into greater detail.

Another broader attempt at dissemination was aimed at empowering user representatives on health councils to press for the implementation of comprehensive PHC. This was done by drawing up an executive summary containing the key results of the study to serve as a guide for health surveillance. It was written as a report with a didactic format to target health-council members, particularly those who are user representatives. The executive summary (Almeida, Giovanella, & Nunan, 2011) presented ways of evaluating PHC at the local level as well as recommendations, with an emphasis on the facilitating factors of and obstacles to care coordination and the implementation of an integrated primary health-care system.

Another lesson that was learned from *RHFA* resulted from working with three different research groups, which directed the study's focus more towards subjects of interest for administrators. Having these three main information sources helped administrators to take stronger ownership of the results and incorporate them into their decision-making processes. The results were also made available for use in domestic political debate with other sectors in order to gain resources to implement the recommendations aimed at facilitating access to necessary medical care.

Finally, in the cases studied, the obstacles that must be surmounted to ensure comprehensive care in Brazil are different in nature: there are hurdles that are financial and organizational (due to system fragmentation), as well as obstacles that stem from insufficient supply (Conill, 2008). Nonetheless, the results of our studies indicate that investing in strengthening the ESF as the preferred gateway to effective care integrated within the health care system has the potential to reorganize the system and guarantee the universal right to health. Given that the central focus of our research was universal and equitable access to health care as a social right, the main findings are primarily related to the principles and scope of PHC in terms of striving for equity and expanding access to health care and other services that are essential for health.

ACKNOWLEDGMENTS

We thank the users, professionals, and managers of the Unified Health System (SUS) as well as our survey participants in Brazil. We would also like to thank the Canadian Global Health Research Initiative and the Brazilian Ministry of Health for the research funding.

REFERENCES

Almeida, P.F., Giovanella, L., Mendonça, M.H.M., & Escorel, S. (2010, Feb). Desafios à coordenação dos cuidados em saúde: estratégias de integração entre níveis assistenciais em grandes centros urbanos. *Cadernos de Saúde Pública, 26*(2), 286–98. http://dx.doi.org/10.1590/S0102-311X2010000200008 Medline:20396844

Almeida, P.F., Giovanella, L., & Nunan, B.A. (2011). *Atenção primária integral à saúde: Indicadores para avaliação*. Rio de Janeiro: Saúde de Familia.

Boerma, W.G.W. (2007). Coordination and integration in European primary care. In R.S. Saltman, A. Rico, & W.G.W. Boerma (Eds.), *Primary care in the driver's seat? Organizational reform in European primary care* (pp. 3–21). Berkshire: Open University Press.

Conill, E.M. (2008). Ensaio teórico-conceitual sobre APS: Desafios para organização de serviços básicos e da Estratégia Saúde da Família em centros urbanos no Brasil. *Cadernos Saúde Pública*, 24(Sup1), S7–S27.

Giovanella, L., Escorel, S., Mendonça, M.H.M., Escorel, S., Almeida, P.F., Andrade, C.L.T., & Teixeira, C.P. (2009). *Estudos de caso sobre a implementação da Estratégia Saúde da Família em grandes centros urbanos. Relatório final.* (Online) Retrieved from http://www6.ensp.fiocruz.br/repositorio/sites /default/files/arquivos/BeloHorizonte.pdf

Haggerty, J.L., Reid, R.J., Freeman, G.K., Starfield, B.H., Adair, C.E., & McKendry, R. (2003, Nov 22). Continuity of care: A multidisciplinary review. *BMJ (Clinical Research Ed.)*, 327(7425), 1219–21. http://dx.doi.org /10.1136/bmj.327.7425.1219 Medline:14630762

Haggerty, J.L., Yavich, N., Báscolo, E.P., & Grupo de Consenso sobre un Marco de Evaluación de la Atención Primaria en América Latina. (2009, Nov). Un marco de evaluación de la atención primaria de salud en América Latina. *Revista Panamericana de Salud Pública*, 26(5), 377–84. Medline:20107688

Labonté, R., Sanders, D., Baum, F., Schaay, N., Packer, C., Laplante, D., & Pooyak, S. (2009). Aplicación, efectividad y contexto político de la atención primaria integral de salud: resultados preliminares de una revisión de la literatura mundial. *Revista Gerencia y Políticas de Salud, Bogotá (Colombia)*, 8(16), 14–29.

Macinko, J., Guanais, F.C., Souza, M.F.M. (2006, Jan). Evaluation of the impact of the Family Health Program on infant mortality in Brazil, 1990–2002. *Journal of Epidemiology and Community Health*, 60(1), 13–19. http://dx.doi .org/10.1136/jech.2005.038323 Medline:16361449

Macinko, J., Souza, M.F.M., Guanais, F.C., & Simões, C.C.S. (2007, Nov). Going to scale with community-based primary care: An analysis of the family health program and infant mortality in Brazil, 1999–2004. *Social Science & Medicine*, 65(10), 2070–80. http://dx.doi.org/10.1016/j.socscimed.2007.06 .028 Medline:17689847

Starfield, B. (2002). *Atenção primária: Equilíbrio entre necessidades de saúde, serviços e tecnologia.* Brasília: Unesco/Ministério da Saúde.

Starfield, B., Shi, L., & Macinko, J. (2005). Contribution of primary care to health systems and health. *Milbank Quarterly*, 83(3), 457–502. http://dx.doi .org/10.1111/j.1468-0009.2005.00409.x Medline:16202000

Terraza Núñez, R., Vargas Lorenzo, I., & Vázquez Navarrete, M.L. (2006, Nov–Dec). La coordinación entre niveles asistenciales: Una sistematización de sus instrumentos y medidas. *Gaceta Sanitaria*, 20(6), 485–95. http://dx .doi.org/10.1157/13096516 Medline:17198628

14 Comprehensive Primary Health Care Models and Strategies in Argentina

MARIO ROVERE, ANA FUKS, ANALÍA
BERTOLOTTO, EUGENIA BAGNASCO,
AND ANDREA JAIT

Background

This study focused on the lessons learned and shortcomings observed in the development and implementation of primary health care (PHC) strategies in the Argentine Republic. It is based on a review of two illustrative yet very different sites. The first site is a shanty town located in the heart of one of the most sought-after neighbourhoods of the city of Buenos Aires. This *"villa miseria,"* one of more than 20 in the national capital city, is known as Villa 31. It is highly visible and has been populated over time by foreign and internal migrants. The second site is the department of General Güemes in the northern province of Salta. It consists of a set of three rural municipalities of varying degrees of urbanization, built around primary industries such as sugar and tobacco processing and low-skilled labour such as that in cement manufacturing and rail workshops. The area has also experienced a high degree of political and economic instability. The two sites were chosen because both had a long history of health programs and experienced radical policy changes under different political regimes, alternating between social democracy and populism, with both leaving marks on local PHC.

The goal of this study was to unmask the stark political and ideological contradictions that have arisen in the PHC field over the last 30 years in Argentina. We based our study on the following assumptions:

- Over time, Argentina developed (as did many other countries in the region) specific health strategies to tackle rural and tropical diseases, especially in agricultural and oil-rich areas. The country also faced health challenges from urban poverty and shanty towns in its big cities, brought on by fast and disordered growth.

- The implementation of PHC at the height of the military dictatorship in Argentina had a "sterilizing" effect on its most social and political components, which persists in some aspects to this day. This effect was reinforced by the adoption of neoliberal policies that promoted selective or highly focused PHC and weakened integrated initiatives within the health-care sector.

Research Questions and Methods

The study's initial questions were aimed at testing these assumptions. To this end, the study sought to answer the following:

- Is there a difference between the selective PHC models encountered at these two sites, one being a rural model inspired by the Rockefeller Foundation and the other being an urban intervention inspired by a classic European public health model?
- Is there a correlation between the different PHC strategies and PHC models implemented in Argentina between 1978 and 2010?
- Are the practices of health-care teams today still influenced by these political models?
- Are these influences consciously perceived by the health-care team?
- Is the health sector ready to implement CPHC?

To answer these questions, a combination of methods was used.

Semistructured interviews with key informants

A total of 35 key informants were identified in both localities. These informants were health workers who had developed their PHC practice during the period covered in this study. Questions were drafted and tested with an initial sample of informants and reformulated accordingly. The selection of informants included professionals from different disciplines (social workers, nutritionists, speech therapists, and physicians), different strata (health workers and administrative personnel), and different ranks (from former ministers to hospital and program directors). A number of members of the Movement of Priests for the Third World (*Movimiento de Sacerdotes para el Tercer Mundo*) also formed part of the cluster of informants for Villa 31. Through these interviews, we were able to establish how Argentina's volatile history left marks on modern-day PHC in the country.

The final phase of the study consisted of an in-depth analysis of issues related to the creation of training models for first-level health workers. Questions discussed with key informants included

- How are we training newer generations of health workers?
- Who are the innovators?

As part of the process designed to answer these questions, we held a symposium with presentations on diverse PHC training, research, and management models that have been implemented in the province, the city of Buenos Aires, and other areas of the country. This was done in order to understand Argentina's PHC strategy, draw parallels between the models being implemented, and create an intersectoral framework linked to health-care centres.

Focus groups

Focus-group discussions (FGDs) were also conducted with a total of 82 experts in the training of health professionals. The purpose of these FGDs was to include the viewpoints of future health workers, thereby reflecting on the difficulties and obstacles already anticipated in training models, particularly in the residency training of different professionals on the health-care teams who partly or exclusively work in community settings.

Literature review and testing of the first theoretical framework

In parallel with the key informant interviews and FGDs, we continued to search for reference materials and resources that allowed us to broaden, assess, and elaborate on the results and findings that arose from the responses of informants. This in turn facilitated the revision of our assumptions and initial hypotheses. It also enabled us to conceptually, politically, and historically contextualize the gathered data, which were analysed and debated during our team meetings. With the help of El Agora[1] team members who had direct knowledge of the localities

---

1 El Agora is a not-for-profit organization based in Argentina that aims to strengthen (inter alia) citizenship, democratization, the right to health, urban development, and governance by fostering community dialogue and participation.

being studied, the theoretical framework was strengthened by defining the tools to be used and adjusting the study's methodology. We developed and used an analytic tool to assess the material garnered from the interviews. This process helped us to identify the key components of PHC history in Argentina and pare down the interviews without decontextualizing the informants' responses.

Results and Analysis

PHC has been an ambiguous reference framework in Argentina, given that it is not, nor has it been, a political priority for the public health sector in the country. The Argentine health-care model historically has been focused on hospitals, and successive reforms were dictated by a logic that related primarily to political discussions (federal vs. unitary systems) and discussions on how to fund the health-care model (public health system vs. insurance system).

Attempts at implementing universal health insurance failed, the net result being an increase in private sector health care during the period studied. PHC became less important in a clearly hospital-centric model as reduced spending by the public health sector helped to expand privately provided free-market medicine. Our two case studies, however, were exceptions. General Güemes in the North of the country saw a great deal of economic innovation with one such sector exploiting the production of sugar. The region also suffered from an endemic outbreak of malaria, which led to the introduction of tropical medicine, specifically with the founding of the Regional Hospital of the North for *"palúdicos"* (malaria sufferers) in 1925.

Our second site was born from large waves of immigration to Buenos Aires in the first decades of 20th century as a result of the 1929 international economic crisis. As a consequence of massive immigration, rural areas soon exceeded their capacity to settle new populations, leading to the generation of shanty towns in port cities. This was the case for Villa 31, the oldest shanty town in the capital city, established in the 1930s. It was first occupied by Polish and Italian migrants and more recently by Bolivians, Paraguayans, and internal migrants from the northern provinces of the country.

In the case of the North and the department of General Güemes, the presence of tropical diseases, combined with the strong economic interest of American investments in industrial crops and oil wells in the region, brought the presence of the Rockefeller Foundation and its sanitary public health programs. The region's antimalarial hygiene policy of the 1920s could be explained, in part, by the socioeconomic context oriented to the protection of the rural workforce in sugar cane and cotton production. It was also based in local scientific advances and the American influence on sanitary matters, principally through the Rockefeller Foundation (Alvarez, 2010, p. 76).

Once malaria was under control in the 1950s, a heavy burden of other avoidable diseases led to continuation of the same strategy as a more expansive rural health program. This program began in the northern province of Jujuy in 1965 and, after a period of scepticism over its outcomes, it demonstrated its capability to improve health indicators at low cost:

> ... The antimalarial strategy ran throughout the rural health program which, after 1978, was renamed the PHC Program. [It included] local cartography, home by home visits, use of the population census, "vistos" (documents registering every visit), health education, detection of suspect illnesses, strict supervision of health workers as a local brigade – though we did not know it at the time, everything evoked the military models [of PHC] used to eradicate Yellow Fever in Havana in the very beginning of the 20th century. (Rovere, 2010, p. 191)

Turning to our second case, Buenos Aires has operated as both a welcoming entrance and control system for immigrants entering as new workers since the late nineteenth century. The *"hotel de los inmigrantes"* (migrant hotels) were overwhelmed, and the *"conventillos"*[2] operated as a reservoir of labourers (as needed) and a system of police control for undesirable migration. Shanty towns around the city's port area arose as temporary measures to face critical housing and employment shortages for these new migrants. The main health considerations of necessity followed earlier European urban public health models, with an emphasis on housing and sanitary conditions, including potable-water supply, garbage treatment, and sewage disposal. These health interventions sometimes flourished with government sympathy or complicity but, in a sort of a "political pendulum," were intermittently followed by another government that looked to eradicate them, usually through violent means.

---

2 *"Conventillos"* were precarious collective housing structures in which each family rented a room and shared the bathroom and the kitchen with other families.

Villa 31 suffered particularly from this pendulum sway for more than 80 years. It is in a strategic location close to the river port, in an area bounded on one side by one of the city's three railroad terminal stations serving the North and West provinces of the country, and on the other by the city's sole long-distance bus station. In the 1970s, Villa 31 had a population estimated at 25,000. In the mid-1970s, the Argentinian military government tried to eradicate the shanty town. It concluded a treaty with the Bolivian military government to deport Bolivian citizens to that country. Thousands of people were moved by force, in military trucks. No more than 50 families were able to successfully resist. Some resettlement began with the fall of the military government in 1983, and, by 2010, Villa 31 had a population of 26,492.

Our historical study focused on the period from 1976 to 2000, observing the main consequences of the extreme political swings in Argentina on PHC and broader health governance. In brief, the Argentinian delegates at the Alma-Ata meeting on PHC were part of a military dictatorship (1976–83); this was followed by the democratic election of a social democratic party (1984–9), which tried to reduce poverty by introducing an extensive national nutritional program (PAN) supported by a framework of human rights. This, in turn, was followed by the election of a neoliberal government (1989–99) that adopted selective health policies which were strongly influenced by international financing organizations such as the World Bank, the IMF, and the Inter-American Development Bank. Figure 14.1 shows the trend in the infant mortality rate (a key marker for both health and socioeconomic status) over this period in our two study sites.

District of General Güemes

Salta province (in which is located the department of General Güemes) had since 1978 implemented selective PHC, inspired by the earlier malaria campaign in the area and the strong influence of the Rockefeller Foundation. The trend line suggests, however, that the most effective reduction in infant mortality occurred after 1983 under a new political context that created a better environment for CPHC, with an emphasis on regulated (mandatory) social participation and intersectoriality. One key informant who worked in Salta from 1983 to 1987 described the transition over this period in the province. He traced some of the dynamics back to Dr. Carlos Alvarado, who had been a fellow of the Rockefeller Foundation and who had led the malaria-eradication

Figure 14.1 Infant mortality rates in two Argentinian districts (1980–2011)

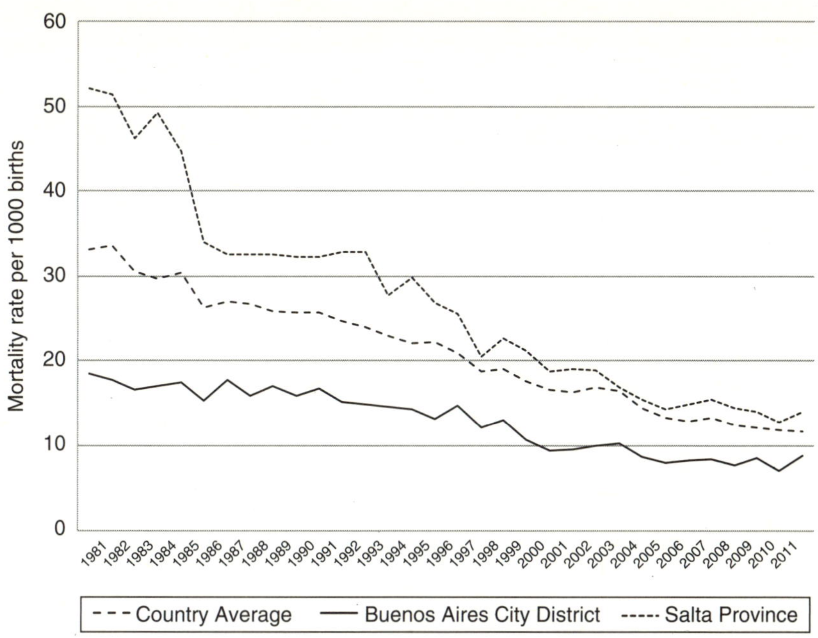

Source: National Statistic and Census Institute of Argentina

campaign in the 1950s before becoming director of the global malaria program at the WHO headquarters in Geneva (1958–64):

> Alvarado designed the action [in Salta] to solve four or five big problems … the diseases that were preventable by vaccines. The vaccines were available but just for people who lived close to the hospital. Tuberculosis was endemic. Malnutrition affected more than 40% percent of children below 5 years.

Our key informant spent time working in Honduras and Nicaragua, before returning to Salta in 1978, where he wanted to apply his newly acquired knowledge in rural health. As he continued,

> In 1983 … we wanted to extend the PHC program so that it would reach at least 50% of the population who were the most vulnerable. This means the rural population and those who lived in the poorest neighborhoods in

the big cities. They had access neither to services nor to health information. They didn't know how to react in emergencies.

As our interviewee further explained, the main difference between "before and after 1983" was the political framework for PHC, which extended the health coverage (especially in big cities) but at the same time included regulated social participation in the program (a council of neighbours could select and remove the community health worker [CHW]) and to embed PHC as a central component of public health policy. Over time, the PHC dimension as a comprehensive strategy was better understood by CHWs, who noted that PHC could not be limited to a cluster of effective measures, no matter how universal the coverage for these measures might be. A CHW supervisor told us,

> We are not the Primary Health Care; we know that we are just a program. But we have considerable influence in the management of care. We visit monthly every house, each of us contacts 200 to 300 children six times every year, we know the nutritional level, the local determinants of health of every family, whether they can access health care or if they are refused by the health services. We act in their health advocacy.

Villa 31

In the case of Villa 31, this shanty town lived under the varying pressures of, and policy responses to, economic and labour contexts. Under the neoliberal era, the local and national government tried to eradicate it. During the social democratic era, despite an improved labour market, there was political mistrust owing to suspicions that the community was a nest for illegal drug commerce and crime. But it was the marks of the earlier military government that were most frequently mentioned by various interviewees, especially the images of bulldozers demolishing the local health centres, which occurred in the 1970s and reoccurred again during the neoliberal democracy of the 1990s. Our key informant for the history of this area recalled:

> The health center was embedded in the middle of the Villa in front of the chapel and the soccer field … An ambulance from Hospital Fernandez [the closest public hospital] came and went without any patrol guard, there was a good security environment. All the time, patients, physicians and residents came and went with ease. All this was destroyed in July 1976. They

[the military government] took away the medicine boxes, scales, nebulizers, blood pressure monitors and stretchers, and demolished the health center.

Through different interviews we found that the health coverage for this population then became a marginal activity of public hospitals, sometimes with and sometimes without local physical facilities but always with health professionals (general physicians, residents, pediatricians, nurses, or social workers). In some cases these health professionals performed their tasks simply as a job; but in many cases they became personally involved in local social and political processes related to community self-organization, the Catholic Church's missions that were influenced by liberation theology, or progressive political parties. But in the 1990s, the political policy once again resembled that of the military government regime; the aim was to eradicate Villa 31. In response, every health initiative was characterized as a legitimation of the population's legal rights and demands. But this created tensions for CHWs and leaders alike, as a social worker active in the 1990s explains:

The unique clear order [from the government] was that we shouldn't work with community leaders. It was an additional cause of conflict for us, they [the government] wanted to negotiate with them, outside the Villa. Our team spirit was diluted. We could only rely on the good will of some professionals or on the nurse residents who remained in place until 2001. They would organize in some way the community work. They undertook many social [organizing] activities while carrying out their day to day work on vaccines campaigns, nutrition controls, milk supply and community canteens.

In both sites, we could perceive the consequences of the political processes in terms of PHC practices: first, an attempt on the part of the military dictatorship (1976–83) to erase the political components from the PHC agenda; second, a social democratic attempt (1984–9) to return them to more comprehensiveness; and third, a neoliberal policy effort (1989–2001) to reduce the PHC agenda to a basic package of highly selected and focused health interventions. During the first and third periods, both regimes oversaw the removal of economic, social, demographic, and cultural determinants from the analysis of health needs and in the formulation of health interventions.

To address the last goal of our study, we developed a set of interviews to explore the social and political conditions for a jump to CPHC in Argentina. Through these we learned of a short-lived but significant and influential experience developed in Buenos Aires Province between 1987 and 1989: ATAMDOS, or Ambulatory and Home Care Program. The program saw the creation of interdisciplinary health teams, each one responsible for 300 families, actively looking for health problems in real-time scenarios while promoting wide community participation. In a brief part of our interview with one of the actors in the ATAMDOS program, we asked about the new skills needed for the future health workers, to which he replied,

> … they must generate competencies to be part of the community … they must be integrated in the community with all the intercultural skills that it demands … the ATAMDOS health team members felt pride in being part of a health project, a political project.

During this study, we felt the strong influence of "good practices," not just in its outcomes, but at the same time as a formative experience for future leadership in a health-transformation process. The influence of this program extended beyond its geographic territory and was the source of innovation in PHC, both in Villa 31 and in General Güemes.

Discussion

Although not explicit in the interviews cited here, the study found that a main shortcoming of the PHC framework used in Argentina was that its strategies were not defined when it was first adopted. Vagueness and imprecision were favoured to reach consensus, and the players and interests at stake as well as the potential conflicts and allies were not clearly identified. PHC, instead, was organized according to different approaches that were sometimes complementary and at other times contradictory, with each one claiming to be "the authentic PHC." These contradictions can be grouped into two extremes: on the one hand, strategies that aimed to improve health indicators, and, on the other hand, strategies that sought to improve income distribution, quality of life, and health determinants. Between these two poles, we found an endless list of different conceptions of PHC, some of which sought to combine PHC components in different ways.

The political dimensions of PHC (such as social participation, inter-sectoriality, and interculturality) were not fully developed in either of the localities studied: neither in General Güemes (where the institutional continuity of a program with roots in the community could have facilitated it), nor in the troubled and, at times, heroic Villa 31. Despite being localities with high levels of political mobilization, none of the defining components of PHC became part of the daily practices of the health teams or of the community. In fact, the absence of these components was not even perceived as a shortcoming in the health-care models of these localities. A health worker interviewed in the department of General Güemes described how "in 1978, when PHC began ... one condition was stipulated: no community participation." Between 1983 and 1989 (the social democratic era), the community was recognized as a participant and empowered as an actor that deserved social accountability and that could elect and remove community workers. After this period, as the same interviewer continued, [even in democratic times] " ... in the 1990s ... the PHC strategy began to change dramatically. It lost its fundamental essence, which was community involvement ... " The subtext was that the same health workers were either subversive and dangerous or positive health and community promoters, depending of the moment of the Argentinian political pendulum.

A similar mistrust of health professionals by the political regime was found to exist in Villa 31 as well. Various key interviewees confirmed that there were health workers among the 30,000 people disappeared by the military dictatorship, but, at the same time, as one key informant reported, "the only clear principle of the 1990s was that health professionals were not to work openly with community representatives." A few health workers who held on to the ideology of community participation would break from the norm and work with the community, but they would do so voluntarily, in solitude, and at their own risk.

Over time, most health-policy officials in the country assumed a technocratic attitude to adapt to the political pendulum. Sometimes they were pushed to employ tactics of repression, discipline, and regulation of PHC practices, and other times they were asked to promote social and health-worker participation. Only those practices not perceived as "deviant" or "dangerous" to the goals of the health policy of the time were allowed to develop and deemed "politically correct." These practices shaped health-worker habits that have given rise to a certain self-discipline that today still defines what first-level health personnel may or may not do.

In both sites, despite experiencing significant political mobilization at the community level, health teams were prevented from fostering community participation, interdisciplinarity in health services, or intersectoral cooperation – all key elements in a CPHC model. These more political components of PHC were either absent or were extremely restricted, regulated, and standardized so as to sterilize or curb their potential for social change. The particular combination of political components resulted in distinct ways of practising and thinking about PHC in each locality and each period.

In follow-up discussions involving individuals with knowledge of PHC history across the whole of the country, and drawing from the history of our two cases, our analysis of the comprehensive versus selective polarity of PHC deepened. Through historical reconstruction, we were able to characterize a number of initiatives that gave rise to health-intervention prototypes that, after Alma-Ata, merged under the new generic name of PHC. The following models were identified (Figure 14.2):

- A model inspired by the fight against vectors that was initially designed by military forces. We call this model the "Epidemiological-Military Approach."
- A model of social advancement specifically targeting poor women. This approach is characterized by moralist overtones and promotes certain guidelines for sexuality and parenting. We call this model the "Missionary Approach."
- A model inspired by the decentralization of certain medical interventions. We call this model the "Satellite-Hospital Approach."
- A model of self-management, often a result of the isolation or absence of the state, or of the inability of a country or the international aid community to respond. We call this model the "Political and Participatory Approach."

We found that the health care models present in our two case studies do not reflect any pure form of these approaches. However, they can be characterized by the almost paradigmatic predominance of some of their elements in their origins, resulting in a mixed model. This mixed model could be useful in characterizing PHC in General Güemes: how it was born as a prototype of the "Epidemiological-Military Approach" but became more comprehensive, incorporating a "Political and Participatory Approach." It could also be used to characterize how Villa 31 was born as a "Satellite-Hospital Approach" but, with health professionals involved, came to include elements of a "Missionary Approach," as well as aspects, at times, of the rather dangerous "Political and Participatory

Figure 14.2 Four health-care models in Argentina

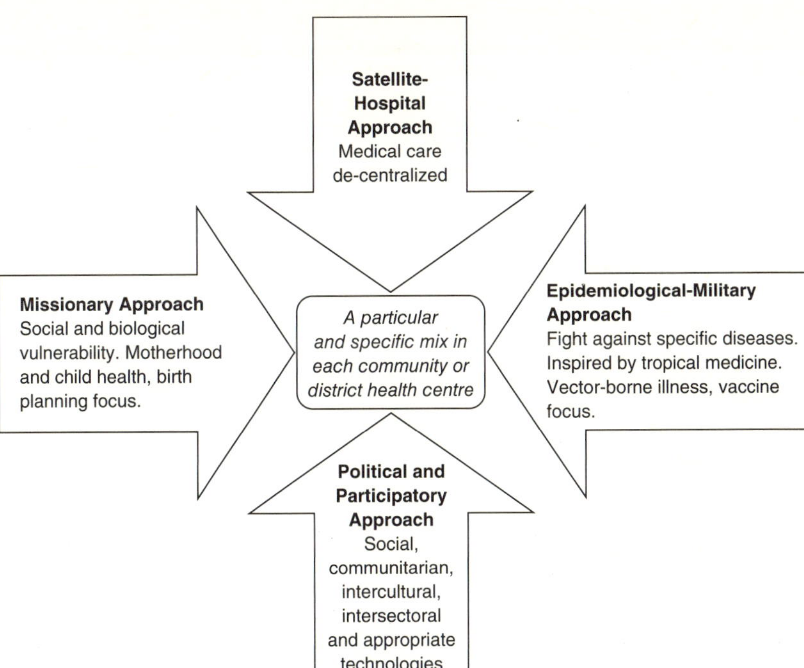

Approach." But the most promising use of this schematic, we suggest, is the possibility to redefine the concept of CPHC in Argentina so as to create a new synthesis that encompasses the most validated and useful features of the four models.

One of the challenges this endeavour will face is that, over the three decades of our study period, PHC strategies based on empowered CHWs did not obtain wide recognition and support in the public health sector, no matter how strong the evidence of their contribution to improved health indicators. At the time of writing, there still is no national recognition or legitimation of the *"agentes sanitarios"* whether it be their educational training, careers, stability of work, or pay. Only a few Argentinian provinces have taken some initiative for change.

Although PHC never obtained status as a key concept of the agenda to reform health systems in the country, Argentina, after a huge economic and political crisis in 2001, launched two programs with greater orientation towards PHC, financed by international credits from the World Bank and the Inter-American Development Bank. One is called REMEDIAR. It focuses on guaranteeing access to a basket of basic medicines in all the Centros de Atención Primaria de Salud (CAPS), the PHC centres, of the country. This reinforces the idea, however, that PHC is essentially "primary medical care" absent its social and participatory dimensions. The other program is called Plan Nacer, superficially a maternal-child health insurance program created in response to the increased national infant mortality rates in 2002 and 2003. After this, a third program financed by the Inter-American Development Bank was launched in 2004 to increase educational training and support for the professional staff working in the CAPS.

Conclusion

Our study enabled us to have a better understanding of the history of PHC in Argentina, not as an academic outcome but as a means to better understand the political processes that underpin CPHC good practices. The study allowed us to envision the necessary set of conditions that would facilitate the adoption of a CPHC model in Argentina. At the very beginning of our research, we emphasized the role of the military government and its responsibility for creating enduring marks that dissuaded health workers from taking risks and promoting a community participation process. We understood that, in addition, an erratic and contradictory political pendulum incentivized a technocratic professional attitude and simultaneously discouraged social or community involvement.

Health workers and communities together with other stakeholders, such as social movements, unions, and academic institutions, could stop the political pendulum and use the experience of the best historical practices in PHC to consider and to guarantee health as a key component of human and social rights existing internationally, as well as within Argentinian policy. Looking forward toward a prospective analysis for CPHC in our country, we contacted educators and educational-program leaders at different levels (graduate, postgraduate, professional residences, and public health) to explore the necessary links between health services and educational innovations. Health leaders and authorities must not be just technically competent but must also be accountable for ensuring policies that create the conditions to allow the communities to fully exercise their right to health. This necessitates both community-responsive, decentralized health services and actions that address key determinants of health located in other sectors. As noted above, neither of these fundamental attributes of PHC had been consistently or fully applied in the study sites. However, some good practices were noted that could be viable "seeds of the future"; one in particular was that of preparing a new workforce, informed and able to form a strong partnership with communities. The growth of these seeds requires good soil: stable health governance that is based in partnership and social participation, and the full involvement of health in developing processes at local as well as at national levels.

REFERENCES

Alvarez, A.C., ed. (2010). *Entre muertes y mosquitos: El regreso de las plagas en la Argentina siglos XIX y XX*. Buenos Aires: Ed Biblos.
Rovere, M. (2010). Epilogue. In A. Alvarez (Ed.), *Entre muertes y mosquito: El regreso de las plagas en la Argentina siglos XIX y XX* (pp. 210–15). Buenos Aires: Ed Biblos.

15 Constructing a Comprehensive Primary Health Care System in Guarjila, El Salvador: 1987–2007

MARIA ARGELIA DUBÓN ABREGO, DAGOBERTO MENJÍVAR LÓPEZ, EDUARDO ESPINOZA FIALLOS, AND CHRISTA BAATZ

Introduction

This study focused on the community health-care system that emerged in the 1980s during the civil war against the military dictatorship in one of the most troubled areas in northern El Salvador: the department of Chalatenango. This site served as an important stage for organizing communities and revolutionary forces.

The objectives of this study were to

1 describe and analyse the development of the community health-care system in Guarjila, El Salvador, during the period 1987–2007;
2 identify the characteristics of community residents and their role in the Guarjila community health system;
3 determine the contextual facilitating and limiting factors that had an impact on the system's development;
4 describe the processes of organization, community participation, decision making, intersectoral action (ISA), the delegation of responsibilities, equity, sustainability, and civic oversight as well as health-impact indicators; and lastly
5 establish the facilitating and limiting factors in the system's development along with their impact on the National Health System (*Sistema Nacional de Salud*) in order to identify transferable lessons that can help revitalize CPHC at a national scale.

Background

In the 1970s, El Salvador became engulfed in a political and social conflict that was based on a broad movement comprising labourers, poor rural farmers, students, and professionals. This conflict culminated in civil war in the 1980s, after democratic spaces had been destroyed by the military dictatorship and social demands had been brutally repressed. This people's war ended with the signing of peace accords in 1992, after which the nation embarked on a long process of recovery. During that time, democratic spaces that had been previously banned by the military and political elite began to open up to the public. The Farabundo Martí National Liberation Front (*Frente Farabundo Martí para la Liberación Nacional, FMLN*), the highest representative of the working class that led the armed uprising against the military dictatorship, became a political party. It began to run candidates in elections and systematically win local legislative and mayoral seats across the country.

Community health care was unknown in El Salvador prior to the Declaration of Alma-Ata; the church had provided some medical services, but they did not fall under the framework of PHC. After the peace declaration of 1992, the government implemented high-impact vertical and selective programs such as immunization, breastfeeding, oral rehydration, growth checks for children, and family planning.

The department of Chalatenango, which is located in the north of the country along the border with Honduras, is, at 1,957 square kilometres, the country's largest department, one of the least populated, and among the five poorest, with largely marginalized communities and unreliable basic services. The northeastern region of the department, where the community of Guarjila is located, encompasses several municipalities that are classified as extremely poor and which saw some of the heaviest fighting during the Salvadoran armed conflict. Chalatenango represents 3.3% of the national population (201,702 inhabitants). In 2008, nearly 24% of its population lived in extreme poverty, and just over 33% lived in relative poverty, for a total poverty rate of 57%. This rate exceeded the national average of 43% for the same year (Programa de las Naciones Unidas para el Desarrollo [PNUD], 2010), with Chalatenango ranking fourth worst among the 14 Salvadoran departments in terms of extreme poverty, and fifth in terms of total poverty.

The region is mountainous and rocky and the land is difficult to cultivate due to its relatively infertile soil. The corn, bean, and rice harvests have never been sufficient for subsistence, and thus residents have been forced to migrate periodically to other parts of the country to work as day labourers. In addition, there is a high level of emigration abroad, particularly to the United States, whose government continuously deports Salvadoran immigrants. Nevertheless, the stream of illegal emigrants – mostly young people – steadily continues, given that they perceive emigration as practically the only option available to improve their living conditions.

The Guarjila community is a canton in a rural area of the Chalatenango municipality, located 8 kilometres east of the city. It has a population of 1,762 residents, more than half of whom are women. Similar to other poor and rural communities throughout the country, the majority of residents subsist on agriculture, livestock, and remittances from family members.

The conflict

The residents of Guarjila and other communities in the area took part in the social movement organized during the popular uprising against the nation's military dictatorship between 1980 and 1992. Many of these communities gained organizing experience during the social movements of the 1970s. Thus the poor rural farmers of northeastern Chalatenango were able to self-govern their small communities when the government withdrew from the area, collectively resolving pressing issues related to health, education, food, and other daily necessities with the scant resources available to them.

Baatz (1994, 1998) explains the emergence of community health care in these communities in the 1980s amid the civil war. She argues that the roots of the community health-care system's development in northeastern Chalatenango can be found in the process of organizing and raising awareness among the masses of poor rural farmers (organized communities) that began in the 1960s and continued into the 1970s.

In 1998, a study carried out with the support of the European Union's INCO program (International Scientific Cooperation Activities) identified 86 local innovative health-care systems that implemented CPHC to varying degrees. Among these was the community health care system in Guarjila, which has been the subject of numerous graduate and postgraduate theses (Dubón & Menjívar, 2013; Espinoza, Elias, & Villalta, 2000; Barten, Espinoza, De Vos, & Perez, 2008; Baatz, 1998). In 2006, the Pan American Health Organization (PAHO) recognized Guarjila's health-care team as "Everyday Heroes" for its important work and achievements in improving the community's health based on comprehensive care in accordance with the principles of CPHC.

Research Questions

To address the research objectives concerning the evolution of these "everyday heroes" and the creation of a comprehensive PHC model, a number of specific questions were identified:

- What was the context in which the health-care system was built in the Guarjila community between 1987 and 2007?
- What are the essential characteristics of the community, what changes have taken place in the living conditions of its residents, and what have been the perceived changes in health over the last 20 years?
- What were the organizational and social participation processes involved in building the community health-care system?
- What were the facilitating and limiting factors in the development process?
- What were the defining moments that enabled the community health-care system to survive over time?
- What has facilitated or impeded the community health-care system's influence on the National Health System?
- What evidence demonstrates that the community health-care system falls under the scope of CPHC?

Methods

A retrospective historical study was conducted consisting of a systematic review and assessment of the experiences in the community health-care system with three main areas of focus: the historical process of building the system, community empowerment, and health-impact indicators. Primary sources of information included community leaders, organized groups, health-care teams, and decision-making bodies in the community. Secondary sources of information included documents pertaining to the community health-care system, operational plans, reports, previous studies, audiovisual materials, and publications that reference communities in postwar El Salvador.

Using a participatory action research approach, qualitative data were obtained through in-depth interviews with key community actors and focus groups with community members. Prompting questions were formulated within these areas of focus, and categories and subcategories of analysis were identified, to reconstruct the historical memory of the community health-care system's creation and development. A literature review and desk study were also undertaken using sources from both within and outside the community. The study was conducted by researchers who had lived in the target community for more than 30 years, providing them with in-depth local historical knowledge as well as familiarity with community members. Findings of the study were shared with community members in a day-long workshop, during which different groups provided testimony or dramatic representations of the history and impacts of the community health system they had created.

Results

From 1981 to 1987, the residents of Guarjila took refuge in the Mesa Grande refugee camp in Honduras, which housed more than 11,000 refugees. They returned to their community in October 1987 with the support of social organizations, nongovernmental organizations, the Catholic Church, other churches, and international organizations such as the United Nations High Commissioner for Refugees, the International Committee of the Red Cross, and Doctors Without Borders.

Between 1987 and 1990, a large part of the repopulated communities organized teams of health promoters that had been trained in the refugee camps by Doctors Without Borders. These health promoters attended to the population's basic health-care needs and war injuries, both in the refugee camp as well as upon return to their communities. In this context, the Guarjila community built a basic health-care infrastructure and organized a health-care team that had greater capabilities than other neighbouring communities, thereby becoming a referral centre for the community health-care network serving the northeastern communities of Chalatenango during the war and subsequent to the 1992 peace accords.

Midway through 1993, the Ministry of Health (MoH) began gradually to install health posts administered by personnel from outside the community. In this way, community health promoters were slowly displaced from the area that they had served for many years as they sought to improve the health of their communities. Guarjila residents rejected the MoH's attempts to absorb the community health-care system into its service network because it privileged a curative approach to health care and marginalized social participation and other components of CPHC.

Guarjila's health-care system was built by the community during the troubled years of the Salvadoran armed conflict. The organizational capacity of the community was made evident by the board of directors, the highest organized representative body of the community, and by local teams and committees in the areas of health care, education, water, agriculture, women, youth, the war-disabled, and other population groups. Community members organized themselves to progressively improve their basic living conditions. They built a potable-water system, housing, and latrines; they developed their own food-production system; and they created an education model with teachers from the community. They also developed a health-care model with community health-care workers, mainly health and rehabilitation promoters, midwives, and groups of volunteer women. This emphasis on community organization allowed for residents' problems to be addressed by way of ISA (involving all community governance sectors) and involved the majority of residents in the decision-making process. Solidarity and the constant pursuit of equity are reflected in numerous community processes.

The community actively participated in different interventions led by the health-care team and took up the cause of health-care as its own, defending it against several attempts at cooptation by outside actors, including the state. The health-care team's work has progressively changed from medical care focused on the treatment of disease and war injuries to the incorporation of preventive care and health promotion, to subsequently adopting an approach focused on gender, human rights, and social determinants of health (SDH).

The extensive community infrastructure built by the residents attests to the work of the community. Some of the most notable community projects include a large school that houses more than 500 students, a community health centre that includes the Ana Manganaro Clinic and a rehabilitation centre, a community centre, a furniture shop, store and cafeteria, workshops, a house museum, and a community radio station. Residents also built a potable-water system that continues under local administration to this day. All these projects were financed with money from foreign donors, but the community provided all the labour. Government investment at the national and regional level was rather low.

These community initiatives resulted in improvements in living conditions; for example, 94% of residences qualify as livable (decent) housing, 98% have potable water, and 95% have electricity. The houses and services were all built with community labour.

Health impacts

The main health outcomes perceived by the residents fall under the categories of prevention, health education, and the adoption of healthy behaviours, particularly in basic sanitation and personal hygiene; treatment of water for human consumption; reduction and treatment of gastrointestinal illness and parasites, respiratory infections, and sexually transmitted diseases; reduction of self-medication; early and ongoing doctor appointments; and improvements in eating habits.

Among all the indicators measuring the impact of the community's actions on health, the absence of maternal and infant mortality in Guarjila from 1997 to the time of this report is the most striking. This is particularly so when compared to national figures: the maternal mortality rate in 2012 was reported to be 0.42 per 1,000 live births (Quandl database, 2015), and the infant mortality rate in the same year was 14 per 1,000 live births (Quandl, 2015). One hundred percent of pregnant women participated in prenatal care, both in health-care facilities and at home, receiving an average of six check-ups. This is considerably higher than the national average reported in 2008 of 78.3% of women receiving four or more prenatal-care visits (Quandl, 2015). Early birth registration (before 12 weeks) reached 90.5% in Guarjila, which is below the national average of 98.5% (Quandl, 2015). At the close of this study, 100% of deliveries took place in a second-level hospital. The only comparable national PAHO figure dates from 2009 and reports that 84.9%of deliveries were attended trained personnel (PAHO, 2015).

Child health care was expanded to include 100% of children under 5, in accordance with El Salvador's Integrated Management of Childhood Illness strategy (IMCI), with a full vaccination series according to the child's age (Cordero, Salgado, & Drasbeck, 2004, p. 15). Guarijla was no exception. In addition, undernutrition was not found in children under 5 at the time of this study. With respect to family planning, 40% of women of childbearing age used a temporary or permanent method of birth control, which is far below the national average of 72%, the year 2008 being the most recent figure available for contraceptive prevalence (Quandl, 2015). Finally, the crude birth rate in Guarjila was 14.4 per

1,000 inhabitants, lower than the national average of 20.2 (2012 figure in Quandl, 2015) and half of the department's figure of 31 per 1,000 inhabitants.

There were factors that limited the development of the health-care system, notably the systematic isolation of the community by different state entities, discrimination against the community health workers by government health workers, and dependence on funding from international supporters. All these factors forced the community to fund the system, which in turn limited universal access. However, despite the lack of adequate financial resources, the health-care team fulfilled its commitment to the residents with few exceptions.

Discussion and Conclusion

The Guarjila health-care system was built thanks to the community's extensive efforts. Organization, community participation, and ISA action empowered residents and thus were instrumental in advancing the health-care system and were essential determinants for the integral development of the community.

The experiences gained during the popular uprising in terms of organization and participation imbued the residents with a high level of awareness and allowed them to think of the community as a collective project. This mindset enabled community projects, especially the health-care system, to survive. Moreover, the mostly local health-care team upheld its commitment to local residents and continued to exercise leadership, becoming agents of change in the community and positively impacting its members, thereby improving health indicators. This finding, while specific to this community, nonetheless speaks to the importance of having health-care teams live and work in the communities they serve. An intersectoral approach, understood as the actions of different organized groups across the community, facilitated greater community participation. The health-care system was built thanks to a broad effort by the community. Organization, community participation, and ISA to health empowered residents and were instrumental in developing and sustaining the health-care system, and in improving other health determinants related to the integral development of the community (e.g., housing, potable water, education, and electricity).

The health-care team's work progressively moved away from a disease-centred model of care to a comprehensive approach focusing on gender, human rights, and action on the SDH – a testament to the dynamism of the community. The health-care team played an instrumental role in becoming agents of change in the fight against the causes of injustice afflicting the community. Current health indicators bear out the system's success and its relevance is reflected in the health-care reform presently underway in El Salvador, which is modelled on Guarjila's health-care system.

The systematization of the health-care experience in Guarjila described in this chapter shows that it is possible to work on advancing CPHC as it was originally conceived: a system that can be immersed in the integral development of the community, in which health constitutes a fundamental component of development, and in which the leadership role of the community is encouraged, thereby raising its level of "social awareness" (Espinoza, 2002).

Guarjila's experience demonstrated that an organized community possesses considerable capacity to resolve problems and initiate its own social development. Moreover, the Guarjila experience attests to the fact that projects are successful provided that the community participates in their design, development, and management. This was seen in how the population progressively solved its own challenges regarding the basic conditions of life. For instance, they constructed a potable-water system, houses, and latrines. They developed their own food-production system, created an educational model popular with teachers, and a health model with community agents promoting health and training midwives and groups of volunteer women. These initiatives demonstrate significant communal direction and involvement by an array of community members, forming teams and local committees that represented health, education, water, agriculture, women, young people, the military, and the disabled. Decision making involved the majority of the community through these organized groups, and together they ensured an intersectoral approach to resolving community problems. In this context of solidarity and constant search for equity, the community assumed responsibility for their health experience and defended it against multiple attempts of cooptation.

REFERENCES

Baatz, C. (1994). *Testimonio sanitario de una vivencia real y cierta: "La lucha de El Salvador por su dignidad* (Unpublished doctoral dissertation). University of El Salvador, El Salvador.

Baatz, C. (1998). *Capacidad resolutiva de comunidades rurales que cuentan con promotores (as) de salud en Chalatenango y Morazán* (Unpublished master's thesis). University of El Salvador, El Salvador.

Barten, F., Espinoza, E., De Vos, P., & Perez, R. (2008). *Rescate de experiencias locales innovadoras en salud en El Salvador y Nicaragua durante el periodo 1980 – 1995.* Research supported by the European Commission. INCO-DEV Program.

Cordero, D., Salgado, R., & Drasbeck, C. (2004). *An analysis of the IMCI implementation process in four countries of Latin America.* Arlington, VA: BASICS II for the United States Agency for International Development and the Pan American Health Organization.

Dubón, A., & Menjívar, D. (2013). *La construcción del sistema comunitario de salud de Guarjila: Sistematización de una experiencia de Atención Primaria de Salud Integral en El Salvador, durante el período de 1987–2007* (Unpublished master's thesis). University of El Salvador, El Salvador.

Espinoza, E.A. (2002). *Health and sustainable development in the Third World: A goal that is ever more distant. Vak Review: Visions on Health and Sustainable Development.*

Espinoza, E.A., Elias, M.A., & Villalta, E.V. (2000). *El sistema local de salud (silos) de la zona norte de San Salvador 1992–1997: Una experiencia innovadora en salud* (Research report). El Salvador: University of El Salvador.

Pan American Health Organization. (2015). El Salvador Country Profile. Retrieved from http://www.paho.org/hq/index.php?option=com_content &view=article&id=3227&Itemid=2408

Programa de las Naciones Unidas para el Desarrollo [PNUD] (2010). *Informe anual PNUD El Salvador 2010.* Antiguo Cuscatlán, El Salvador: Author. Retrieved from http://www.pnud.org.sv/2007/component/option,com _docman/task,cat_view/gid,176/Itemid,99999999/

Quandl. (2015). El Salvador Health Data. Retrieved from https://www.quandl .com/collections/el-salvador/el-salvador-health-data

16 Conclusion: Is There a Future for Comprehensive Primary Health Care?

RONALD LABONTÉ, DAVID SANDERS,
CORINNE PACKER, AND NIKKI SCHAAY

Our global research program on the revitalization of comprehensive primary health care (CPHC) strongly suggests that the answer to our concluding chapter's title question is "Yes, provided that the sociopolitical context is favourable and visionary leadership is present." Just as the structured narrative review in Chapter 2 noted that most attempts at CPHC were still partial, the new studies undertaken in our research program (most of which are described in the chapters or the section introductions of this book) provide evidence of PHC that is still somewhat fragmented and not yet fulfilling its potential. But every study also found suggestions of its increasing promise and clear indications of the directions programs must take to achieve greater comprehensiveness.

We begin this final chapter by drawing from a synthesis article that examined the different projects for examples of where some of the intended outputs and outcomes of CPHC first postulated in Chapter 1 of this book were being achieved, even if only partially. In doing so, we draw attention to particular studies for the implications they bring forward that represent challenges to or opportunities for a broader, global revitalization of CPHC. We conclude by commenting on what the changes in the landscape, from the time we began our study, portend for CPHC – the shift from PHC to a discourse of universal health coverage (UHC), the arrival of the post-2015 Sustainable Development Goals, expansion of interest in the "Health in All Policies" (HiAP) approach to health-systems reform, and the increasing influence of private-public partnerships on health-system financing and reform. These initiatives are occurring in the context of continuing dominance of neoliberal economics that has escalated wealth inequalities, promoted austerity policies, and challenged the ability of states to build sustainable public-health systems modelled on CPHC principles.

What We Found

Our project was premised on an idealized model of CPHC that proposed six interrelated outcomes:

1 increased equity in access to health care and other services/resources essential to health;
2 reduced community vulnerabilities through increases in community empowerment;
3 reduced exposures to risk through improvements in social and environmental determinants of health;
4 improved community participation and increased political capabilities of marginalized population groups;
5 increased intersectoral policy actions on the social and economic determinants of health; and
6 improved population health outcomes and health equity.

As Table 1.1 in Chapter 1 noted, most of the studies generated at least some findings related to the six outcomes noted above, and that defined our global research program.[1] Taking each briefly in turn:

1. Increased equity in access to health care and other services/ resources essential to health

Our research program considered this output as the baseline for CPHC: necessary, but insufficient in the absence of actions specifically related to the other outputs below. Findings generally noted that the PHC services were successful in improving access. Although few of the projects specifically analysed the equity dimension (e.g., did access disproportionately increase for those in greatest need?), all of the PHC services being studied were targeted at areas or population groups experiencing both need and relative disadvantage.

Some projects were more specific in their targeting, such as the Men's Health Program/Ingkintja in Central Australia, which recognized an equity gap in their services for Aboriginal men. An important – and potentially transferable – lesson was that access for men (a group frequently neglected in PHC programs that emphasize maternal and child health)

---

1 The following six syntheses include excerpts from Labonté, Sanders, Packer, & Schaay, 2014. We thank the journal for allowing us to reproduce them.

did not improve until the program shifted from a vertical service for sexually transmitted infections to one that incorporated broader social determinants of health (SDH) and practical supports for daily living. The Health Extension Program in Ethiopia, described in two of the chapters in this book, has focused much of its attention on improving maternal, neonatal, and child health through the deployment of paid health extension workers (HEWs) as part of the formal public health system. Although the program has shown positive results for improved access to family planning, antenatal care (ANC), and HIV testing, it has been less successful in increasing women's use of health facilities for skilled birth attendance. Understanding why many women still choose not to use health facilities for childbirth remains a challenge for the national government and not just for the particular regions (Tigray and Jimma) in our study.[2] Most of the other projects similarly showed improved access, even in the case of the ASHA program in North Bihar, which had limited CPHC outcomes but which did increase pregnant women's access to health facilities. But as with the negative finding about health-facility births in Ethiopia, most of our studies also documented ongoing shortcomings in improved access, often related to cost and underfunding of services, geographic barriers, and/or inadequate cultural sensitivity.

2. Reduced community vulnerabilities through increases in community empowerment

There is a large body of health-promotion literature on community empowerment and capacity-building that distils to improving the knowledge, analytical skills, local leadership, internal and external resource mobilization, and organizing abilities of disadvantaged communities (Labonté, 1993; Labonté & Laverack, 2001; Laverack & Labonté, 2000; Mihanda, Likofata, & Lusi, 2013). The evidence-informed argument this literature presents is that improvement in these capacity (or empowerment) domains reduces vulnerabilities to disease threats by increasing

---

2 It is also now the focus of a new follow-up implementation study (2015–19) with one of our Ethiopian teams (Jimma): An Implementation Study of Interventions to Promote Safe Motherhood in Jimma Zone, Ethiopia, IDRC No. 108028–002. One of the interventions being studied is provision of fully equipped maternal waiting areas at health facilities, providing women for whom distance is a barrier with a home-like environment in which they can stay when they are near term. Such waiting areas are exemplary of the "other services/resources" to which CPHC reforms must attend.

both material and psychosocial resources for health (Manandhar et al., 2004). Most projects manifested some efforts in this direction.

In the case of the Kenyan project, sites that had implemented a community strategy approach (which emphasized identification of and action by the public health system on health concerns raised by community members) outperformed other sites on such key outputs as ANC and use of insecticide-treated nets. The longer the exposure to this approach, and the more thorough its community engagement, the better the outputs. Other projects similarly demonstrated different facets of empowerment, notably for Aboriginal populations in Australia and for women in many of the projects in other regions. The Safe Motherhood project in DRC, for example, emphasized not only ANC and safe delivery through development of "solidarity groups," but also women's economic empowerment (albeit at a local scale). The ASHA program in North Bihar, India, presented an interesting paradox, insofar as the ASHAs (poor women in rural communities) identified their roles as offering some forms of empowerment for themselves, yet the lack of training or support for their largely voluntary efforts meant that their capacity to work towards greater empowerment of community members was largely inefficient.

Several of the other projects similarly noted simultaneous strengths (or possibilities) and weaknesses in PHC contributions to empowerment. Although many of the community-based PHC services emphasized peoples' rights and entitlements, this was sometimes compromised by low literacy rates or lack of knowledge among CHWs of their role in promoting such rights, as was the case with the ASHA study, but also with CHWs in two of three sites in the South Africa study. These findings raise critical issues regarding the training of and support for CHWs, which we address under the theme of community participation (below).

3. Reduced exposures to risk through improvements in social and environmental determinants of health

Although policy discourse on SDH has gained momentum following the work of the World Health Organization (WHO) Commission on Social Determinants of Health (WHO Commission on Social Determinants of Health & WHO, 2008), the importance of action on SDH has existed in the health-promotion literature since the 1980s. It is also referenced in the 1978 Alma-Ata Declaration itself, though not in the same terms and with an emphasis on local environmental determinants, such as improved sanitation and potable water, and community development more generally. Several instances of modest interventions on SDH were documented by the research projects, some reflecting more traditional environmental actions and others incorporating local economic-development initiatives.

Sometimes the improvements in SDH were subtle, where programs helped to break down gender or social-class stigmas (an important finding in the DRC study) or provided income or nonfinancial resources to CHWs coming from the poorest communities (such as found with the ASHA program). Most of the projects in low-income countries included efforts to improve sanitary conditions and potable-water access, often through the efforts of CHWs. This was noted most strongly in those projects in which CHWs were paid and employed as formal workers within the public health system (Ethiopia, Iran, and the community HEWs in the Kenya program, who are responsible for supervising voluntary CHWs at a village level); in Iran's case, this largely followed gendered lines along which male *behvarz* worked primarily on sanitary and environmental health issues, while female *behvarz* emphasized maternal and child health interventions.[3] Food-security initiatives also existed in some projects, notably in Kenya, where household poultry raising and crop diversification increased following the community strategy program; but suffered neglect in others, as found in the Bangladesh study and attributed to poor levels of community engagement.

Some of the strongest examples of actions on SDH came from the Australian Aboriginal projects, in which Aboriginal control over the governance of these CPHC services combined with the generally severe deficits in SDH for this population to incentivize actions extending well beyond access to health care. As the VAHS report in this book noted, "Aboriginal people have been one of the driving forces behind the CPHC agenda in Australia," embodying an activism to improve health status by acting on the social factors that affect health. The same held true for the small community example, Guarjila, in El Salvador, which implemented and self-governed a comprehensive set of health,

---

3 A subsequent study that examined the (voluntary) CHW program in Afghanistan, which similarly deployed both male and female CHWs working in local villages, found the same gendered pattern of responsibilities, reflecting strong patriarchal cultural norms; see Najafizada, Labonté, & Bourgeault, 2014.

education, sanitation, rehabilitation, housing, and other infrastructure projects. These examples speak to how CPHC, in its structure, staffing, and the extent to which it actively engages communities retains enormous potential to challenge structurally embedded health inequities.

One weakness cutting across most projects, however, was the localized nature of their SDH initiatives. This was not unique to low-income countries, as our structured narrative literature reviews found; and attests to the difficulties local communities often experience in gaining access to the higher-level economic and policy decisions that condition and constrain their local community efforts. We return to this topic in our discussion of intersectoral action (ISA) for health.

4. Improved community participation and increased political capabilities of marginalized population groups

Few aspects of PHC have received as much study or commentary as that of community participation, as much of the literature reviewed in Chapter 2 recounts. Participation by community members is regarded as an axiomatic feature of PHC and is generally assumed to occur through the work of CHWs. This was clearly the case in our project's own suite of studies, in which CHWs and community engagement were dominant features marked either by the positive impact of CHWs' presence (e.g., in Kenya, Ethiopia, Iran, El Salvador, and Aotearoa/ New Zealand) or the implications of their absence or underdevelopment (e.g., in North Bihar, Bangladesh, and South Africa).

The term CHW, of course, is generic and covers a wide range of health workers with differing roles and relationships with the formal health system, differentiated by the extent of their training, remuneration, scope of practice and status, and the degree of their community management and accountability. Within our own studies some CHWs were reasonably well trained and employed as paid members of the public health system, while others were volunteers with only minimal financial or other forms of support (Sanders, Labonté, Packer, & Schaay, 2012). Early on in efforts to "roll out" comprehensive PHC (Walt, 1990), warnings were made about using volunteers to substitute for underfunded public health programs; indeed, in sub-Saharan Africa the majority of CHWs remain unsalaried, often leading to high attrition rates affecting program quality, a problem also found in other regions (e.g., South Asia) that continue to rely on voluntary or underpaid CHW labour. The inequitable gendered dimension of this reliance (that most

CHWs are women, are frequently underresourced, underpaid, or unpaid, and not formally recognized by the health system) has long been noted, and is seen as a barrier to improving maternal and child health, particularly in the low-income, low-resource settings in which they often work (Langer et al., 2015).

These historical limitations of CHW programs do not negate the positive experiences and personal benefits accrued by volunteer CHWs (such as community esteem or exposure to other income-generating opportunities), or the contributions (if often only small) they make to the health and well-being of community members (Leon et al., 2015), a point emphasized in one of the South African cases. A more recent study of Kenyan CHWs further emphasized the agency expressed by these unpaid, voluntary health workers, despite a lack of resources constraining their efforts (Oliver, Geniets, Winters, Rega, & Mbae, 2015). The self-organization of ASHAs in our North Bihar study, and their desire both to receive better training and support and to be remunerated for their labour, further attests to an important dynamic in CHW activism. It is perhaps not surprising, then, that CHWs in some South African provinces have recently and successfully petitioned the government for better pay and binding work contracts (Gonzalez, 2014), echoing comments made by CHWs in several of our studies: the need for their recognition as a formal and paid cadre of health workers.

Just as our studies examined the broader empowerment role of CHWs, and not just their service-delivery function, our initiative emphasized community participation as a "political capability," with some, but not all, projects showing some movement in this direction. Participation by communities in PHC, however, remained problematic in many of the projects, sometimes being seen primarily as voluntary labour (the construction of latrines in Ethiopia) or as passive recipients of health-education messaging (Bangladesh).

A common structure for both empowerment and participation in PHC is presumed to be community health committees (CoHCs) that, among other tasks, are intended to manage CHWs and their work and to engage with CHWs around broader social and environmental health concerns. But CoHCs were often nonexistent or nonfunctional, with little or no support or training in supervising CHWs. Moreover, whether CHWs had received sufficient training to develop the skills and capacities to act as social animateurs engendering community actions on broader health determinants was moot, with one exception being the Iranian *behvarz* program.

Most of our studies identified the importance of structures for community participation (whether within health systems or through local governments), yet several found that even when such structures existed, they were not used. This was partly attributed to political dysfunction (as in two of the South African cases), but also to the assumption that poor people in poor living conditions would "volunteer" their unpaid labour. The Kenyan study underscored the importance of dedicating some of the time of paid community health extension workers to supporting the work of local community committees – community participation is not a cost-free endeavour.

In 2013, a new initiative hosted by the Columbia University Earth Institute was launched with the goal of supporting scale-up of "one million community health workers" (One Million Community Health Workers, 2016), In this current scale-up, an emphasis on "task-shifting" to lower-level health cadres, together with the current dominance of cost/benefit analyses in UHC scale-up, to which we return later in this chapter, could detract from the role of CHWs as "social animateurs" helping communities to engage more fully with political institutions around SDH and further entrench the "vertical" program delivery of selected technical interventions This development, while having great potential to rapidly improve coverage of basic health care, risks instrumentalizing the role of CHWs, echoing the caution expressed in the seminal paper "The Village Health Worker – Lackey or Liberator?" (Werner, 1977).

More fundamentally, and reflecting findings from the Latin American literature review in Chapter 2, the Argentinian study documented how participatory approaches to PHC were undercut by 15 years of military dictatorship and the adoption of neoliberal economic policies. Without an ideologically and economically supportive government, effective and politically capable forms of community participation will remain underdeveloped or, at best, "below the radar" to avoid confrontation with unsupportive political forces.

5. Increased intersectoral policy actions on the social and economic determinants of health

The Alma-Ata Declaration recognized the importance of intersectoral action for health (IAH) such as education, sanitation, and safe water. Evidence of health-system engagement in IAH was found in several of our projects and was closely linked with community mobilization on SDH. HEWs in Ethiopia, for example, despite being constrained by a lack of IAH at higher health-system governance levels, created strong links with the educational and agricultural sectors.

As found in other studies (e.g., Kenya, Ethiopia, and Iran), CHWs quickly became the "go to" people at the local level for linking across public service sectors, embodying much of the original vision of Alma-Ata. This was true even in the high-income country studies reviewed in Chapter 2 and could be considered a generalizable finding. Although structures for local-level ISA sometimes existed, fragmentation within local government services (in two of the South African cases, and in the Brazilian study on family health teams' links to higher levels of care), together with a general lack of support for community-based organizations, often rendered these structures ineffectual.

The lack of IAH at higher governance levels was also problematic in most of our studies, an exception being Iran, where the creation of *beh-varz* councils in 2006 is seen as a conduit for raising local IAH issues to these levels.[4] The same year also saw Iran create IAH structures at both the national and local levels ("Councils on Health and Food Security") (Khayatzadeh-Mahani, Sedoghi, Mehrolhassani, & Yazdi-Feyzabadi, 2015), with the need for both horizontal collaboration within levels and vertical collaboration between levels commonly reflected in new academic scholarship on IAH (Carey & Crammond, 2015; Leppo, Ollila, Peña, Wismar, & Cook, 2013; McQueen, Wismar, Lin, Jones, & Davies, 2012).

Returning to the centrality of CHWs in enabling local-level IAH, CHWs' earnings are based on specific activities (e.g., immunizations, clinic visits, as found in the ASHA program), which became a disincentive for any work related to community mobilization or ISA. It was also one of the reasons why the ASHAs began advocating for a salary rather than pay-for-performance scheme and reinforces the caution raised earlier about CHWs being considered merely inexpensive service-delivery workers. In other instances, IAH efforts were weakened by a lack of any guidelines from more senior government levels on the obligations sectors have for mutual cooperation. Exceptions again existed with the Aboriginal projects, where community control and "ownership" was given particularly strong emphasis, alongside clear mandates for

---

4 Although these councils are not a focus of this chapter, a discussion on their origin and potential IAH role can be found in the full report of the Iran study, available here: http://globalhealthequity.ca/webfm_send/100

CPHC staff to advocate with, and on behalf of, community members across relevant sectors and governance levels.

6. Improved population health outcomes and greater health equity

Given the short duration and limited budgets for our studies, few of the projects were able to capture health-outcome measures, much less attribute changes in such measures to the CPHC components they were studying. Most projects focused instead on changes in health-system outputs, which, as noted above, generally showed positive gains. Some findings directly generated or assessed by our projects, however, included declines in rural infant mortality following the introduction of CHW programs, and better health indices where programs were more comprehensive in scope than in areas where services were more fragmented. This finding was similar to that generated by our structured literature review.

Conclusion: Is There a Future for CPHC?

As noted at the outset of this chapter, the global discourse on health systems has shifted from a concern with PHC and SDH to one of "universal health coverage," now one of the targets of the 2015 Sustainable Development Goals (SDGs).[5] On the one hand, the SDGs present an enormous opportunity for CPHC, since the 17 goals are predicated on a "whole-of-government" responsibility: the goals are to be seen as integrated, interrelated, and indivisible. This approach certainly affords an opening for health workers committed to CPHC principles to push for an IAH approach in their own work. This is how the UHC goal within the SDGs was seen in *Tracking Universal Health Coverage: First Global Monitoring Report*, released by the WHO and the World Bank in 2015 (WHO, 2015a), and is generally given a supporting nod in most statements about UHC. At the same time, and as many commentators have cautioned, there is a risk that the overwhelming ambition of the

---

5 We note, however, that what public health advocates describe as "social determinants of health" are embodied in most of the "nonhealth" Sustainable Development Goals. Nonetheless, the absence of any reference to SDH in the health goals weakens the support health systems should be providing to intersectoral action on SDH, a weakness found in our structured literature review of PHC and persisting in the set of studies recounted in this book.

SDGs will see sectors slip back more firmly into their silos, rather than the reverse. Although initiatives on SDH and HiAP (as the term for IAH has now been rebranded) still define part of the WHO's ongoing work program, there is clearly a comfortable acceptance of the UHC goal being the health sector's main contribution to the SDGs. As WHO Director-General Margaret Chan stated in the WHO's 2015 report on the SDGs,

> In health the target on universal health coverage (UHC) provides the platform for integrated action across all 13 health targets. Rather than being seen as one target among many, it is my belief that UHC should be seen as the linchpin of the health development agenda, not only underpinning a more sustainable approach to the achievement of the other health targets, but allowing for a balance between them. (WHO, 2015b)

This emphasis on UHC perforce demands some exploration of what is meant by it and whether it poses the risk to CPHC that some contend.

First mooted by the WHO in 2005, UHC is defined as "ensuring that all people can use the promotive, preventive, curative, rehabilitative and palliative health services they need, of sufficient quality to be effective, while also ensuring that the use of these services does not expose the user to financial hardship" (WHO, 2015c). This apparent alignment with the original Alma-Ata Declaration (with the new addition of palliative health services) is initially reassuring, but is marginalized by the emphasis the WHO then places on financing and services, stating that UHC

> ...embodies three related objectives:
> - equity in access to health services – those who need the services should get them, not only those who can pay for them;
> - that the quality of health services is good enough to improve the health of those receiving services; and
> - financial risk protection – ensuring that the cost of using care does not put people at risk of financial hardship. (WHO, 2015c)

Concern with financing is important, and that was noted in many of our studies; and the UHC discourse does acknowledge the importance of public financing in achieving health objectives. But rather than affirming the state's role in providing health services, thereby overcoming market failures in private financing and provision, many powerful proponents of UHC envision a pluralist model in which private markets and providers (albeit supported by public financing) coexist with public provision (People's Health Movement, Medact, Health Action International, Medico International, & Third World Network, 2014, Chap. B:1). This "new public management" model creates opportunities for private profit making in health systems, usually defended on the basis that the private sector is more efficient and effective in service delivery.

One example of this model has been the proliferation of "public-private partnerships" (PPPs), which have taken two forms. The first has been the dramatic growth since 2000 in "global health partnerships," which bring public and private actors together in initiatives that channel increasing amounts of health assistance to low- and middle-income countries (e.g., the Global Alliance for Vaccines and Immunization, and the Global Fund to Fight AIDS, Tuberculosis and Malaria). With the parallel growth in private philanthropies (e.g., the Bill & Melinda Gates Foundation), private actors are increasingly defining health systems' programs and functions in countries still relying on donor assistance, particularly in the world's poorest countries. The emphasis of most of these funding programs on treatment and products to address specific diseases "has the effect of deflecting the focus from environmental and social determinants and from effective prevention activities and thus from comprehensive PHC" (Sanders, Baum, Benos, & Legge, 2011). The second form of PPPs are "private financing initiatives," wherein private investors front the initial capital for new health facilities' construction (and may also contract with governments to undertake all aspects of facility operations for a defined number of years) in return for guaranteed returns on investment, often as high as 20% to 25%. Although usually associated with hospitals, PPPs are also being used and promoted for construction and management of primary health-care facilities (Baig, Panda, Das, & Chauhan, 2014; European Investment Bank, 2015; Pal & Pal, 2009). Experiences with this model have generally been disastrous, with governments spending far more over the long-term than they would otherwise if they had borrowed the necessary capital and undertaken facilities construction and management directly (Pollock, 2014a, 2014b). The high cost of private financing initiatives, especially in low-income countries, can substantially drain government revenues that would otherwise support PHC programs, as Oxfam's recent study of the World Bank's private-public partnership model for a new hospital in Lesotho found (Marriott, 2014). A 2015 European Parliament policy report on the contribution of private financing for development was equally damning, finding that

> PPPs are by far the most expensive way to fund projects. Equally important, the cost is often non-transparent and not accountable to auditors, parliaments or civil society groups. Similarly, debt sustainability assessments do not currently take account of this cost as these are treated as off-budget transactions, and PPPs have also tended to be very high risk financing. (Griffiths, Martin, Pereira, & Strawson, 2014)

Moreover, managing a "mixed market" in health care (where social or private insurance schemes and private providers or facilities "compete" with tax-funded public insurance schemes and facilities) generates enormous public and private transaction costs compared to health systems that are primarily publicly financed and provided (People's Health Movement, Medact, Health Action International, Medico International, & Third World Network, 2014, Chap. B:1), again draining resources that could go into creating a more integrated health system based on comprehensive PHC principles. This problem was highlighted in several of our projects (notably Colombia and Argentina).

The potential threat that PPPs could pose to a renewal in CPHC cannot be overstated. Not only are such partnerships increasingly ubiquitous within the UN family of agencies and assumed to be essential in moving forward on health, social, environmental, and development goals; they are also seen as essential elements in future health-system strengthening (Taylor & Christian, 2016) and for achieving UHC (Kapilashrami, 2016).

Even if UHC remains primarily a public affair, the present focus in UHC on financial barriers (Reich et al., 2016) could detract from strengthening health systems' capacities to contribute meaningfully to actions affecting SDH (WHO, 2015d). That is, there has been a shift from debates about how services should be provided to how they should be financed; and from the comprehensiveness of a health system to coverage of specific – often curative – services (Waitzkin, 2016). This is evident in much of the literature now focusing on how UHC can promote a "pro-poor" universalism by prioritizing service coverage for the poor first, then universalizing with time (Bump et al., 2016). Although prioritizing the poor is an important health-equity goal, emphasizing service coverage captures only the first of the six outcomes of CPHC while introducing administrative costs in determining who is "poor enough" to be targeted (Cotlear, Nagpal, Smith, Tandon, & Cortez, 2015). It also surrenders to a general discourse of "scarcity" in health resources, captured in two of the preambular articles in the 2016 Bangkok Statement on Priority-Setting for Universal Health Coverage:[6]

> 2. Recognizing that universal health coverage will require difficult trade-offs between expanding priority services, including more people, and reducing out-of-pocket payments, and the fact that *demand for health services may be infinite while resources are limited and donor contributions are declining in some settings* …
>
> 5. Recognizing the need for more explicit priority-setting considering fairness and equity, and *based on cost-effectiveness with respect to health outcomes*, while also incorporating due consideration of financial protection, ethical principles, social values, political feasibility, and public health security [emphases added]. (Prince Mahidol Award Conference, 2015)

What these statements leave unquestioned is *why* resources are limited, or how the cost-effectiveness metric (not that anyone should be in favour of cost-ineffectiveness) is likely to lead to a focus on the "low hanging fruits" of selective interventions for which discrete costs and outcomes can be easily measured. As another recent World Bank study on "bottom-up" UHC experiences described, many governments are using financing "stepping stones" in their push for UHC, including voluntary insurance schemes, autonomous programs for the poor only, and parallel private insurance or copayments for services beyond a basic package (Cotlear et al., 2015). Although the World Bank study implies that these are only partial "steps" towards what UHC should be, there are worrisome echoes of the "interim strategy" that was selective PHC just a year after Alma-Ata's comprehensive declaration, justified on economic and political grounds (Walsh & Warren, 1979). Rather than being a short-term transitional fix, and with the few exceptions noted in Chapter 2 and in some of the contributions to this book, selective PHC continues to dominate global health funding.

It is the excuse of "resource scarcity," however, that cuts to the most fundamental challenge to CPHC and to the likelihood that UHC could

---

6 The statement was issued on behalf of the ministers of health and participants at the 2016 Prince Mahidol Awards Conference (PMAC). The annual PMAC has become an important venue for discussions on global health and health systems reform.

become cemented in a "stepping stone" incompleteness. As Chapter 2 discussed, with particular reference to CPHC studies in the Latin American region, and as several of the projects in this book referenced, the backdrop to efforts to implement CPHC has been the four-decade dominance of a neoliberal globalization. On the one hand, this period has witnessed huge declines in infant and child mortality attributed to the global diffusion of effective low-cost interventions and the "trickle-down" health benefits of economic growth in many low-income countries. On the other hand, this period has seen the development of huge health and wealth inequalities, a decline in economic product going to labour relative to capital, weakened labour rights and high unemployment, the rise of speculative finance creating global financial crises, and policies of "austerity" in response to such crises that resemble the discredited structural adjustment programs of the 1980s and 1990s, all of which threaten the global health gains made in earlier decades (People's Health Movement, Medact, Health Action International, Medico International, & Third World Network, 2014; Labonté & Stuckler, 2016). Another and vitally important outcome of this neoliberal period has been a marked decline in the public revenue (taxation) share of global economic product as countries engage in tax competition to attract foreign direct investment, marginal rates on high-income earners slide downwards, and transnational corporations avail themselves of tax havens and transfer-pricing to contribute ever smaller portions to the public purse:

> … using monetized (constant dollars) value of the Global Economic Product and the amount captured by the effective global tax rate, the amount of private capital falling outside the bounds of taxation jumped from $28 trillion in 2004 to $58 trillion in 2012, more than doubling in just 8 years. (Labonté & Stuckler, 2016)

The simple bottom line is that we are not living in an era of scarcity but of massive inequality. We would not argue that all private wealth should be taxed, or that financing for health systems should be considered unbound and infinite if for no other reason than public investments in SDH (e.g., housing, climate-change mitigation, food security, and many other of the goals identified under the SDG umbrella) are probably even more critical than health care to improve health and health equity. But neither should advocates of CPHC passively accept the discourse of resource constraints, without questioning *why* those constraints exist and whether they are even necessary.

As Chapter 1 described, the broader global political and economic context – a New International Economic Order – was raised, at the time of Alma-Ata, as crucial to implementing CPHC. If the current context seems inimical to an effective revitalization of CPHC, our research and the findings of our teams nonetheless offer a cautiously optimistic signal that PHC reforms in several countries are indeed moving in the direction of greater comprehensiveness, even amidst a plethora of globally driven and vertical disease initiatives. These reforms are acknowledging (and initiating some actions on) SDH, and are making efforts (albeit sometimes weak) to engage communities on broader issues of health equity and the delivery platforms and sociopolitical conditions that facilitate it. Moreover, our studies' results also confirm the importance (noted by respondents in most of our studies) of a horizontal approach to PHC that incorporates ISAs on SDH and broad forms of community participation.

As part of their study remits, each of our research teams reviewed critically the reports on PHC literature (Chapter 2) pertinent to their region, to fill in any gaps (drawing extensively from the grey literature) and to elaborate on the specific historical and contemporary contexts in which their findings of PHC reforms were situated. Their final reports contain detailed contextual analyses, across which a consistent theme – one consonant with our structured literature reviews – stands out: the importance of political commitments to health equity and to health reform policies that clearly identify primary care, community participation, and ISA as essential health-system components. These overarching conclusions from the synthesis of our wide range of studies have been confirmed in two key and influential publications: the *Lancet* series on PHC (McCoy et al., 2011) and the World Health Report of 2008 (WHO, 2008). These reports among others (see, e.g., Barten & Sanders, 2009) identify political commitment and its translation into participatory, comprehensive, and integrated health systems as a common set of attributes in those countries where progress in health has been most impressive. It is this political commitment to the ethos of CPHC that remains most important to its revitalization today.

Whether or not this commitment materializes remains a matter of conjecture. Nonetheless, and based upon the efforts recounted by the case studies in this book, we remain cautiously optimistic that the ideals of CPHC will continue to be a force in the health system reforms of many countries, for the simple reason that CPHC offers an efficient, effective, and equitable means of improving peoples' health. Stated somewhat differently: it is an idea too powerful to disappear.

REFERENCES

Baig, M.B., Panda, B., Das, J.K., & Chauhan, A.S. (2014). Is public private partnership an effective alternative to government in the provision of primary health care? A case study in Odisha. *Journal of Health Management, 16*(1), 41–52. http://dx.doi.org/10.1177/0972063413518679

Barten, F., & Sanders, D. (2009). Retos contextuales a la revitalización de la atención primaria de la salud: Algunas lecciones de África y de América Latina. In F. Barten, M. Rovere, & E. Espinoza (Eds.), *Salud para todos una meta posible, pueblos movilizados y gobiernos comprometidos en un nuevo contexto global, construyendo prioridades para la investigación en APS con la sociedad civil* (pp. 267–78). Buenos Aires: IIED – América Latina Publicaciones.

Bump, J., Cashin, C., Chalkidou, K., Evans, D., González-Pier, E., Guo, Y., …, Yamey, G., & Participants at the Bellagio Workshop on Implementing Pro-Poor Universal Health Coverage. (2016, Jan). Implementing pro-poor universal health coverage. *Lancet Global Health, 4*(1), e14–e16. http://dx.doi.org/10.1016/S2214-109X(15)00274-0 Medline:26700794

Carey, G., & Crammond, B. (2015, Mar). Action on the social determinants of health: Views from inside the policy process. *Social Science & Medicine, 128,* 134–41. http://dx.doi.org/10.1016/j.socscimed.2015.01.024 Medline:25616195

Cotlear, D., Nagpal, S., Smith, O., Tandon, A., & Cortez, R.A. (2015). *Going universal: How 24 developing countries are implementing universal health coverage reforms from the bottom up.* Washington, DC: The World Bank. http://dx.doi.org/10.1596/978-1-4648-0610-0.

European Investment Bank (2015). Primary care centres PPP. Retrieved from http://www.eib.org/projects/pipeline/2014/20140692.htm

Gonzalez, L.L. (2014, Mar 28). Health dept. to pay community health workers, renew contracts. *Health-e News: The South African Health News Service.* Retrieved from http://www.health-e.org.za/2014/03/28/department -health-pay-workers-issue-new-contracts/

Griffiths, J., Martin, M., Pereira, T., & Strawson, T. (2014). *Financing for development post-2015: Improving the contribution of private finance.* Brussels: Directorate-General for External Policies Policy Department, European Parliament. Retrieved from https://europa.eu/eyd2015/sites/default/files/users/maja .ljubic/expo-deve_et2014433848_en.pdf

Kapilashrami, A. (2016). Private sector heterogeneity and universal health coverage. *Global Health Check*. Retrieved from http://www.globalhealthcheck.org/?p=1851

Khayatzadeh-Mahani, A., Sedoghi, Z., Mehrolhassani, M.H., & Yazdi-Feyzabadi, V. (2015, Jun 18). How health in all policies are developed and implemented in a developing country? A case study of a HiAP initiative in Iran. *Health Promotion International*, dav062. http://dx.doi.org/10.1093/heapro/dav062 Medline:26092852

Labonté, R. (1993). Health promotion and empowerment: Practice frameworks. *Issues in Health Promotion Series* (HP-10-0102). Toronto: Centre for Health Promotion and Participation.

Labonté, R., & Laverack, G. (2001). Capacity building in health promotion, part 2: Whose use? And with what measurement? *Critical Public Health*, *11*(2), 129–38. http://dx.doi.org/10.1080/09581590110039847

Labonté, R., Sanders, D., Packer, C., & Schaay, N. (2014, Aug 21). Is the Alma Ata vision of comprehensive primary health care viable? Findings from an international project. *Global Health Action*, *7*(0), 24997. http://dx.doi.org/10.3402/gha.v7.24997 Medline:25150030

Labonté, R., & Stuckler, D. (2016, Mar). The rise of neoliberalism: How bad economics imperils health and what to do about it. *Journal of Epidemiology and Community Health*, *70*(3), 312–18. http://dx.doi.org/10.1136/jech-2015-206295 Medline:26424847

Langer, A., Meleis, A., Knaul, F.M., Atun, R., Aran, M., Arreola-Ornelas, H., …, & Frenk, J. (2015, Sep 19). Women and health: The key for sustainable development. *Lancet*, *386*(9999), 1165–210. http://dx.doi.org/10.1016/S0140-6736(15)60497-4 Medline:26051370

Laverack, G., & Labonté, R. (2000, Sep). A planning framework for community empowerment goals within health promotion. *Health Policy and Planning*, *15*(3), 255–62. http://dx.doi.org/10.1093/heapol/15.3.255 Medline:11012399

Leon, N., Sanders, D., Van Damme, W., Besada, D., Daviaud, E., Oliphant, N.P., …, & Doherty, T. (2015, Mar 12). The role of "hidden" community volunteers in community-based health service delivery platforms: Examples from sub-Saharan Africa. *Global Health Action*, *8*(0), 27214. http://dx.doi.org/10.3402/gha.v8.27214 Medline:25770090

Leppo, K., Ollila, E., Peña, S., Wismar, M., & Cook, S. (2013). *Health in all policies. Seizing opportunities, implementing policies*. Helsinki: Ministry of Social Affairs and Health.

Manandhar, D.S., Osrin, D., Shrestha, B.P., Mesko, N., Morrison, J., Tumbahangphe, K.M., …, & Costello, A.M., & Members of the MIRA Makwanpur trial team. (2004, Sep 11–17). Effect of a participatory intervention with women's groups on birth outcomes in Nepal: Cluster-randomised controlled trial. *Lancet, 364*(9438), 970–9. http://dx.doi.org/10.1016/S0140-6736(04)17021-9 Medline:15364188

Marriott, A. (2014). *A dangerous diversion: Will the IFC's flagship health PPP bankrupt Lesotho's Ministry of Health?* Policy Paper, Oxfam Briefing Notes, Consumers Protection Association (Lesotho) and Oxfam International.

McCoy, D., Labonté, R., Walt, G., Sanders, D., Ram, R., Luppe, T., …, & Dare, L. (2011, May 28). The IHP+: A welcome initiative with an uncertain future. *Lancet, 377*(9780), 1835–6. http://dx.doi.org/10.1016/S0140-6736(11)60774-5 Medline:21621714

McQueen, D.V., Wismar, M., Lin, V., Jones, C., & Davies, M. (2012). Intersectoral governance for health in all policies: Structures, actions and experiences. Observatory Study Series. European Observatory on Health Systems and Policies. Retrieved from http://www.euro.who.int/__data/assets/pdf_file/0005/171707/Intersectoral-governance-for-health-in-all-policies.pdf

Mihanda, R.B., Likofata, J.R., & Lusi, G.J. (2013). Contribution of safe motherhood solidarity groups in using and accessing maternity services during a period of armed conflict. *Health, 5*(7), 1085–91. http://dx.doi.org/10.4236/health.2013.57146

Najafizada, S.A., Labonté, R., & Bourgeault, I.L. (2014, Dec 01). Community health workers of Afghanistan: A qualitative study of a national program. *Conflict and Health, 8*(26),1-16. http://dx.doi.org/10.1186/1752-1505-8-26 Medline:25904976

Oliver, M., Geniets, A., Winters, N., Rega, I., & Mbae, S.M. (2015, May). What do community health workers have to say about their work, and how can this inform improved programme design? A case study with CHWs within Kenya. *Global Health Action, 8,* 27168–84. http://dx.doi.org/10.3402/gha.v8.27168 Medline:26004292

One Million Community Health Workers (2016). Community health workers: Bridging the gap to universal health coverage. Retrieved from http://1millionhealthworkers.org/

Pal, R., & Pal, S. (2009). Primary healthcare and public-private partnership: An Indian perspective. *Annals of Tropical Medicine and Public Health, 2*(2), 46.

People's Health Movement, Medact, Health Action International, Medico International, & Third World Network. (2014). *Global Health Watch 4: An Alternative World Health Report.* New York/London: Zed Books. Retrieved from http://www.ghwatch.org/node/45484

Pollock, A. (2014a, Aug. 15). NHS privatisation keeps on failing patients despite a decade of warnings. *The Guardian.* Retrieved from https://www.theguardian.com/commentisfree/2014/aug/15/nhs-privatisation-failing-patients-warnings

Pollock, A. (2014b). Submission to health committee enquiry: Public expenditure on health and social care. Retrieved from http://www.allysonpollock.com/wp-content/uploads/2014/11/AP_2014_Pollock_HealthCommittee PublicExpenditure.pdf

Prince Mahidol Award Conference. (2015). Draft Bangkok statement on priority-setting for universal health coverage. Retrieved from http://pmaconference.mahidol.ac.th/index.php?option=com_content&view=article&id=758&Itemid=

Reich, M.R., Harris, J., Ikegami, N., Maeda, A., Cashin, C., Araujo, E.C., …, & Evans, T.G. (2016, Feb 20). Moving towards universal health coverage: Lessons from 11 country studies. *The Lancet, 387*(10020), 811–16. http://dx.doi.org/10.1016/S0140-6736(15)60002-2 Medline:26299185

Sanders, D., Baum, F.E., Benos, A., & Legge, D. (2011, Aug). Revitalising primary healthcare requires an equitable global economic system - now more than ever. *Journal of Epidemiology and Community Health, 65*(8), 661–5. http://dx.doi.org/10.1136/jech.2009.095125 Medline:19955097

Sanders, D., Labonté, R., Packer, C., & Schaay, N. (2012). Dimensiones comunitarias de la atención primaria integral en salud. *Saúde em Debate, 36*(94), 473–81. http://dx.doi.org/10.1590/S0103-11042012000300018

Taylor, R.M., & Christian, J. (2016). The role of public-private partnerships in health systems strengthening: Workshop summary 2016. Forum on Public-Private Partnerships for Global Health and Safety. Retrieved from http://www.nap.edu/catalog/21861/the-role-of-public-private-partnerships-in-health-systems-strengthening http://dx.doi.org/10.17226/21861

Waitzkin, H. (2016). Universal health coverage: The strange romance of *The Lancet,* MEDICC, and Cuba. *Social Medicine (Social Medicine Publication Group), 9*(2), 93–7.

Walsh, J.A., & Warren, K.S. (1979, Nov 1). Selective primary health care: An interim strategy for disease control in developing countries. *New England Journal of Medicine, 301*(18), 967–74. http://dx.doi.org/10.1056/NEJM197911013011804 Medline:114830

Walt, G. (1990). *Community health workers in national programmes: Just another pair of hands?* Milton Keynes: Open University Press.

Werner, D. (1977). The village health worker: Lackey or liberator? Presented at International Hospital Federation Congress, Tokyo, Japan.

WHO. (2008). *Primary health care: Now more than ever.* Geneva: WHO Press.

WHO. (2015a). *Tracking universal health coverage: First global monitoring report.* Geneva: WHO Press.

WHO. (2015b). *Health in 2015: From MDGs, Millennium Development Goals to SDGs, Sustainable Development Goals.* Geneva: WHO Press.

WHO. (2015c). *Health financing for universal coverage.* Geneva: WHO Press.

WHO. (2015d). *Anchoring universal health coverage in the right to health: What difference would it make?* Policy brief. Geneva: WHO Press.

WHO Commission on Social Determinants of Health & WHO. (2008). *Closing the gap in a generation: Health equity through action on the social determinants of health: Commission on Social Determinants of Health final report.* Geneva: WHO, Commission on Social Determinants of Health.

Contributors

Abera Asefa Deressa holds an MSc in nursing. He is currently deputy head of Jimma Zone Health Office, Ministry of Health, in Jimma, Ethiopia. He is involved in implementing health programs as well as research with various institutions. His key role is to help translate research results into program modifications.

Berardo Augusto Nunan is a general practitioner, specialist in public policy and strategic management in health care. He is director of Unified Health System Improvement School of the Department of Health of Distrito Federal, Brasília, Brazil.

Christa Baatz (1943–2015) was a German citizen who settled in El Salvador in the 1980s. She obtained her Master of Public Health and Doctor of Medicine at the University of El Salvador, and became director of the Ana Manganaro Clinic in Guarjila. She passed away on 17 April 2015, but her work in the rural communities of the department of Chalatenango is a legacy of unwavering struggle for justice and equity.

Eugenia Bagnasco is a psychologist who previously worked in an interprofessional training program in the first level of care in Berisso, Argentina. Currently Eugenia Bagnasco works in a gender-oriented program of the Ministry of Health of Buenos Aires to prevent domestic violence.

Fran Baum is a Matthew Flinders Distinguished Professor and the director of the Southgate Institute for Health, Society and Equity and at Flinders University. She is a member of the Coordinating Committee and Advisory Council of the People's Health Movement – a global network of health activists (www.phmovement.org). She is a fellow of the Academy of the Social Sciences in Australia and of the Australian Health Promotion Association. She is a past national president and life member of the Public Health Association of Australia. She also served as a commissioner on the World Health Organization's Commission on the Social Determinants of Health from 2005 to 2008. Fran Baum is one of Australia's leading researchers on the social and economic determinants of health. She leads research projects that are considering a wide range of aspects of health inequities and social determinants of health. Her book, *The New Public Health,* is widely used as a public health text.

Yemane Berhane is a medical doctor with a PhD in Epidemiology and Public Health from Umeå University, Sweden. His public health research interests include maternal/child health, infectious diseases, and noncommunicable diseases. From 1993 to 2006 he contributed to the development of the Butajira Health and Demographic Surveillance System in Ethiopia. He has been teaching since 1992, first at Addis Ababa University and later at Addis Continental Institute of Public Health in Ethiopia. He is a founding fellow of the Ethiopian Academy of Sciences. He has also served as the president of the Ethiopian Public Health Association (1995–9); associate vice president for Research and Graduate Studies at Addis Ababa University (2001–2); regional director for Measure Evaluation Anglophone Africa Training on Monitoring and Evaluation of Health Programs (2005–6); member of the WHO/AFRO Technical Advisory Group on Measles Control in Africa (2005–present); and chair of the Global Evaluation and Monitoring Network for Health (GEMNet-Health, 2012–14).

Analía Bertolotto is a psychologist with a Master's degree in Public Health. Previously, she worked in an interprofessional training program in the first level of care in Berisso. Today, she works as a consultant in human resources development in the Ministry of Health of Buenos Aires and as a professor at La Matanza National University.

Richard Bitwe Mihanda is a medical doctor specializing in pediatrics in DRC, with a PhD in medical science from Brussels Free University (ULB) in Belgium. He has a strong interest in safe motherhood and maternity services, which has led him to mentor trainees at HEAL Africa. In the past he worked as an instructor in pediatrics and head of the pediatric department at the University of Kisangani, Goma Campus, and was medical director of the Provincial Hospital of North Kivu. From 2009 to 2014 he was dean of the Faculty of Medicine, University of Goma, where he is now vice rector in charge of academic affairs.

Roman Blanco is a medical doctor with a passion for combining appropriate ICT systems and learning in science. He leads the efforts of "Digital Campus" to develop and promote new technologies and learning methods in higher educational institutions and health systems in emerging countries. With more than 20 years of experience in educational and health science projects, he has worked through constant technological advances incorporating them into low-resource settings.

Jack Buong is a community health and development specialist with 11 years of experience in strengthening health systems, health institutions, community health strategy, research and training. He possesses extensive hands-on experience in capacity building in leadership, management, and governance in development and health systems. He is a core facilitator and researcher in health system strengthening in the devolved county health structures in Kenya.

Anil Cherian is currently director of the National Institute of Health Sciences Jonglei which trains various cadres of health workers for South Sudan. He is a pediatrician from India who worked for more than 20 years with poor and oppressed communities in North India, which eventually led to his involvement in community health and development. He has a Master's in Public Health from the University of Philippines Manila, specializing in epidemiology, and later studied health economics at the University of York, UK. He has also been actively involved in public health research and his primary area of interest relates to inequities in health.

Geert-Jan Dinant is a professor in family medicine. His research focuses on frequently occurring diseases in primary care, with a special interest in diagnostic research. He has undertaken several research projects in many different parts of the world; Ethiopia in particular.

Maria Argelia Dubón Abrego is a medical doctor with a Master's degree in Public Health. She was director of the Primary Health Care Program of El Salvador's Ministry of Health and is currently director of health for El Salvador's Central Region. Since her youth, she has been committed to promoting community health and primary health care in her country.

Eduardo Antonio Espinoza Fiallos, M.D., is a former dean of the University of El Salvador (UES) and founder of the University's Master of Public Health program. From 1999 to 2007 he was secretary of National and International Relations of UES. Since 2009, he has been deputy minister for health policy of the Ministry of Health of El Salvador. He also remains a member of the academic staff of the International People's Health University (IPHU).

Patty Fidelis de Almeida is a professor at the Health Planning Department at Federal Fluminense University (UFF) in Niterói, Brazil. Her research interests include evaluation of primary health care policies, programs, and services.

Ana Fuks is a phono-audiologist with a Master's degree in Public Health. She has worked for more than a decade as coordinator of the postgraduate program of residence in the Ministry of Health of Buenos Aires City District. Today she is a professor at La Matanza National University.

Jameela George is the executive director of the Centre for Bioethics, India. She received her medical degree from India, certificate in missions from All Nations Christian College, U.K, and a diploma in community health from Jamkhed, India. She has been providing primary health care in rural India for 13 years. She has led a number of community programs, including a vibrant adolescents' development program, an extensive female-adult-literacy program, and "mothers-in-law" groups. She developed a self-sustaining referral system to facilitate safe delivery for those living in the sub-Himalayan Mountains. After obtaining her Master's degree in International Research Bioethics from Monash University, she became the manager of research and bioethics. Her research interests include adolescents, the elderly, and livelihoods.

Lígia Giovanella is senior researcher in the Health Management and Planning Department of the National School of Public Health, Oswaldo Cruz Foundation (Ensp/Fiocruz), Rio de Janeiro, Brazil. Her research interests include international health-care systems comparisons, health reforms, and primary health care.

Jane Goudge, director of the Centre for Health Policy, University of the Witwatersrand, South Africa, has been conducting research in the field of health systems and policy for 16 years. Themes in her research include access to health care, the role of community health workers in improving access to care, governance within district health systems, implementation processes around major reforms, and health-care financing to achieve universal coverage.

Clementine Gwoswar is the Migori County nursing officer and has more than 15 years of experience in health-systems management. As a research user she has been involved in the implementation of the community strategy for the implementation of the essential care for health, which is the Kenyan version of CPHC. She also has been involved in scaling up efforts in more than six devolved health units (counties) in Kenya.

Gholamreza Heidari is the ex-chair of the board and chancellor of Boushehr University of Medical Sciences and Health Services in Iran. He received his Doctor of Dental Medicine degree from Southwestern University in the Philippines and PhD from Tehran University, Iran. He has extensive experience in public health at national and international levels, including technical advisor to WHO in Afghanistan in 2004, consultant to IPPF (International Planned Parenthood Federation) in South Asia Regional Office in HIV/AIDS and Adolescent Health, director general in the Center for Network Development and Health Promotion in the Iranian Ministry of Health, project manager of UNFPA in Iran, and vice chair and secretariat of Country Coordination Mechanism for the Global Fund. More recently he has been appointed as a member of the Finance and Operational Performance Committee in the Global Fund, Geneva.

Jinneth Hernández Torres is a medical doctor with an MSc degree in Health Systems. Currently she is working as a national professional of systematization at the Pan American Health Organization office in Colombia. Her areas of interests involve evaluation of public health programs, health systems, and primary health care.

Anwar Islam holds a PhD in Sociology from the University of Alberta, Canada. He has had a long professional career with the International Development Research Centre and the former Canadian International

Development Agency. He also served the Community Health Sciences Department at the Aga Khan University in Karachi, Pakistan, as associate professor and head of the Health Systems Division, as well as the James P Grant School of Public Health at BRAC University in Dhaka, Bangladesh, as professor and director. Presently, he is an adjunct professor with the School for International Development and Global Studies, University of Ottawa, Canada, and adjunct scientist and consultant with the International Centre for Diarrheal Disease Research in Dhaka, Bangladesh.

Andrea Jait has a degree in communication sciences and a postgraduate residence in health education. She works at the National Ministry of Health and is a professor with La Matanza National University.

Sara Javanparast is a senior research fellow at the Southgate Institute for Health, Society and Equity, Flinders University, Australia. She received her medical degree from Tehran University of Medical Sciences, Iran, and worked for eight years in the Iranian Ministry of Health and primary health care system, where when she was involved in the national planning and implementation of primary health care policies, community health workers program, and child health programs. Sara did her PhD at Flinders University, focusing on the contribution of comprehensive primary health care in addressing social determinants of childhood malnutrition. She is involved in a wide range of research projects including primary health care and health system research, child health, and nutrition.

Taufique Joarder holds a PhD from Johns Hopkins Bloomberg School of Public Health. He is an assistant professor at James P Grant School of Public Health, BRAC University, Dhaka, Bangladesh; and an adjunct assistant professor at Johns Hopkins Bloomberg School of Public Health, Baltimore, Maryland, USA.

Vandana Kanth is a medical doctor with a Master's degree in Public Health. She is a community health physician who works as community health director of the Duncan Hospital in East Champaran District of North Bihar, which is part of the Emmanuel Hospital Network of hospitals in North India. Her work is focused on mental health, advocacy, HIV/AIDS, disability, gender-based violence, and prevention of slavery.

Dan Kaseje is professor of public health at the Great Lakes University of Kisumu. He has been involved in promoting CPHC throughout the world for about 30 years, has undertaken action-oriented research in the field, and published a number of papers during this period. He also has led several networks for CPHC, such as the Christian Medical Commission (a pioneer of PHC pre-dating Alma-Ata), International Federation of the Red Cross, Africa Action Network for Health (AfriCAN), Universities in Solidarity for the Health of the Disadvantaged (UNI-SOL), and Social Aspects of HIV-AIDS Alliance (SAHARA).

Yohannes Tewelde Kifle is a specialist in public health. He has nearly 25 years of experience in comprehensive nursing care, health-systems strengthening and management, and community-based health interventions. He managed the Tigray Health Bureau, advised the Tigray Regional State on epidemic preparedness and management, and has been regional maternal and child health coordinator for the Clinton Health Access Initiative, and regional manager for the Ethiopian Network for HIV/AIDS Care and Support. He is a PhD candidate at the University of South Africa (UNISA).

Ronald Labonté holds a Canada Research Chair in globalization and health equity and is professor in the Faculty of Medicine, University of Ottawa, as well as in the Faculty of Health Sciences, Flinders University of South Australia. His work focuses on the health equity impacts of contemporary globalization. From 2005 until 2008 he chaired the Globalization Knowledge Network for the World Health Organization's Commission on the Social Determinants of Health, some of the work of which is published in the book *Globalization and Health: Pathways, Evidence and Policy* (Routledge, 2009). Present research interests include health equity impacts of comprehensive primary health care reforms, health worker migration, medical tourism, global health diplomacy, and globalization and tobacco control. Prior to his research on globalization and health, he worked as a health promotion consultant and wrote and consulted extensively on community development, empowerment, policy advocacy, and other facets of community health. He has authored or edited more than 20 books, 150 book chapters and monographs, and 250 articles in peer-reviewed journals on topics ranging from health promotion, empowerment, and community development to globalization-related health determinants and health in foreign policy. In 2015 he was made an Honorary Fellow in the Faculty of Public Health (UK), and received the R.D. Defries Award and honorary life membership, the two highest awards of the Canadian Public Health Association.

John Liddle served as the director of the Central Australian Aboriginal Congress from 1981 to 2001. During this time his contribution to Aboriginal comprehensive primary health care was widely recognized by his peers. He has been a regular contributor to national policy fora. Since 2004 he has managed the innovative Aboriginal Male Health Program – Ingkintja, a nationally recognized comprehensive primary health care service for Aboriginal males in the central Australian region.

Jean Robert Likofata is a physician and public health specialist with 18 years of experience strengthening health systems on behalf of government organizations and NGOs throughout DRC. For more than a decade, Dr. Likofata worked as a physician throughout the country, in positions spanning all levels of the health system. From 2006 to 2008, Dr. Likofata worked for the World Health Organization as the epidemiologist responsible for emergencies and humanitarian action in the Equateur Province of DRC. Dr. Likofata received a degree in Medicine, Surgery, and Childbirth and a Master's of Public Health, both from the University of Kinshasa. He is a trainer who is fluent in French and Lingala.

Gwendolyn (Lyn) J. Lusi founded, along with her husband, HEAL Africa, a charity that provides medical and social care services in Goma, in eastern Congo. She earned her Master's degree in Human Resource Development and training and became the organization's program director, specializing in supporting women victims of violent rape. She developed HEAL Africa into not only a training centre for young Congolese doctors, but also a place capable of healing and supporting victims of rape and violence. Lyn Lusi died of cancer in 2012 in Goma, at the age of 62.

Jorge Martínez Collantes is a mathematician with an MSc degree in Statistics, an MSc degree in Applied Mathematics and a PhD in Statistics. He is research scientist and associate professor at the National University of Colombia where he has also served as dean of the Faculty of Science and director of the Department of Mathematics and Statistics. He is member of the Colombian Academy of Exact, Physical and Natural Sciences, and his main areas of interest are multivariate analysis, regression and correlation, and applied probability and statistics.

Araya Abrha Medhanyie holds a PhD and is assistant professor of public health at the School of Public Health at Mekelle University, Ethiopia. He has over a decade of work experience in teaching, research, and community service. His research interests include reproductive, maternal, neonatal, child, and adolescent health, as well as health-care innovation, and health systems. He has implemented mobile health technologies to improve the efficiency of health extension workers. He is member of the research advisor council for the Ethiopian Federal Ministry of Health. In that role, he routinely sits at the table with policymakers involved in improving maternal and child health in the country. He is founding member of the Ayder Enlightenment Forum. Currently, he serves as the interim Director of the Research Center for Maternal, Adolescent, Reproductive Health and Child health (MARCH) at Mekelle University.

Dagoberto Menjívar López is a medical doctor with a Master's degree in Public Health. He is the coordinator of the "MicroRed de Salud" initiative as well as the community health program "Unidad Comunitaria de Salud Familiar Especializada" in Guarjila, Chalatenango, El Salvador. He is also an adjunct professor in the Master of Public Health program at the University of El Salvador.

Sudhakar Narayan Morankar holds a PhD in medical anthropology. He is a professor in the Health Education and Behavioural Sciences Department at Jimma University and has approximately 40 years of international experience in research, teaching, training in development issues. He has conducted several research projects in social and economic development, and health (malaria, TB, HIV/AIDS, STDs, diarrhoeal diseases, leprosy, reproductive health, and health systems). His interests lie in global health, social, and behavioural-change communication for health and development, as well as evidence translation.

Paola Andrea Mosquera Méndez is a psychologist with a specialization in epidemiology, an MSc degree in Social Policy and a PhD in Epidemiology and Public Health. Currently she is working at the Division of Epidemiology and Global Health at Umeå University, Sweden, as a postdoc researcher. During the last six years she has been analyzing the implementation of the primary health care strategy of Bogotá and its contributions to reducing health inequalities. Her postdoctoral research focuses on exploring how to apply a life-course approach to analyze socioeconomic inequalities in cardiovascular health in Sweden. Her research interests involve social epidemiology, evaluation of public health policies, measurement of health inequalities, and the application of an equity lens to public health interventions.

Nonhlanhla Nxumalo is a researcher at the Centre for Health Policy, University of the Witwatersrand, South Africa, and has eight years of experience in the field of health systems and policy. Her interests include access to health care and human resources for health. She is involved in research that focuses on the improvement of governance and leadership in district health systems, and her work on community health workers continues to be one of the areas of focus in her research on primary health care. She is involved in the teaching of the Master of Public Health program, both as a facilitator and module coordinator. She supervises and co-supervises Masters and PhD students, respectively.

Corinne Packer is senior researcher at the University of Ottawa. She has authored two books on reproductive health and international human-rights law and is coeditor of the volume *Globalization and Health: Pathways, Evidence and Policy* as well as associate editor of a volume on humanitarian assistance. She has written numerous articles and book chapters on diverse subjects, such as the migration of health professionals, the African Union, Roma women, and comprehensive primary health care.

Clive Rosewarne is a research and community development worker with more than 20 years of experience working with Aboriginal people in central and South Australia on health, community and environmental justice issues. He has published on alcohol issues, primary health care system reform, and Aboriginal health and history. He is a currently a higher degree by research student at La Trobe University Melbourne.

Mario Rovere is a physician, specializing in public health with a trainee in International Health in PAHO/WHO. He has worked as a health officer in the PHC program at local subnational and national levels in Argentina and as a regional consultant in human resources development for PAHO. Today he works as vice dean in the Health Sciences Department at La Matanza National University.

David Sanders, professor and founding director of the School of Public Health at the University of the Western Cape (UWC), South Africa, is a specialist pediatrician qualified in public health. He has been an academic in the medical schools of the Universities of Zimbabwe and Natal. He has 35 years of experience in health policy and program development in Zimbabwe and South Africa, having advised governments, NGOs, and UN agencies in primary health care, child health and nutrition, and health human resources. He has published extensively in these fields as well as on structural adjustment and development aid, having authored three books, more than 40 chapters and monographs, and 160 articles in peer-reviewed journals. He is internationally recognized as an advocate for child health, primary health care, and health equity in Africa, and is frequently a plenary speaker at national and international meetings. In 2012 he received an Honorary Doctorate from the University of Cape Town for his contribution to the global policy of Primary Health Care, and in 2014 the Public Health Innovation and Lifetime Achievement (PHILA) Award of the Public Health Association of South Africa. He is Co-Chair of the Global Steering Council of People's Health Movement.

Nikki Schaay contributes to the teaching activities of the School of Public Health, University of the Western Cape, South Africa, by convening a core Master's of Public Health module on comprehensive primary health care and facilitating a course on community participation. She has contributed to a number of reviews of home and community-based services in the Western Cape and is currently involved in a participatory action learning research project that aims to strengthen various aspects of district management and leadership within a subdistrict in the city of Cape Town.

Mark Spigt is a health scientist. He currently holds academic positions at Maastricht University (Netherlands), Tromsø University (Norway), and Mekelle University (Ethiopia), with an international research line focusing on innovation in primary care and on pragmatic research methodology.

Liz Thomas has been involved in research into urban health for a number of years, with a special interest in the social determinants of health equity. She has an academic and hands-on background in urban development and health. She has contributed to national policy on the social determinants of HIV with a focus on the spatial variation of the overlapping factors that result in spatial variation in HIV infection between and within districts. Based at the WITS Centre for Health Policy, she has been involved in the supervision of a number of PhDs. She has also conducted research into the social determinants of health as the director of the University of Fort Hare's Hunterstoun Centre, located in Hogsback in the Eastern Cape, South Africa.

Aftab Uddin is the senior manager and head of the Technical Training Unit of the International Centre for Diarrhoeal Disease Research in Bangladesh.

Román Rafael Vega Romero holds a PhD in health care administration from University of Hull, UK. He is full professor at the Pontificia Universidad Javeriana (Bogotá), with expertise in social policy, primary health care, and public health.

Gai Wilson, senior research fellow, University of Melbourne, has collaborated with Indigenous communities, utilizing participatory action research and community development methods to identify their health-development priorities and the strategies required to address them. She has been a founding member of women's health services and networks, a member of government advisory committees, and has published with WHO, the *International Journal of Public Health*, *Critical Public Health*, and the *Australian and New Zealand Journal of Public Health*.

Mirkuzie Woldie is a medical doctor with a Master in Public Health degree specializing in health services management. He currently serves as an associate professor of health policy and management with the College of Health Sciences of Jimma University. He has published more than 40 peer-reviewed research papers on various topics relating to the Ethiopian health system. Dr. Woldie's research interests include health-systems research, infectious diseases, and utilization of research evidence for policy and practice.

Index